Balmore Park
Health Visitors

Doshis'
A to Z Series on Syndromes

Edited by

Sachin M Doshi
Resident in Ophthalmology
GSMC and KEM Hospital Mumbai

Sanket M Doshi
MD Pathology
LTMMC and Sion Hospital Mumbai

Ankur M Doshi
Resident in Orthopaedics
SIOR Pune

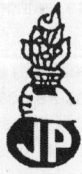

JAYPEE BROTHERS
MEDICAL PUBLISHERS (P) LTD
New Delhi

Published by

Jitendar P Vij
Jaypee Brothers Medical Publishers (P) Ltd
EMCA House, 23/23B Ansari Road, Daryaganj
New Delhi 110 002, India
Phones: +91-11-23272143, +91-11-23272703, +91-11-23282021,
+91-11-232456-72
Fax: +91-11-23276490, +91-11-23245683   e-mail: jpmedpub@del2.vsnl.net.in
Visit our web site: www.jaypeebrothers.com

Branches
- 202 Batavia Chambers, 8 Kumara Kruppa Road
  Kumara Park East, **Bangalore** 560 001, Phones: +91-80-22285971,
  +91-80-22382956, +91-80-30614073   Tele Fax : +91-80-22281761
  e-mail: jaypeebc@bgl.vsnl.net.in
- 282 IIIrd Floor, Khaleel Shirazi Estate, Fountain Plaza
  Pantheon Road, **Chennai** 600 008, Phone: +91-44-28262665,
  +91-44-28269897   Fax: +91-44-28262331
  e-mail: jpmedpub@md3.vsnl.net.in
- 4-2-1067/1-3, Ist Floor, Balaji Building, Street No.6, Ramkote Cross Road,
  Hyderabad 500 095, Phone: +91-40-55610020, +91-40-24758498
  Fax: +91-40-24758499   e-mail: jpmedpub@rediffmail.com
- 1A Indian Mirror Street, Wellington Square
  Kolkata 700 013, Phone: +91-33-22451926 Fax: +91-33-22456075
  e-mail: jpbcal@cal.vsnl.net.in
- 106 Amit Industrial Estate, 61 Dr SS Rao Road
  Near MGM Hospital, Parel, **Mumbai** 400 012
  Phones: +91-22-24124863, +91-22-24104532, +91-22-30926896
  Fax: +91-22-24160828   e-mail: jpmedpub@bom7.vsnl.net.in

Doshis' A to Z Series on Syndromes

© 2005, Sachin M Doshi, Sanket M Doshi, Ankur M Doshi

All rights reserved. No part of this publication should be reproduced, stored in a retrieval system, or transmitted in any form or by any means: electronic, mechanical, photocopying, recording, or otherwise, without the prior written permission of the editors and the publisher.

> This book has been published in good faith that the material provided by editors is original. Every effort is made to ensure accuracy of material, but the publisher, printer and editors will not be held responsible for any inadvertent error(s). In case of any dispute, all legal matters to be settled under Delhi jurisdiction only.

First edition: **2005**

ISBN 81-8061-416-6

Typeset at   JPBMP typesetting unit
Printed at   Replika Press Pvt. Ltd.

to
Our Parents
Mrs Jyoti M Doshi
Mr Mahasukhlal J Doshi

Preface

"A Man Attains Excellences by Devotion to Duty"

Dear Friends,

The basic concept of bringing this book to you all is to help you all, to have a comprehensive and latest information on various important topics covered by us at an instant of time. This work of ours is brought out with view of helping the entire medical fraternity, as reference book for undergraduates, postgraduates, residents, teaching faculty members as well as to the practitioners, as vast data of various topics is covered and compiled by us.

All the topics covered by us are very important from the examination point of view. We intend to make this book a first hand reference book.

Sachin M Doshi
Sanket M Doshi
Ankur M Doshi

Structure of the Book

This book titled as *Doshis' A to Z Series on Syndromes* where 14 important topics are covered such as syndromes, diseases, disorders, maneuvers etc. Where all existing informations about an individual topic from alphabet. A to Z are covered, say for example, all existing syndromes from letter A to letter Z are covered under the syndrome section.

Information is given in short but important aspects are covered in precise.

Pattern of Usage of the Book

The book is made very much user-friendly. The concept of using this book is—whenever any specific information about a topic covered is required enter the main menu of that topic and screen for the alphabet from which the desired information is required and you will have that information.

With these we hope this book will prove your best companion now and forever and help you in difficult times.

Acknowledgements

We would like to express sincere thanks and deep gratitude to our teachers and friends for their continuous support, encouragement and positive inputs in bringing about first edition of this book.

We would like to sincerely thanks the following people.
- Our parents who are toiling even today for us.
- Our friends for their continuous support.
- Mr JP Vij, a dynamic and versatile personality, CMD of Jaypee Brothers Medical Publishers, New Delhi for his mature understanding and giving us a chance to bring out the first edition of this book.
- Associates of Jaypee Brothers for their continuous help and inputs.

Contents

1. Syndromes *1*
2. Diseases *102*
3. Disorders *209*
4. Signs *218*
5. Tests *259*
6. Maneuvers *370*
7. Methods *374*
8. Pressures *406*
9. Procedures *409*
10. Phenomena *410*
11. Paralyses *423*
12. Operations *434*
13. Triads *455*
14. Factors *457*
    Appendix *477*

1
Syndromes

Syndrome: It's a set of symptoms which occur together; the sum of signs of any morbid state; a symptom complex. In genetics, a pattern of multiple malformations thought to be pathogenetically related.

Aarskog s., Aarskog-Scott s., an X-linked syndrome characterized by ocular hypertelorism, anteverted nostrils, broad upper lip, peculiar scrotal "shawl" above the penis, and small hand, called also faciogenital dysplasia and faciodigitogenital syndrome.

Aase s., a familial syndrome characterized by mild growth retardation, hypoplastic anemia, variable leukocytopenia, triphalangeal thumbs, narrow shoulder, and late closure of fontanels, and occasionally by cleft lip, cleft palate, retinopathy, and web neck. A recessive mode of inheritance has been suggested.

Abercrombie's s., amyloid degeneration—degeneration with deposition of lardacein in the tissues; it indicates impairment of nutritive function, and is seen in wasting disease.

Abstinence s., (DSM-III-R) a substance specific organic brain syndrome that follows the cessation of use or reduction in intake of a psychoactive substance that had been regularly used to induce a state of intoxication. (DSM-III-R) includes specific withdrawal syndromes for alcohol, amphetamines or similarly acting sympathomimetics, cocaine, nicotine, opioids and sedatives, hypnotics or anxiolytics called also substance withdrawal, withdrawal symptom or syndrome.

Achard s., arachnodactyly associated with receding mandible and joint laxity limited to the hands and feet.

Achard-Theirs s., an association of diabetes, hirsutism, and other masculinizing features in postmenopausal women resulting from overproduction of adrenocortical androgens.

Acquired immunodeficiency s., Acquired immune deficiency s. (AIDS), an epidemic transmissible retroviral disease due to infection with human immunodeficiency virus (HIV), manifested in severe cases as profound depression of cell-mediated immunity, and affecting certain recognized risk groups, including homosexual or bisexual males, intravenous drug abusers, hemophiliacs and other blood transfusion recipients, female sexual contacts of males in at risk groups, and newborn infants of individuals at risk for AIDS. The criteria established by the Centers for Disease Control for the diagnosis of AIDS (CDC/AIDS) comprise: the presence of reliably diagnosed disease that is at least moderately indicative of an underlying defect in cell-mediated immunity (e.g. Kaposi's sarcoma in an individual less than 60 years of age, or Pneumocystis pneumonia or other life threatening opportunistic infection), occurring in the absence of known cause of underlying immunodeficiency or of any other host defence defects reported to be associated with that disease (e.g. iatrogenic immunosuppression of lymphoreticular malignancies) AIDS-related complex (ARC), a complex of signs and symptoms representing a less severe form of HIV infection than classic AIDS, characterised by chronic generalized lymphadenopathy associated with fever, weight loss, prolonged diarrhea, minor opportunistic infections cytopenias, and T-cells abnormalities associated with AIDS: considered by some authorities to be pre-AIDS, although the proportion of cases that will progress to the full blowen disease is unknown.

Acute brain s., acute organic brain s., see organic brain s.

Acute radiation s., a syndrome caused by exposure to a whole body dose of over 1 gray of ionizing radiation. Symptoms, whose severity and time of onset depend on the side of the dose, include erythema, nausea and vomiting, fatigue, diarrhea, fever, petechiae, bleeding from the mucous membranes, reduction in the number of lymphocytes, granulocytes, and platelets, gastrointestinal hemorrhage, epilation, hypotension tachycardia, and dehydration; death may occur within hours or weeks of exposure.

Adair-Dighton s., see under van der Hoeve's s.

Addisonian s., see under Adams-Stokes disease.

Addisonian s., the complex of symptoms resulting from adrenal insufficiency; see Addison's disease.

Adie's s., a syndrome consisting of a pathological pupil reaction (tonic pupil), the most important elements of which is a myotonic condition on accommodation; the pupil on the affected side contracts on near vision more slowly than does the pupil on the opposite side, and it also dilates more slowly. The affected pupil does not usually react to direct or indirect light, but it may do so in an abnormal fashion. Certain tendon reflexes are absent or diminished, but there are neither motor or sensory disturbances, nor demonstrable changes indicative of disease of the nervous system. Called also Holmes-Adie s.

Adiposogenital s., a condition characterized by adiposity of feminine type and genital hypoplasia associated with lesions of hypothalamus called also Fröhlich s.

Adrenogenital s., hyperfunction of the adrenal cortex, associated with any of five enzymatic defects, that results in pseudohermaphroditism and virilism in the female, usually evident at birth, and precocious sexual development (epiphyseal syndrome) in the male, usually not appearing until three or four years after birth; the clinical findings are due to deficient production of cortisol and consequent hypersecretion of pituitary ACTH, resulting in excessive production of androgen. Called also congenital adrenal hyperplasia.

Adult respiratory distress s. (ARDS), fulminant pulmonary interstitial and alveolar edema, which usually develops a few days after the initiating trauma, thought to result from a massive sympathetic discharge due to brain injury or hypoxia and from increased capillary permeability. Called also shock lung.

Afferent loop s., chronic partial obstruction of the proximal loop of duodenum and jejunum after partial gastrectomy and gastrojejunostomy, resulting in duodenal distension, pains, and nausea following ingestion of food.

Aglossia adactylia s., see under hypoglossia adactylia s.

Ahumada-del Castillo s., a nonpuerperal triad consisting of galactorrhea, amenorrhea, and low gonadotropin secretion.

Aicardi's s., a syndrome affecting female infants, characterized by agenesis of the corpus callosum, large discrete areas of chorioretinopathy, spasms and tonic seizures, and mental retardation.

Alajouanine's s., symmetric lesions of the sixth and seventh cranial nerves with bilateral facial paralysis and bilateral lateral rectus palsy of the eyeball, associated with bilateral clubfoot.

Albright's s., Albright-McCune-Sternberg s., polyostotic fibrous dysplasia—[a disease of bone marked by thinning of the cortex and replacement of the bone marrow by gritty fibrous tissue containing bony spicules producing pain, disability, and gradually increasing deformity. Only one bone may be involved (monostotic fibrous dysplasia), with the process later involving several or many bones (polystotic fibrous dysplasia). When associated with melanotic pigmentation of the skin and endocrine disorders, it is known as Albright syndrome], patchy dermal pigmentation and endocrine dysfunction. Called also Albright's disease and McCune-Albright s.

Aldrich's s., see Wiskott-Aldrich s.

Alezzandrini's s., unilateral tapetoretinal degeneration followed by facial vitiligo and poliosis on the same side, sometimes associated with deafness.

"Alice in Wonderland" s., a delusional state manifested by depersonalization, disturbance of body image, alteration in the sense of the passage of time, and other delusions or illusion, it may be associated with schizophrenia, epilepsy, migraine, disease of the parietal lobe, hypnogogic states, or the use of hallucinogenic states.

Allemann's s., the association of double kidney and clubbed finger's sometimes associated with facial asymmetry and degeneration of various motor nerves.

Alport's s., a hereditary disorder characterized by progressive sensorineural hearing loss, progressive pyelonephritis or glomerulonephritis and, occasionally, ocular defects. It is transmitted as an autosomal dominant trait.

Alstroms s, an autosomal recessive syndrome of retinitis pigmentosa with nystagmus and early loss of central vision, deafness, obesity, and diabetes mellitus.

Amnesic s., see amnestics s.

Amnestic s. (DSM III-R), an organic mental disorder characterized by impairment of memory, both anterograde and retrograde amnesia, occurring in a normal state of consciousness, i.e, the syndrome does not include memory impairment seen in dementia or delirium. Disorientation, confabulation, and a lack of insight into the memory deficit are often present but are not invariable features. The most common cause is thiamine deficiency associated with chronic alcohol abuse (alcohol amnestic disorder, Wernicke-Korsakoff syndrome), but the syndrome may result from any pathological process causing bilateral damage to certain structure in the medial-temporal lobe and dience-phalon (e.g. the hippocampal formations, mamillary bodies, and dorsal medial nuclei of the thalamus), Causes include head trauma, brain tumors, infarction, cerebral hypoxia, carbon monoxide poisoning, and herpes simplex encephalitis. Called also amnesic s., amnestic confabulatorys., dysmnesic s., and Korsakoff's s.

Amnestic confabulatory s. see amnestic s.

Amniotic infection s. of Blane, a syndrome in which fetal sepsis follows swallowing and at times aspiration of contaminated amniotic fluid.

Amyostatic s., see Wilson's disease

Andersen's s., bronchiectasis, cystic fibrosis of the pancreas, and vitamin A deficiency.

Angelucci s., excitable temperament, palpitation, and vasomotor disturbance in patients with vernal conjunctivitis.

Anorexia-cachexia s., a systemic response to cancer occurring as a result of a poorly understood relationship between anorexia and cachexia, manifested by malnutrition, weight loss, muscular weakness, acidosis, and toxemia. The basis of the anorexia may be multifactorial severe metabolic disturbance that contributes to the development of cachectic wasting, which in turn reinforces the anorexia by the release from the tumor of a anorexigenic humoral product that stimulates the satiety center in the hypothalamus producing appetite loss.

Anterior abdominal walls s., continuous pain in the anterior abdominal wall, affecting either the left or right lower quadrant or the superior margins of the upper quadrant area; etiology unknown.

Anterior chamber cleavage s., a term for several types of mesenchymal dysgenesis affecting neural crest derivatives in the iris, trabeculum and cornea. In ascending severity these disorders are; posterior embryotaxon, Axenfeld's anomaly, Axenfeld's syndrome Rieger's anomaly, and Rieger syndrome.

Anterior cord s., localized injury to the anterior portion of the spinal cord, characterized by complete paralysis and hypalgesia and hypesthesia to the level of the lesion, but with relative preservation of posterior column sensations of touch position, and vibration.

Anterior cornual s., muscular atrophy due to lesions of the anterior horns of the spinal cord.

Anterior tibial compartment s., rapid swelling, increased tension, pain, and ischemic necrosis of the muscles of the anterior tibial compartment of the leg; the skin becomes glossy, erythematous and edematous as the necrosis occurs. The cause is unknown, but usually there is a history of excessive exertion.

Anticholinergic s., the central and peripheral effects produced by overdosage or abnormal reaction to clinical dosage of anticholinergic drugs, e.g., atropine, phenothiazines, antihistamines, and tricyclic antidepressants; signs and symptoms include anxiety, delirium, disorientation, hallucinations, seizures, tachycardia, hyperpyrexia, mydriasis, vasodilation, gastric and urinary retention, and decreased salivary sweat, bronchial and nasopharyngeal secretions, etc.

Anton's s., denial of, and usually unawareness of one's own blindness, with resort to confabulation, as seen in cortical blindness due to bilateral infarction of occipital lobe.

Anxiety s., the physical symptoms accompanying anxiety, such as palpitation of the heart, rapid and shallow respiration, sweating, pallor, and a feeling of panic.

Aortic arch s., any of group of disorders leading to occlusion of the arteries arising from the aortic arch; such occlusion may be caused by atherosclerosis, arterial embolism, syphilitic or tuberculous arteritis, etc. See also pulseless disease.

Apert s., acrocephalosyndactyly-craniostenosis characterized by acrocephaly and syndactyly, probably occurring as an autosomal dominant trait and usually as a new mutation.

Apert's s., acrocephalosyndactyly, see Apert s.

Argentaffinoma s., see carcinoid s.

Arnold's nerve reflex cough s., a reflex cough due to irritation of the area supplied by Arnold's nerve (the auricular branch of the vagus nerve); this area is the posterior and inferior portion of the external auditory canal and the posterior half of the tympanic membrane.

Arnold-Chiari s., a congenital anomaly in which the cerebellum and medulla oblongata which is elongated and flattened, protrude down into the spinal canal through the foramen magnum; it may be associated with many other defects, including spina bifida occulta and meningomyelocele. Called also Arnold-Chiari malformation or s.

Ascher s., blepharochalasis occurring with goiter (adenoma of the thyroid) and redundancy of the mucous membrane and submucous tissue of the upper lip.

Asherman's s., persistent amenorrhea and secondary sterility due to intrauterine adhesions and synechiae, usually occurring as a result of uterine curettage.

Asherson's s., syndrome of dysphagia due to neuromuscular incoordination and achalasia of the cricopharyngeal sphincter with failure of relaxation of the cricopharyngeal muscle during the third stage of swallowing. It causes diversion of liquids into the air passages, precipitating paroxysms of coughing. Called also cricopharyngeal achalasia s.

Asphenia s., see Ivemark's s.

Ataxia-telangiectasia s., a complex hereditary disorder, transmitted as an autosomal recessive trait, characterized by cerebellar ataxia and nystagmus, oculocutaneous telangiectasia, variable degrees of humoral and cellular immunodeficiency with recurrent sinopulmonary bacterial infections, and an increased incidence of lymphoreticular malignancies. There is an increased sensitivity to ionizing radiation caused by a defect in DNA repair. Gonadal hypoplasia, insulin resistance and hyperglycemia, liver function abnormalities, and elevated levels of alpha-fetoprotein and carcinoembryonic antigen are also seen in some patients. Called also Louis-Bar s.,

Auriculotemporal s., the appearance of a red area and of sweating on the cheek in connection with eating; seen in lesions of the parotid gland and due to some involvement of the auriculotemporal nerve.

Autoerythrocyte sensitization s., see painful bruising s.

Autoimmune polyendocrine-candidiasis, s. see Polyendocrine autoimmune disease type 1.

Avellis's., ipsilateral paralysis of vocal cord and soft palate, loss of pain and temperature sensibility in contralateral leg, trunk, arm and neck and in the skin over the scalp; called also ambiguospinothalamic paralysis.

Axenfeld's s., Axenfeld's anomaly (a developmental anomaly consisting of posterior embryotoxon and iris processes to Schwalbe's ring) with glaucoma and with defective development of the corneoscleral trabecular meshwork and other angle structures. See also anterior chamber cleavage s.

Ayerza's s., pulmonary hypertension with dilatation of the pulmonary arteries, related to disease of the lungs; formerly attributed to syphilis.

Baastrup's s., kissing spines—a condition in which the spinous processes of adjacent vertebra are in contact.

Babinski's s., the association of cardiac and arterial disorders with chronic syphilitic meningitis, tabes dorsalis, paralytic dementia, and other late syphilitic manifestations.

Babinski-Fröhlich s., see Adiposogenital s.

Babinski-Nageotte s, a syndrome due to multiple lesions affecting the pyramidal and sensory tracts, the cerebellar peduncle, and the reticular formation, and marked by contralateral hemiplegia and hemianesthesia (usually only of the pain and temperature senses), ipsilateral hemiasynergia, hemiataxia, and Horner's syndrome.

Babinski-Vaquez s., see Babinski's s.

BADS s., a syndrome whose acronym stands for black locks oculocutaneous albinism, and deafness of the sensorineural type; oculocutaneous albinism—a human albinism occurring in ten types all distinguished in their incidence and genetic, biochemical, and clinical characteristics but having in common varying degrees of decreased melanotic pigments of the skin, hair and eyes, hypoplastic foveas, photophobia, nystagmus, and decreased visual acuity.

Bafverstedt's s., lymphocytoma cutis a manifestation of cutaneous lymphoid hyperplasia, seen especially in women, characterized by skin lesions ranging from a solitary plaque or nodule to several regionally localized lesions, preferentially resemble malignant lymphoma, but some have a tendency toward spontaneous resolution, sometimes with recurrence. Exposure to sunlight insect bites and mechanical trauma have been implicated as causative factors.

Balint's s., cortical paralysis of visual fixation, optic ataxia, and disturbance of visual attention, with preservation of spontaneous and reflex eye movements. The parietooccipital lesions are bilateral.

Baller-Gerold s., an autosomal recessive syndrome characterized by craniosynostosis and radial aplasia. Called also craniosynostosis-radial aplasia s.

Bannwarth's s., the European term for the meningopolyneuritis that may occur in Lyme disease.

Banti's s., congestive splenomegaly. seen Banti's disease.

Bardet-Biedl s., an autosomal recessive disorder characterized by mental retardation, pigmentary retinopathy, obesity, polydactyly, and hypogonadism; clarify with Lawrence Moon s. and Biemond's s., II.

Barlow s., see Mitral valve prolapse s.

Barraquer-Simons s., partial lipodystrophy (a condition occurring especially in females in the first decade of life, characterized by the loss of subcutaneous fat, usually beginning on the face and gradually extending to the chest, neck, back, and upper extremities, giving the lower part of the body an apparent, and possibly real, adiposity of the buttocks, thighs and legs. Some affected patients develop insulin-resistant diabetes mellitus, triglyceridemia, and renal disease). Called also Barraquer's or Simons' disease.

Barré-Guillain s., acute febrile polyneuritis, i.e. rapidly progressive ascending motor neurone paralysis of unknown etiology, frequently following an enteric or respiratory infection. An autoimmune mechanism following viral infection has been postulated. It begins with paresthesias of the feet followed by flaccid paralysis and weakness of the legs, ascending to the arms, trunk and face, and is attended by slight fever, bulbar palsy, absent or lessened tendon reflexes, and an increase in the protein of the cerebrospinal fluid without corresponding increase in cells.

Barrett's s., peptic ulcer of the lower esophagus, often with stricture, due to presence of columnar-lined epithelium, which may contain functional mucous cells, parietal cells, or chief cells, in the esophagus instead of normal squamous cell epithelium. Called also Barrett's esophagus.

Bart's s., a form of epidermolysis bullosa dystrophica inherited as an autosomal dominant trait, characterized by congenital localized absence of the skin blister formation as a result of mechanical trauma and nail dystrophy.

Bartter's s., hypertrophy and hyperplasia of the juxtaglomerular cells, producing hypokalemic alkalosis and hyperaldosteronism, characterized by absence of hypertension in the presence of markedly increased plasma renin concentrations and by insensitivity to the pressor effects of angiotensin. It usually affects children. It is perhaps hereditary, and may be associated with other anomalies, such as mental retardation and short stature. Called also juxtaglomerular cell hyperplasia.

Basal cell nevus s., an autosomal dominant syndrome characterized by the development in early life of numerous basal cell carcinomas, occurring in association with abnormalities of the skin (especially an unusual erythematous pitting edema of the hands and feet), bone, nervous system, eyes, and reproductive tract, called also Gorlin's s., Gorlin-Goltz s., nevoid basal cell carcinoma s., and nevoid basalioma s.

Bassen-Kornzweig s, abetalipoproteinemia; familial lipoprotein deficiency (Any of the three of disorders of lipoprotein and lipid metabolism). *Abetalipoproteinemia* caused by defective synthesis of apolipoprotein B is characterized by acanthocytosis hypocholesterolemia, ataxic neuropathy, atypical retinitis pigmentosa with involvement of the macula, and fat malabsorption, and may be treated with vitamin E.

Battered-child s., unexplained or inappropriately explained physical trauma and other manifestations of severe, repeated physical abuse of children, usually by a parent.

Bazex's s., eczematous and psoriasis form lesions on the ears, nose, cheeks, hands, feet, and knees in patients with carcinomas of the upper respiratory and digestive tracts. Called also paraneoplastic acrokeratosis.

Beals' s., congenital contractural arachnodactyly—a form of hereditary bone dysplasia characterised by abnormal length and slenderness of the fingers and toes.

Bearn-Kunkel s., Bearn-Kunkel-Slater s., lupoid hepatitis-chronic active hepatitis with autoimmune manifestations.

Beau's s., asystole-cardiac standstill or arrest, absence of heartbeat.

Beckwith's s., a hereditary disorder marked by extreme cytomegaly of the fetal adrenal cortex, omphalocele, macroglossia, hyperplasia of the kidney and pancreas, Leydig cell hyperplasia, and postnatal gigantism.

Beckwith-Wiedemann s., a congenital autosomal dominant syndrome with variable expressivity characterized by exomphalos, macroglossia, and gigantism, often associated with visceromegaly, adrenocortical cytomegaly, and dysplasia of the renal medulla. Called also EMGs and Exomphalos-macroglossia-gigantism s.

Behçet's s., a chronic inflammatory disorder involving the small blood vessels, which is of unknown etiology, and is characterized by recurrent aphthous ulceration of the oral and pharyngeal mucous membranes and the genitalia, skin lesions, severe uveitis, retinal vasculitis, and optic atrophy. It frequently also involves the joints, gastrointestinal system, and central nervous system. Called also Behçet's disease.

Benedikt s., a syndrome consisting of ipsilateral oculomotor paralysis, contralateral hyperkinesia, contralateral tremor and paresis of the arm and leg, and ipsilateral ataxia; caused by lesions that damage the third nerve and involve the nucleus ruber and corticospinal tract.

Bernard's s., Bernard-Horner s., see Horner's s.

Bernard-Sergent s., diarrhea, vomiting, and collapse characteristic of Addison's disease.

Bernard-Soulier s. (BSS), see under disease.

Bernhardt-Roth s., meralgia paresthetica, see Roth-Bernhardt s.

Bernheim's s., right heart failure with absence of dyspnea or pulmonary congestion, in the presence of gross left ventricular hypertrophy, sometimes attributed to impairment of right ventricular capacity and filling.

Bertolottis s., sacralization of the fifth lumbar vertebra together with sciatica and scoliosis.

Bianchi's s., a sensory aphasic syndrome with apraxia (loss of ability to carry out familiar, purposeful movements in the absence of paralysis or other motor or sensory impairment, especially inability to make proper use of an object) and alexia (a form of receptive aphasia in which there is a loss of the ability to understand written language as a result of a cerebral lesion), seen in lesions of the left parietal lobe.

Biemond s. II, an autosomal recessive disorder characterized by iris coloboma, obesity, mental retardation, hypogonadism and postaxial polydactyly; cf, Bardet-Biedl s. Lawrence Moon s.

Bjornstad's s., an autosomal recessive disorder characterized by congenital sensorineural deafness and pili torti (twisted hair).

Blatin's s., hydatid thrill—a tremulous impulse sometimes felt on palpation of the body surface over a hydatid cyst.

Blind loop s., a syndrome resulting from alterations in the anatomy of the small intestine, as by strictures or after surgery, in which a loop is disconnected from the main stream or when intestinal contents may gain access to it but not readily egress from it; it is associated with bacterial overgrowth, particularly anaerobic organisms, with resultant malabsorption of vitamin B_{12}, statorrhea and anemia.

Bloch-Sulzberger s., incontinentia pigment, see Franceshetti-Jadassohn s.

Bloom s., an autosomal recessive syndrome developing during infancy, consisting of erythema and telangiectasia in a butterfly distribution on the face, photosensitivity, and dwarfism of prenatal onset.

Abnormalities in chromosome structure (sister chromatid exchange q.v.) and in immunoglobulins are present, and there is a high incidence of malignancy, especially leukemia. About one-half of the patients are of Jewish ancestry.

Blue diaper s., a defect of tryptophan absorption in which, because of intestinal bacterial action on the tryptophan, the urine contains abnormal indoles, giving it a blue color. It is similar to Hartnup's disease.

Blum's s., hypochloremic azotemia.

Body of Luys s., hemiballismus—a violent form of motor restlessness involving only on side of the body and being most marked in the upper extremity, resulting from destructive lesion of the hypothalamic nucleus.

Boerhaave's s., spontaneous rupture of the esophagus.

Bonnier's s., a series of symptoms due to lesion of Deiters' nucleus or of the vestibular tracts related thereto; it consists of vertigo, pallor, and various aural and ocular disturbances.

Book's s., see PHC s.,

Borjeson's s., **Borjeson-Forssman-Lehmann s.**, an X-linked syndrome characterized by severe mental retardation, epilepsy, hypogonadism hypometabolism, marked obesity swelling of the subcutaneous tissues of the face, and large ears.

Bouillaud's s., the coincidence of pericarditis and endocarditis in acute articular rheumatism.

Bouveret's s., paroxysmal tachycardia.

Brachial s., a morbid condition resulting from compression or irritation of nerves of the brachial plexus. **Brachmann-de Lange s.**, see de Lange s.,

Bradycardia-tachycardia s., episodic or repetitive tachycardia of short duration followed by transient or protracted heart standstill, sometimes accentuated by quinidine.

Brennemann's s., mesenteric and retroperitoneal lymphadenitis as a sequel of throat infections.

Briquet's s., hysteria (q.v.) especially that characterized by multiple symptoms, many visits to physicians, and often much unnecessary medical treatment; now called somatization disorder.

Brissaud-Sicard s., spasmodic hemiplegia caused by lesions of the pons.

Bristowe's s., a series of ingravescent symptoms characteristic of tumor of the corpus callosum; (1) gradual onset of hemiplegia; (2) association of hemiplegia on one side, vague hemiplegic symptoms on the other, (3) stupor and drowsiness, difficulty of swallowing; and speechlessness; (4) absence of direct implication of the cranial nerves; (5) death from coma.

Brittle bone s., osteogenesis imperfecta—a collagen disorder due to defective biosynthesis of type 1 collagen and generally characterized by brittle, osteoporotic, easily fractured bones. Other defects that may appear include blue sclera, wormian bones, lax joints and dentinogenesis imperfecta.

Brittle cornea s., an X-linked recessively inherited syndrome, characterized by brittle cornea, blue sclera, and red hair.

Brock s., see Middle lobe s.

Brown's vertical retraction s., adhesion of the muscles of the eye in the fetus.

Brown-Séquard s., a syndrome due to damage of one-half of the spinal cord, resulting in ipsilateral paralysis and loss of discriminatory and joint sensation, and contralateral loss of pain and temperature sensation. Called also Brown-Séquard's disease, paralysis, or sign.

Bruns' s., intermittent headache, vertigo, vomiting and visual disturbances on sudden movement of the head, characteristic of cysticercus infection of the fourth ventricle, lesion of the fourth ventricle, or tumors of the midline of the cerebellum and third or lateral ventricles; called also Bruns' sign.

Brunsting's s., a recurrent eruptive syndrome usually affecting middle aged men, in which grouped, vesicular lesions occur about the head and neck, and result in scarring.

Brushfield-Wyatt s., a congenital syndrome consisting of extensive unilateral nevus flammeus, hemianopia affecting the right or left halves of the visual fields of both eyes, contralateral hemiplegia, cerebral angioma, and mental retardation; it is probably related to the Sturge-Weber syndrome.

Buckley's s,. see hyperimmunoglobulinemia E s.

Budd-Chiari s., symptomatic obstruction or occlusion of the hepatic veins, causing hepatomegaly, abdominal pain and tenderness, intractable ascites, mild jaundice; and eventually, portal hypertension and liver failure; the obstruction is caused by thrombi or fibrous obliteration of the veins and has been associated with coagulation disorders, myeloproliferative disorders, invasion of hepatic veins by hepatic, renal, or adrenal carcinoma, and with abdominal trauma. Onset may be acute with death occurring within day in cases of complete occlusion, more often there is chronic course with survival for months or years called also Budd-Chiari disease, Chiari's disease or syndrome and endophlebitis hepatica obliterans. Cf: veno-occlusive disease of liver.

Bulbar s., see Dejerine's syndrome, def 2.

Burger-Griitz s., familial hyperlipoproteinemia, type 1—a recessive trait due to lipoprotein lipase deficiency, is manifested by abdominal pain and vomiting, acute pancreatitis, xanthomas, hepatosplenomegaly and lipemia retinalis.

Burnett's s., see Milk-alkali s.

Burning Feet s., see Gopalan's s.

Buschke Oilendorff s., dermatofibrosis lenticularis disseminata— an autosomal dominant syndrome present at birth or appearing before puberty, characterized by development of connective tissue nevi of the elastic type in association with osteopoikilosis; the skin lesion are manifested as small, firm, yellowish or skin coloured papules or plaques distributed symmetrically, primarily on the lower trunk and extremities.

Bywaters s., see Crush s.

Caffey's s., Caffey-Silverman s., infantile cortical hyperostosis, see Caffey's disease.

Callosal s., an association of symptoms thought to result from a lesion of the corpus callosum.

Camptomelic s., oestochondrodysplasia (see Morquio s) associated with flat facies, bowed tibiae with skin dimpling, hypoplastic scapulae, and short vertebrae.

Canada-Cronkhite s., see Cronkhite-Canada s.

Capgras's s., the delusion that other persons in the patient's environment are not their real selves but doubles.

Caplan's s., pneumoconiosis associated with rheumatoid arthritis radiographycally, multiple spherical nodular lesions with clearly demarcated borders are found throughout both lungs. Called also rheumatoid pneumoconiosis.

Capsular thrombosis s., hemiplegia due to thrombosis of a blood vessels supplying the internal capsule.

Capsulothalamic s., hemiplegia hemianopia, and perverted pain perception due to lesions of the thalamus and internal capsule.

Carcinoid s., a symptoms complex associated with carcinoid tumors (argentaffinoma) and characterized by attacks of severe cyanotic flushing of the skin lasting from minutes to days and by diarrheal watery stools, bronchoconstrictive attacks, sudden drops in blood pressure, edema, and ascites. Symptoms are caused by secretion by the tumor of serotonin, prostaglandins, and other biologically active substance. Called also argentaffinoma s.

Cardiofacial s., a syndrome of congenital heart disease associated with unilateral partial lower facial paresis, the latter being transient or persistent.

Carotid sinus s., syncope sometimes associated with convulsive seizures due to overactivity of the carotid sinus reflex when pressure is applied to one or both carotid sinuses.

Carpal tunnel s., a complex of symptoms resulting from compression of the median nerve in the carpal tunnel, with pain an burning or tingling paresthesias in the fingers and hand sometimes extending to the elbow.

Carpenter's s., acrocephalopolysyndactyly, type II, autosomal recessive, with mental retardation and brachydactyly.

Cat's cry s., see Cri du chat s.

Cat-eye s., cat's eye s., an association of coloboma of the iris and anal atresia; there may also be many other anomalies, including preauricular skin tags or fistulas, hypertelorism congenital heart disease, skeletal abnormalities and renal malformations. It is associated with partial trisomy 22, i.e the presence of an additional, deleted chromosome 22.

Cauda equina s., dull aching pain of the perineum, bladder, and sacrum, generally radiating in a sciatic fashion, with associated paresthesias and are flexic paralysis due to compression of the spinal nerve roots.

Caudal dysplasia s., caudal regression s., failure of formation of part or all the coccygeal, sacral, and occasionally lumbar vertebral units and the corresponding segments of the caudal spinal cord, with resulting neurogenic dysfunction of bowel and bladder. Called also sacral agenesis.

Cavernous sinus s., edema of the conjunctiva, proptosis edema of upper lid and root of the nose, together with paralysis of the third, fourth and sixth nerves, due to thrombosis of the cavernous sinus.

Celiac s., see under disease

Central cord s., injury to the central portion of the cervical spinal cord resulting in disproportionately more weakness or paralysis in the upper extremities than in the lower; pathological change is caused by hemorrhage or edema.

Centroposterior s., syringomyelic dissociation of sensibility and vasomotor disorders, due to lesions of the centroposterior portion of the gray matter of the spinal cord.

Cerebellar s., hereditary cerebellar ataxia.

Cerebrocardiac s., see Krishnaber's disease.

Cerebrohepatorenal s., an autosomal recessive disorder characterized by craniofacial abnormalities, hypotonia, hepatomegaly, polycystic kidneys, jaundice, and death in early infancy and associated with absence of peroxisomes in the liver and kidneys; called also Zellweger s.

Cervical s., a condition caused by irritation or compression of the cervical nerve roots, marked by pain in the neck radiating into the shoulder, arm, or forearm, depending on which nerve root is affected.

Cervical rib s., cervicobrachia s., see scalenus s.

Cestan's s., s. of Cestan-Chenais, an association of contralateral hemiplegia contralateral hemianesthesia, ipsilateral lateropulsion and hemiasynergia, Horner's syndrome, and ipsilateral laryngoplegia, due to scattered lesions of the pyramid, sensory tract, inferior cerebellar peduncle, necleus ambiguous, and oculopupillary center.

Cestan-Raymond s., See Raymond-Cestan s.

Chancriform s., primary extrapulmonary coccidioidomycosis.

Charcot's s., 1. Amyotrophic lateral sclerosis. 2. Intermittent claudi-cation. 3. Intermittent hepatic fever, due to cholangitis.

Charcot-Weiss-Baker s., see Carotid sinus s.,

Charlin's s., pain, iritis, corneitis, rhinorrhea, and tenderness along the nose in eye disturbance of nasal origin.

Chauffard's s., Chauffard-Still s., polyarthritis with fever and enlargement of the spleen and lymph nodes in persons infected with nonhuman tuberculosis.

Chédiak-Higashi s., a lethal autosomal recessive syndrome associated with oculocutaneous albinism, massive leukocyte inclusions (giant lysosomes), histiocytic infiltration of multiple body organs, development of pancytopenia, hepatosplenomegaly, recurrent or persistent bacterial infections, and a possible predisposition to development of malignant lymphoma. Called also Beguez Cesar disease and Chédiak-Higashi anomaly.

Chiari's s., see Budd-Chian s.

Chiari-Arnold s., See Arnold Chiari s.

Chiari-Frommel s., galactorrhea amenorrhea syndrome occurring after pregnancy. Called also Frommel-Chiari s., Chiari-Frommel disease, and Frommel's disease.

Chiasma s., Chiasmatic s., a syndrome indicative lesion affecting the optic chiasma; impairment of vision, limitations of the field of vision, central scotomata, headache, vertigo, and syncope.

Chilaiditi s., 1. Interposition of the colon between the liver and diaphragm. Usually the condition is asymptomatic in adults, but symptoms are evident in children and include vomiting, abdominal pain, anorexia, constipation, aerophagia. Signs include abdominal distension and absence of liver dullness. 2. Hepatoptosis—positioning of liver between liver and diaphragm on X-ray.

Chinese restaurant s. (CRS), a transient syndrome associated with arterial dilatation, due to ingestion of monosodium glutamate, which is used liberally in seasoning Chinese food; it is characterized by throbbing of the head, light headedness, tightness of the jaw, neck, and shoulders, and backache.

Chotzen's s., an autosomal dominant disorder characterized by acrocephalosyndactyly in which the syndactyly is mild and by hypertelorism, ptosis, and sometimes mental retardation. Called also acrocephalosyndactyly type III and Saethre-Chotzen s.

Christian's s., see Hand-Schüller-Christian disease.

Christ-Siemens Touraine s., anhidrotic ectodermal dysplasia—an X-linked disorder or, rarely, an autosomal recessive disorder with full expression in both sexes, characterized by ectodermal dysplasia associated with aplasia or hypoplasia of the sweat glands, hypothermia, or alopecia, anodontia, conical teeth, and typical facies with frontal bossing, midfacial hypoplasia, saddle nose, large chin, and thick lips.

Chronic brain s., chronic organic brain s., see organic brain s.

Churg-Strauss s., allergic granulomatosis angiitis—a form of systemic necrotising vasculitis in which there is prominent lung involvement, generally manifested by eosinophilia, granulomatous reactions, and usually severe asthma; if present cutaneous lesions consist of tender subcutaneous nodules, large ecchymotic plaques, and cutaneous infarct.

Citelli's s., mental backwardness, loss of power of concentration, drowsiness or insomnia, seen in persons with adenoids or sinus infection.

Clarke-Handefield s., congenital pancreatic disease with infatilism; with enlarged liver, bulky fatty stools, and extensive atrophy of pancreas in undersized and underweight child.

Claude's s., paralysis of the third (oculomotor) nerve on one side and asynergia on the other side, together with dysarthria. Called also inferior s. of red nucleus and rubrospinal cerebellar peduncle s.

Claude Bernard-Horner s., see Horner's s.

Click s., a left ventricular abnormality marked by apical midsystolic click and later murmur, with inversion of T waves.

Closed head s., the complex of symptoms characteristic of cerebral injury without cranial penetration.

Clough and Richter's s., anemia in which the red corpuscles exhibit a severe degree of autoagglutination.

Clouston's s., hidrotic ectodermal dysplasia—an autosomal dominant disorder characterized by ectodermal dysplasia associated with dystrophic, hypoplastic, or absent teeth, hypotrichosis, hyperpigmentation of the skin over the joints, hyperkeratosis of palm and soles, and occasionally small teeth with extensive decay.

Cockayne's s., a hereditary syndrome transmitted as an autosomal recessive trait, consisting of dwarfism with retinal atrophy and deafness, associated with progeria, prognathism, mental retardation, photosensitivity.

Cogan's s., nonsyphilitic keratitis with vestibuloauditory symptoms.

Cold agglutinin s., the presence of circulating antibodies, usually IgM, that can agglutinate red cell and do so most efficiently at temperatures below 37°C. The cold agglutinins are directed against three types of polysaccharide red cell antigens. "I antigens," expressed primarily on adult red cells, "i antigens," expressed primarily on cells of fetuses and infants, and "Pr antigens," which unlike I and i antigens, are protease sensitive. The primary clinical manifestations are intravascular hemolysis in exposed extremities and mild hemolytic anemia due to complement fixation, both occurring only upon exposure to cold. There are two major types; chronic cold agglutinin disease of the elderly, a condition with gradual onset and chronic course, and postinfectious cold agglutinin syndrome, usually following *Mycoplasma pneumoniae* infection or infectious mononucleosis and lasting a few months. The syndrome can also develop secondary to malignancy.

Collet's s., Collet-Siecard s., glossolaryngoscapulopharyngeal hemiplegia due to complete lesion of the ninth, tenth, eleventh and twelfth cranial nerves.

Combined immunodeficiency s., deficiency of lymphoid cells that mediate both antibody (B-lymphocytes) and cellular (T-lymphocytes) immunity.

Compartmental s., a condition in which increased tissue pressured in a confined anatomical space causes decreased blood flow leading to ischemia and dysfunction of contained myoneural elements, marked by pain, muscle weakness, sensory loss, and palpable tenseness in the involved compartment ischemia can lead to necrosis resulting in permanent impairment of function.

Compression s., shock with hematuria and oliguria following long continued pressure on a limb, as in bombed buildings.

Concussion s., encephalopathy due to trauma; see Postconcussional s.

Congenital rubella s., transplacental infection (which may or may not be clinically apparent), resulting in various development abnormalities in the newborn infant. They include cardiac and ocular lesions. Deafness, microcephaly, mental retardation, and generalized growth retardation, which may be associated with acute self-limited conditions such as thrombocytopenic purpura anaemia, hepatitis, encephalitis, and radiolucencies of long bones. Infected infants may shed virus to all contacts for extended period of time. Called also rubella s.,

Conn's s., primary aldosteronism that arising from oversecretion of aldosterone by an adrenal cortical adenoma, characterized typically by hypokalemia, alkalosis, muscular weakness, polyuria, polydipsia, and hypertension.

Conradi's s., chondrodysplasia punctate.

Conradi-Hunermann s., an autosomal dominant form of chondrodysplasia punctate, characterized by asymmetric shortening of the extremities and scoliosis; intelligence and life expectancy are normal. The syndrome is also associated with maternal use of warfarin sodium during pregnancy.

Contiguous gene s., any syndrome known to be caused by the involvement of contiguous genes on a chromosome, e.g. aniridia-Wilms' tumor association, which may also have genitourinary tract abnormalities, gonadoblastoma, and mental retardation.

Cornelia de Lange's s., see de Lange's s.

S. of corpus striatum., see Vogt's s.

Costen's s. see temporomandibular dysfunction s.

Costoclavicular s., pain or other difficulties in the arm and/or hand, apparently due to pressure, stretching, or friction on the nerves or vessels at the cervicobrachial outlet.

Cotard's s., paranoia with delusion of negation, a suicidal tendency, and sensory disturbances.

Courvoisier-Terrier s., dilatation of the gallbladder, retention jaundice, and discoloration of the feces, indicating obstruction due to a tumour of the ampulla of Vater.

Couvade s., the occurrences in the mate of a pregnant woman of symptoms that are related to pregnancy, such as nausea, vomiting, and abdominal pain.

Cowden's s., see under disease.

Craniosynostosis-radial aplasia s., see Baller-Gerold s.

CREST s., a form of systemic scleroderma usually less severe than other forms, consisting of calcinosis cutis, Raynaud's phenomenon, esophageal dyfunction, sclerodactyly, and telangiectasia. That in which esophageal dysfunction is not prominent is known as CRST s.

Creutzfeldt-Jakob s., see under disease.

Cricopharyngeal achaladia s., see Asherson's s.

Cri du chat s., a hereditary congenital syndrome characterized by hypertelorism, microcephaly, severe mental deficiency, and a paintive catlike cry, due to deletion of the short arm of chromosome. Called also Cat's cry s.

Crigler-Najjar s., an autosomal recessive form of nonhemolytic jaundice due to the absence of the hepatic enzyme glucuronosyl-transferase. It is chracterized by the presence in the blood of excessive amounts of unconjugated bilirubin and by kernicterus and severe disorders of the central nervous system. Called also congenital hyperbilirubinemia and congenital nonhemolytic jaundice.

S. of crocodile tears, spontaneous lacrimation occurring parallel with the normal salivation of eating. It follows facial paralysis and seems to be due to straying of the regenerating nerve fibers, some of those destined for the sallivary glands going to the lacrimal glands.

Cronkhite-Canada s., allergic granulomatosis angiitis. Called also Canada-Cronkhite s.

Cross s., Cross-McKusick-Breen s., an autosomal recessive syndrome marked by oculocutaneous albinism, microphthalmus, small opaque corneas, oligophrenia with spasticity, high-arched palate, gingival hypertrophy, and scoliosis. Called also Oculocerebral-hypopigmentation s.

CRST s., see CREST s.

Crush s., the edema, oliguria, an other symptoms of renal failure which follow the crushing of a part, especially a large muscle mass; a condition of renal insufficiency leading to uremia, due to necrosis of the lower nephrons, blocking the tubular lumens of this region. The condition is seen after severe injuries especially crushing injuries to muscles.

Cruveilhier-Baumgarten s., cirrhosis of the liver with portal hypertension, associate with congenital patency of the umbilical or paraumbilical veins. It is characterized by hematemesis, ascites, splenomegaly, hypersplenism, esophageal varices, caput medusae, large tortuous veins in the abdominal wall, and a venous hum, often accompanied by a thrill, usually hear over the region of the xiphoid process. Called also Cruveilhir-Baumgarten cirrhosis.

Cryptophthamos s., an autosomal recessive abnormality, characterized by absence of the palpebral apertures, disorganization of one or both ocular globes, malformed ears, cleft palate, laryngeal stenosis, syndactyly, meningoencephalocele, imperforate anus, cardiac defects, and maldeveloped kidneys.

Cubital tunnel s., a complex of symptoms resulting from injury or compression of the ulnar nerve at the elbow, with pain and numbness along the ulnar aspect of the hand and forearm, and weakness of the hand.

Culture-specific s., a form of disturbed behavior highly specific to certain cultural systems and that does not conform to Western nosolgic entities; examples are amok, koro, piblokto, and windigo.

Curtius's., hypertrophy of one side of the entire body or a portion of one side of the body, as of the face; called also hemihypertrophy.

Cushing's s., 1. A condition, more commonly seen in females, due to hyperadrenocorticism resulting from neoplasms of the adrenal cortex or the anterior lobe of the pituitary, or to prolonged excessive intake of glucocorticoids for therapeutic purpose (Cushing's s. medicamentosus or iatrogenic Cushing's s.). The symptoms and signs may include rapidly developing adiposity of the face, neck, and trunk, kyphosis caused by osteoporosis of the spine, hypertension, diabetes mellitus, amenorrhea, hypertrichosis (in females), impotence (in males), dusky complexion with purple markings (striae), polycythemia, pain in the abdomen and backs, and muscular wasting and weakness. When secondary to excessive pituitary secretion of adrenocorticotropin, it is known as Cushing's disease. Called also Cushing's basophilism, and pituitary basophilism. 2. In tumors of the crebellopontine angle and acoustic tumors; subjective noises, impairment of hearing, ipsilateral cerebellar ataxia, and eventually ipsilateral impairment of the sixth and seventh nerves function together with elevated intracranial pressure.

Cushing's medicamentosus, see Cushing's s. def 1.

Cyrix's s., a syndrome due to slipped rib cartilages pressing on the nerves at the interchondral joint, resulting in pain in the region of the cartilage, radiation of pain in the shoulder and arm, or pain similar to that of angina pectoris.

Da costa's s., neurocirculatory asthenia, see functional cardiovascular disease.

Danbolt-Closs s., acrodermatitis enteropathica—a severe gastrointestinal and cutaneous disease of early childhood, due to autosomal recessive disorder of zinc uptake and characterized by a vesicopustulous dermatitis, preferentially located around body orifices and on the head, hands, and feet, with diarrhea, true steatorrhea and loss of hair.

Danlos's s., see Ehlers-Danlos s.

Dandy-Walker s., congenital hydrocephalus due to obstruction of the foramina of Magendie and Lushka.

Debré-Sémélaigne s., autosomal recessive athyrotic cretinism associated with myotonia and muscular pseudohypertrophy. Called also Kocher-Debre-Semelaigne s.

Defibrination s., diffuse intravascular coagulation—a disorder characterised by reduction in elements involved in blood coagulation due to their utilization in widespread blood clotting within the vessels; the activation of clotting mechanism may arise from any of a number of disorders. In the late stages, it is marked by profuse hemorrhaging.

Dego's s., malignant atrophic papulosis; see Dego's disease

Dejerine's s., 1. A syndrome in cortical sensory disturbances characterized by impairment of sensory discrimination (astereognosis), judgement of intensity and recognition of difference. 2. Of bulbar lesions, those in the upper part of the bulb produce paralysis of the twelfth nerve of the side of the lesion and hemiplegia on the opposite side; lesion in the lower part of the bulb cause paralysis of the larynx and soft palate. 3. Symptoms of radiculitis; namely distribution of the pain, motor and sensory defects in the region of the radicular or segmental disturbances of the nerve roots rather than along the course of the peripheral nerve. 4. A syndrome resembling tabes dorsalis, with deep sensibility depressed but tactile sense normal. It is due to lesion of the long root fibers of the posterior column.

Dejerine-Klumpke s., see Klumpke's paralysis.

s. of Dejerine-Roussay, see Thalamic s.

Dejerine-Sottas s., progressive hypertrophic interstitial neuropathy, see Dejerine-Sottas disease.

de Lange's s., a congenital syndrome in which severe mental retardation is associated with many abnormalities, including short stature (Amsterdam dwarf), brachycephaly, low-set ears, webbed neck, carp mouth, depressed bridge of the nose with the end tilted up and forward directed nostrils, bushy eyebrows meeting at the midline, unruly coarse hair growing low on the forehead and neck and flat spade like hands with short tapering fingers. Called also Brachmann-de Lange s., Cornelia de Lange's s., and typus degenerative amstelodamensis.

Dengue shock s., a syndrome affecting principally South-East Asian children, distinguished from classic dengue by hemorrhagic manifestation, including thrombocytopenia and hemoconcentration, and caused by the same serotype of dengue virus. WHO's classification according to severity is grade I, fever, constitutional symptoms, and positive tourniquet test; grade II, grade I plus spontaneous bleeding into skin, gums, gastrointestinal tracts and other sites; grade III, grade II plus circulatory failure and agitation; and grade IV profound shock with undetectable blood pressure and pulse. Dengue shock syndrome comprises grades III and IV. Called also Phillipine d., and Thai hemorrhagic fever.

del Castillo's s., galactorrhea-amenorrhea syndrome not associated with pregnancy.

Dengue-Marfan's., spastic paralysis and mental retardation in association with congenital syphilis.

Depersonalization s., see under disorder.

Depressive s., major depressive episode (DSM III-R), a period of depressed mood with a loss of interest or pleasure in one's usual activities. Associated symptoms of depressive syndrome are appetite or sleep disturbance, change in weight, psychomotor agitation or retardation, difficulty in thinking and concentration, lack of energy and fatigue, feeling of worthlessness, self-reproach, or inappropriate guilt and recurrent thoughts of death or suicide.

De Sanctis-Cacchione s., a hereditary syndrome transmitted as an autosomal recessive trait, consisting of xeroderma pigmentosum associated with mental retardation, retarded growth, gonadal hypoplasia and sometimes with neurologic complications and photosensitivity; called also Xerodermicidiocy.

De Toni-Fanconi s., see Fanconi's s. def 2.

Diamond Blackfan s., congenital hypoplastic anemia—a general term indicating a form of anemia due to varying degrees of erythrocytic hypoplasia without leukopenia or thrombocytopenia.

Diencephalic s., failure to thrive, emaciation, and sometimes nevus unius lateris (a verrucous epidermal nevus, ranging from flesh colored to yellowish-brown, but sometimes more deeply pigmented, and occurring in linear, unilaterally distributed pattern on the extremities, the lesions usually follow the long axis and may be arranged in continuous or broken spiral streaks, band or patches, and on the trunk, they usually have a transverse orientation, as if along the distribution of intercostal nerves).

DiGeorge s., A congenital disorder in which defective development of the third and fourth pharyngeal pouches results in hypoplasia or aplasia of the thymus and parathyroid glands, often associated with congenital heart defects, anomalies of the great vessels, esophageal atresia, and abnormalities of facial structures. Depending on the degree of parathyroid and thymic hypoplasia, there is hypocalcemic tetany or seizures due to lack of parathyroid hormone and deficiency of cell-mediated immunity resulting in increased susceptibility to low grade or opportunistic pathogens, e.g. fungi, viruses, and *Pneumocystis carinii*, called also Thymic aplasia or Hypoplasia and Pharyngeal Pouch syndrome.

Dightons-Adair s., see van der Hoeve's s.

Di Guglielmo s., erythroleukemia—a malignant blood dyscrasias, one of the myeloproliferative disorders, characterized by neoplastic proliferation of erythroblastic and myeloblastic elements, with atypical erythroblasts and myeloblasts in the peripheral blood, and showing a variable (acute and chronic) clinical course.

Donohue's s., leprechaunism—an exceedingly rare and lethal familial condition marked by slow development both physically and mentally, by elfin facies (wide-set eyes and low-set ears, with hirsutism), as suggested by name, and severe endocrine disorders, as indicated by enlargement of clitoris and breasts in females and of the phallus in males.

Down s. a chromosome disorder characterized by a small, antero-posteriorly flattened skull, short, flat-bridge nose, epicanthal fold, short phalanges, widened spaces between the first and second digits of hands and feet, and moderate to severe mental retardation, with Alzheimer's disease developing in the fourth or fifth decade. The chromosomal aberration is trisomy of chromosome 21 associated with late maternal age. Called also Trisomy 21 and nondisjunction; formerly called Mongolism.

Drebach's s., elliptocytosis—a hereditary disorder in which the greater proportion of the erythrocytes are elliptical in shape, and which is characterized by varying degrees of increased red cell destruction and anemia.

Dressler's s., see Postmyocardial infarction s.

Duane's s., a hereditary congenital syndrome in which the affected eye shows limitations or absence of abduction, restriction of adduction, retraction of the globe on adduction, narrowing of the palpebral fissure on adduction and widening on abduction and deficient convergence. It is transmitted as an autosomal dominant trait. Called also retraction s. and Stilling-Turk-Duane's.

Dubin-Johnson s., a familial chronic form of nonhemolytic jaundice thought to be due to defect in the excretion of conjugated bilirubin and certain other organic anions (e.g. sulfobromophthalein) by the liver. It is characterized by the presence of a brown, coarsely granular pigments in the hepatic cells, which is pathognomonic of the condition.

Dubin-Sprinz s., see Dubin-Johnson s.

Dubreuil-Chambardel s., dental caries of the incisors, in most instances only the upper ones, usually appearing during adolescence; within a few years the teeth are irreparably damaged. Some authorities do not consider this syndrome a legitimate entity.

Duchenne's s., the collective signs of bulbur paralysis, see under paralysis.

Duchenne-Erb s., see under paralysis.

Dumping s., a complex reaction thought to be secondary to excessively rapid emptying of the gastric contents into the jejunum, manifested by nausea, weakness, sweating, palpitation, varying degrees of syncope, often a sensation of warmth, and sometimes diarrhea, occurring after ingestion of food by patients who have had partial gastrectomy and gastrojejunostomy. Called also Jejunal s, and Postgastrectomy s.

Duncan's s., see X-linked lymphoproliferative s.

Duplay's s., (obs) subacromial or subdeltoid bursitis; inflammation and calcification of the subacromial or subdeltoid bursa, resulting in pain, tenderness, and limitation of motion in the shoulder.

Dupre's s., the symptoms and signs of meningeal irritation associated with acute febrile illness or dehydration or actual infection of the meninges. Called also Dupre's disease.

Dyke-Davidoff s., a syndrome possibly due to injury to or severe disease affecting one side of the brain during the neonatal period, characterized by mental retardation, asymmetry of the face, and varying degrees of hemiplegia, neurological impairment and atrophy of the side of the body contralateral to the lesion.

Dysmnesic s., see Amnestic s.

Dysplasia oculodentodigitalis s., oculodentodigital dysplasia—a rare hereditary condition transmitted as an autosomal dominant trait, characterized by bilateral microphthalmos, abnormally small nose with anteverted nostrils, hypotrichosis, dental anomalies, camptodactyly, syndactyly, and missing phalanges of the toes.

Dysplastic nevus s., the occurrence of dysplastic nevi in persons with or at risk for familial or nonfamilial malignant melanoma.

Eaton-Lambert s., a myasthenia-like syndrome in which the weakness usually affects the limbs, and ocular and bulbar muscles are spared; there is reduced muscle action potential on stimulation of its nerve but with repetitive stimulation it becomes augmented. It is often associated with oat-cell carcinoma of the lung. Called also Myasthenic s.

Ectopic ACTH s., a condition in which tumors arising from nonendocrine tissue produce ACTH. Depending on its duration, the syndromes may be subtle, resemble true Cushing's disease, but hypokalemic alkalosis and weakness are often the dominant manifestations.

Ectopic-hypercalcemic s., hypercalcemia resulting from ectopic production by a pancreatic islet cell or other (lung, kidney) tumor of a polypeptide with activity like that of parathyroid hormone.

Ectrodactyly-ectodermal dysplasia-clefting s., see EEC s.

Edwards's., see trisomy 18 s.

EEC s., a congenital syndrome inherited as an autosomal dominant trait involving both ectodermal and mesodermal tissues, which consists of ectodermal dysplasia associated with hypopigmentation of the skin and hair, scanty hair and eyebrow, absence of lashes, nail dystrophy, hypo-and microdontia, ectrodactyly, and cleft lip and palate. Called also Ectrodactyly-ectodermal dysplasia-clefting s.

Effort s., neurocirculatory asthenia see Dacosta's s.,

Egg-white s., biotin deficiency—deficiency of biotin has been produced in humans and experimental animals fed uncooked egg-white, such deficiency being due to avidin present in the egg-white, which renders the biotin of the diet unavailable. Manifestation of biotin deficiency in the experimental animals includes paralysis usually of the hind quarters (cows, dogs, rats), dermatitis (rats, pigs, fowl), alopecia (mice, pigs, monkeys) and graying of brown black fur (mice, monkeys) alpha b is the product isolated from the egg yolk, and beta b from the liver.

Ehlers-Danlos s., a group of inherited disorders of the connective tissue, occurring in many types based on clinical, genetic and biochemical evidence, varying in severity from mild to lethal and transmitted genetically as autosomal recessive, autosomal dominant, or X-ray linked recessive traits. The major manifestations include hyperextensible skin and joints, easy bruisability, friability of tissues with bleeding and poor wound healing, calcified subcutaneous spheroids and pseudotumors, and cardiovascular, gastrointestinal, orthopedic, and ocular defects. Called also cutis elastica or hyper-elastica, Danlos s., Danlos or Ehlers-Danlos disease, and elastic or India rubber skin.

Eisenmenger's s., ventricular septal defect with pulmonary hypertension and cyanosis due to right-to-left (reversed) shunt of blood. Sometimes defined as pulmonary hypertension (pulmonary vascular disease) and cyanosis with the shunt being at the atrial, ventricular, or, great vessel area.

Ekbom s., see Restless legs s.

Elfin facies s., see Williams s.

Ellis-van Creveld s., chondroectodermal dysplasia—a chondroplasia occurring in association with defective development of the skin, hair, and teeth, polydactyly and defect of the cardiac septum.

Embryonic testicular regression s., see Vanishing testes s.

EMG s., (acronym for exomphalos-macroglossia-gigantism), see Beckwith-Wiedemann s.

Empty-sella s., a syndrome diagnosed radiologically in which the diaphragm sellae is vestigial, the sella turnica forms an extension of the subarachnoid space and is filled with cerebrospinal fluid, and the pituitary fossa appears to be empty, although the pituitary gland is present in a flattened form. Pituitary hormone secretion may be normal, deficient, or excessive.

Encephalotrigeminal vascular s., the combination of multiple angiomas of the brain and vascular nevi in the trigeminal region.

Epiphyseal s., precocious development of external genitalia and sexual function, precocious abnormal growth of long bones, appearance of signs of internal hydrocephalus, in the absence of all other motor and sensory symptoms indicating a lesion of the pineal body. Called also Pellizzi's s., Pineal s., and macrogenitosomia precox.

Epstein's s., see Nephrotic s.

Erb's s., the totality of signs of myasthenia gravis—a disorder of neuromuscular function due to the presence of antibodies to acetylcholine receptors at the neuromuscular junction; clinically there is exhaustion and fatigue of the muscular system with the tendency to fluctuate in severity and without sensory disturbance or atrophy. The disorder may be restricted to muscle group or become generalized with severe weakness and, in some cases with ventilatory insufficiency. It may affect any muscle of the body, but especially those of the eye, face, lips, tongue, throat, and neck.

Erythrocyte autosensitization s., see Painful bruising s.

Euthyroid sick s., the simulation of hypothyroidism as assessed by thyroid-function tests in a euthyroid patient suffering from systemic illness.

Evans's s., acquired hemolytic anemia and thrombocytopenia.

Exomphalos-macroglossia-gigantism s., see Beckwith-Wiedemann syndrome.

Extrapyramidal s., any of a group of clinical disorders characterized by abnomal involuntary movements, including parkinsonism, athetosis, and chorea.

Faber's s., hypochromic anemia.

Faciodigitogenital s., see Aarskog-Scott s.

Fallot's s., see Fallot disease.

Fanconi's s., 1. A rare recessive disorder, with a poor prognosis, characterized by pancytopenia hypoplasia of the bone marrow, and patchy brown discoloration of the skin due to the disposition of melanin, and associated with multiple congenital anomalies of the musculoskeletal and genitourinary systems. Called also Fanconi's pancytopenia, pancytopenia-dysmelia s., congenital hypoplastic anemia, constitutional infantile panmyelopathy, fanconi's anemia, and congenital pancytopenia. 2. A general term for a group if diseases marked by dysfunction of the proximal renal tubules, with generalized hyperaminoaciduria, renal glycosuria, hyperphosphaturia, and bicarbonate and water loss; the most common cause is cystinosis (q.v.) but it is also associated with other genetic disease and occurs in idiopatic and acquired forms. When unassociated with cystinosis, the disorder is also called de Toni-Fanconi syndrome.

Farber s., Farber-Uzman s., see Farber disease.

Favre-Racouchot s., nodular elastoidosis of Favre-Racouchot—actinic elastosis occurring chiefly in elderly men, in which giant comedones, pilosebaceous cysts, and large fold of yellow and furrowed skin are seen in periorbital region.

Felty's s., a combination of chronic (rheumatoid) arthritis, splenomegaly, leukopenia pigmented spots on the skin of the lower extremities, and other inconsistent evidence of hyperplenism, namely, anemia and thrombocytopenia.

Feminizing testes s., see Testicular feminization s.

Fertile eunuch s., a syndrome of eunchoidism, with variable secondary sexual development, associated with normal spermatogenesis, normal levels of follicle-stimulating hormone, and variably low levels of luteinizing hormone.

Fetal alcohol s., a syndrome of altered prenatal growth and morphogenesis occurring in infants born of women who were chronically alcoholic during pregnancy; it includes maxillary hypoplasia, prominence of the forehead and mandible, short palpebral fissures, midophthalmia, epicanthal folds, severe growth retardation mental retardation, and microcephaly.

Fetal face s., see Robinow's s.

Fetal hydantoin s., a symptom complex characterized by poor growth and development with craniofacial and skeletal abnormalities, produced by prenatal exposure to hydantoin analogues, including phenytoin.

Fevre-Languepin s., popliteal webbing associated with cleft lip and palate, fistula of the lower lip, syndactyly, onychodysplasia, and pes equinovarus. Called also popliteal pterygium s.

Fiessinger-Leroy-Reiter's s., see Reiter's syndrome.

First arch s., malformations including macrostomia, hemignathia, and deformities of the external ear, resulting from an inhibitory process occurring toward the seventh week of embryonic life and affecting the facial bones derived from the first branchial arch.

Fitz Hugh-Curtis s., perihepatitis occurring as a complication of gonorrhea in women, marked by fever, upper quadrant pain, tenderness and spasm of the abdominal wall, an occasionally by friction rub over the liver.

Floppy infant s., a congenital myopathy of infants, characterized clinically by hypotoria an muscle weakness. The pathologic changes in skeletal muscle include numerous eosinophilic intranuclear crystals, characteristic crystal morphology, myofibrillar fragmentation, sarcoplasmic crystals, and expansion of the Z bands.

Floppy valve s., See Mitral valve prolapse s.

Focal dermal hypoplasia s., a hereditary congenital syndrome of extensive ectodermal and mesodermal dysplasia, chiefly of skin and bones, with linear or serpiginous patches (especially on the buttocks and thighs), telangiectases, pigmentation, and orificial papillomas, often with syndactyly, oligodactyly, or adactyly. An X-linked dominant trait, lethal in male, is believed responsible. Called also Goltz's and Goltz-Gorlin s.

Forbes-AI bright s., galactorrhea-amenorrhea syndrome not associated with pregnancy, usually a pituitary tumor is present.

Forsius-Eriksson s., an X-linked ocular albinism differing from the Nettleship type in that the males show hypoplastic foveas, axial myopia, and protanomaly and the females show slightly defective color discrimination and latent nystagmus, but no mosaic pigment pattern in the fundus. Called also ocular albinism, OA_2, Forsius-Eriksson type ocular albinism, and Aland eye disease.

Foster kennedy s., see Kennedy's s.,

Four-day s., respiratory distress syndrome of newborn; so called because the infant usually recovers or dies within four days.

Foville's s., a syndrome similar to the Millard-Gubler syndrome (q.v.), except that, in addition to paralysis of the outward movement of the eye, there is paralysis of conjugate movement.

Fragile X s., an X-linked syndrome associated with fragile site on the long arm of the X chromosome at q 27-28, associated with mental retardation, enlarged testes, high forehead, big jaw, and long ears in most males and mild mental retardation in many heterozygous females. In some families, unaffected transmitting males have occurred.

Franceschetti s., mandibulofacial dysostosis—a hereditary disorder occurring in two forms the complete form (Franceschetti s,) is characterized by antimongoloid slant of the palpebral fissures, coloboma of the lower lid, micrognathia and hypoplasia of the zygomatic arches and microtia. It is transmitted as and autosomal dominant trait. The incomplete form (Treacher Collins s.) is characterized by the same anomalies in less pronounced degrees. It occurs sporadically, but and autosomal dominant mode of transmission is suspected.

Franceschetti-Jadassohn s., an autosomal dominant disorder characterized by the presence of slate-gray to brown reticular pigmentation beginning after infancy without preceding inflammatory changes, and associated with palmoplantar hyperkeratosis, vasomotor changes with hypohidrosis, and yellowing of the dental enamel. Called also chromatophore, nevus of Naegeli, Naegeli syndrome and Naegeli's incontentia pigmenti.

Francois s., see oculomandibulofacial s.

Freeman-Sheldon s., craniocarpotarsal dystrophy—a congenital anomally transmitted as an autosomal dominant trait, consisting of characteristic flattened mask like facies, microstomia; the lips protruding as in whistling; deep set eyes with hypertelorism; camptodactyly with ulnar deviation of the fingers; and talipes equinovarus.

Frey's s., see Auriculotemporal s.

Friderichsen-Waterhouse s., see Waterhouse-Friderichsen s.

Friedmann's vasomotor s., a train or cycle of symptoms due to a progressive subacute encephalitis of traumatic origin, including a sense of fullness in the head, headache, vertigo, irritability, insomnia, easy fatigability, and defect of memory.

Frohlich's s., adiposogenital dystrophy, see Adiposogenital s.

Froin's s., a condition of the lumbar spinal fluid consisting of a transparent clear yellow color (xanthochromia), with the finding of large amounts of protein, rapid coagulation, and the absence of an increased number of cells. It is seen in certain organic nervous diseases in which the lumbar fluid is cut off from communication with the fluid in the ventricles. Called also Loculation s.

Frommel-Chiari s., see Chiari-Frommel s.

Fuchs's s., unilateral heterochromia, fine keratic precipitates, and secondary cataract.

Functional prepubertal castrates., see Vanishing testes s.

G s., see Hypertelorism-hypospadias s.

Gailliard's s., dextrocardia from retraction of lungs and pleura to the right.

Gaisbock's s., stress polycythemia, see Osler's disease, Vanquez's disease.

Galactorrhea-amenorrhea s., amenorrhea and galactorrhea associated with increased levels of prolactin usually produced by a pituitary adenoma.

Ganser's s., the giving of approximate answers to questions, commonly associated with amnesia, disorientation, perceptual disturbances, fugue, and conversion symptoms.

Gardner's s., familial polyposis of the large bowel (with malignant potential), supernumerary teeth, fibrous dysplasia of the skull, osteomas, fibromas, and epithelial cysts.

Gardner-Diamond s., painful bruising s.

Gasser's s., see Hemolytic-uremic s.

Gay bowel s., an assortment of sexually transmitted bowel and rectal diseases affecting homosexual males, caused by a wide variety of infectious agents.

Gee-Herter-Heubner s., the infantile form of nontropical sprue, see adult celiac disease.

Gelineau's s., narcolepsy.

General dysphoria s., a group of psychological problems associated with discrepancy between the physical sex assignment and the psychological gender identity.

General adaptation s., the total of all non-specific systemic reactions of the body to long-continued exposure to systemic stress.

Gernardt's s., bilateral abductor paralysis of the vocal cords causing inspiratory dyspnea.

Gerlier's s., see Gerlier's disease.

Gerstmann's s., a combination of finger agnosia, right-left disorientation, agraphia, acalculia, and often constructional apraxia, due to a lesion in the angular gyrus of the dominant hemisphere.

Gianotti-Crosti s., a generally benign and self-limited disease of young children representing a primary natural infection with hepatitis B virus, characterized by the appearance of crops of monomorphous, usually nonpruritic dusky or coppery red, flat-topped, firm papules forming a symmetrical eruption on the face, buttocks, and limbs, including the palms and soles, and associated with malaise, low-grade fever, and few other constitutional symptoms. Called also Acrodermatitis papulosa infantum, infantile papular acrodermatitis and papular acrodermatitis of childhood.

Giant Platelet s., see Bernard-Soulier disease.

Gilbert s., an inborn error of bilirubin metabolism, probably autosomal dominant, a benign elevation of unconjugated bilirubin with no liver damage or hematologic abnormalities. Called also constitutional hepatic dysfunction, familial cholemia, hyperbilirubinemia I, constitutional hyperbilirubinemia, familial non-hemolytic jaundice, and Gilbert cholemia or disease.

Gilles de La Tourette's s., a syndrome of facial and vocal tics with onset in childhood, progressing to generalized jerking movements in any part of the body, with echolalia and coprolalia; once thought to have an unfavorable prognosis but recently shown to be responsive to treatment with butyrophenones.

Glioma-polyposis s., see Turcot s.

Glaucagonoma s., a glucagon-secreting tumor of the alpha cells of the pancreas (glucagonoma) occurring in association with increased serum levels of glucagon, mild diabtes mellitus, weight loss, anemia, glossitis, stomatitis, angular cheilitis, blepharitis, and necrolytic migrating erythema (q.v).

Goldenhar's s., oculoauriculovertebral dysplasia, see OAV s.

Goltz s., focal dermal hypoplasia.

Goods's s., immunodeficiency with thymoma.

Goodman s., acrocephalopolysyndactyly, type IV—congenital heart defects, clinodactyly, campylodactyly, and ulnar deviation, but with unimpaired intelligence, is autosomal recessive.

Goodpasture's s., glomerulonephritis associated with pulmonary hemorrhage and circulating antibodies against basement membrane antigens, a condition occurring most frequently in young men and usually having a course of rapidly progressing renal failure with hemoptysis, pulmonary infiltrates, and dyspnea, Cf: anti-glomerular basement membrane antibody disease, under disease.

Gopalan's s., a symptom complex resulting from malnutrition, with signs suggestive of riboflavin deficiency, a burning sensation in the extremities, a feeling of "pins and needles" in the distal parts, and hyperhidrosis.

Gorlin's s., 1. See Basal cell nevus s. 2. See Gorlin-Chaudhry-Moss s.

Gorlin-Goltz s., see Basal cell nevus s.

Gouge-rot-Carteaud s., confluent and reticulated papillomatosis

Gougerot-Nulock-Houwer s., see Sjorgren's s.

Gowers s., Vasovagal attack—a transient vascular and neurogenic reaction marked by pallor, nausea, sweating, bradycardia, and rapid fall of arterial blood pressure which, when below a critical, results in loss of consciousness and characteristic electroencephalographic changes. It is most commonly evoked by emotional stress associated with fever and pain.

Gradenigo's s., palsy of the sixth nerve and unilateral headache in suppurative disease of the middle ear, caused by involvement of the abducens and trigeminal nerves by direct spread of the infection.

Graham Little s., a syndrome characterized by the presence of cicatricial patches of alopecia of the scalp with prominent follicular plugging and follicular keratoses involving the trunk and extremities, sometimes associated with noncicatricial alopecia of the axillae, pubes, trunk, and extremities.

Gray s., a potentially fatal condition seen in neonates, particularly premature infants, due to a reaction to chloramphenicol, characterized by an ashen gray cyanosis, listlessness, weakness, and hypotension.

Gray spinal s., muscular atrophy, syringomyelic disturbances of sensation, and vasomotor troubles due to lesions of the gray matter of the spinal cord.

Greig's s., ocular hypertension—a condition characterized by abnormal increase in the interorbital distance, often associated with cleidocranial or craniofacial dystosis, and occasionally accompanied by mental deficiency.

Griscelli s., an albinoidism of autosomal recessive inheritance, marked by hypomelanosis, frequent pyogenic infection, hepatosplenomegaly. Neutro and thrombopenia and possible immunodeficiency. Called also hypopigmentation immunodeficiency disease.

Gronblad-Strandberg s., angioid streaks in the retina together with pseudoxanthoma elasticum of the skin.

Gruber's s., see Meckel's s.

Guillain-Barre s., acute febrile polyneuritis, see Barre-Guillian s.

Gunn's s., unilateral ptosis of the eyelid, with the association of movements of the affected upper eyelid with those of the jaw. Called also Jaw-winking s.

Gustatory sweating s., see Auriculotemporal s.

Hadefield-Clarke s., Clarke-Hadefield s.

Hakim's s., normal-pressure hydrocephalus.

Hallemann-Streiff s., Hallermann-Streiff-Francois., see oculomandibulofacial s.

Hallervorder-Spatz s., a hereditary disorder characterized by marked reduction in the number of the myelin sheaths of the globus pallidus and substantia nigra, with accumulations of iron pigment. Progressive rigidity beginning in the legs, choreoathetoid movements, dysarthria, and progressive mental deterioration. Transmitted as an autosomal recessive trait, it usually begins in the first or second decade, with death usually occurring before the thirtieth year. Called also Hallervorden-Spatz disease, status dysmyelinatus, and status dysmyelinisatus.

Hamman's s., pneumomediastinum.

Hamman-Rich s., idiopathic pulmonary fibrosis—chronic inflammation and progressive fibrosis of the pulmonary alveolar walls, with steadily progressive dyspnea, resulting finally in death from oxygen lack or right heart failure.

Hand-foot-and-mouth s., see under disease.

Hand-foot-uterus s., a congenital syndrome consisting of small feet with unusually short great toes, abnormal thumbs, and, in females, duplication of the genital tract.

Hand-Schüller-Christian s., the triad of exophthalmos, diabetes insipidus, and bone destruction, sometimes found in Langerhans' cell granulomatosis.

Hand-shoulder s., reflex sympathetic dystrophy of the upper extremity; see under dystrophy.

Hanhart's s., a congenital syndrome characterized chiefly by severe micrognathia, high nose root, small eyelid fissures, low-set ears, and variable absence of digits or limbs, usually below the elbow or knee.

Hanot's s., see Hanot's disease.

Hanot-Chauffard s., hypertrophic cirrhosis with pigmentation and diabetes mellitus.

Harada's s., bilateral diffuse exudative choroiditis and retinal detachment occurring in association with headache, vomiting, an increase of lymphocytes in the cerebrospinal fluid, and temporary or permanent deafness; alopecia, vitiligo, and poliosis may be transient features. Called also Harada's disease Cf: Vogt-Kayanagi s.

Hare's s., see Pancoast's s., def 1.

Harris s., hyperinsulinism due to organic endogenous factors, such as insulinoma, manifested by hypoglycemia, weakness, perspiration, jitteriness, tachycardia, mental confusion, and disturbances of vision. Hartnup s., see under disease.

Hayem-Widal s., hemolytic anemia.

Heart hand s., see Holt-Oram s.

Heerfordt's s., an occasional manifestation of sarcoidosis consisting of enlargement of the parotid and lacrimal glands, anterior uveitis, bell's palsy and fever. Called also Heerfordt's disease and uveoparotid fever.

Heidenhaim's s., a rapidly progressive degenerative disease manifested by cortical blindness presenile dementia, dysarthria, ataxia, athetoid movements, and generalized rigidity.

Hemangioma-thrombocytopenia s., see Kasa-Bach-Merritt s.

Hemohistioblastic s., reticuloendotheliosis (hyperplasia of reticuloendothelial tissue).

Hemolytic-uremic s., a rare syndrome of unknown etiology occurring mainly in children under 4 years of age, characterized by renal failure, microangiopathic hemolytic anemia, and severe thrombocytopenia and purpura.

Hemopleuropneumonic s., dyspnea, hemoptysis, tachycardia, and fever, with dullness at the base of the chest and tubular respiration over the middle zone of the chest; indicative of pneumonia and hydrothorax in puncture wounds of the chest.

Hench-Rosenberg s., palindromic rheumatism—a condition in which there are repeated episodes of arthritis and periarthritis without fever and without producing irreversible changes in the joints.

Henoch-Schonlein s., see Schonlein-Henoch disease.

Hepatorenal s., functional renal failure, oliguria, and low urinary sodium concentration, without pathological renal changes, associated with cirrhosis and ascites or with obstructive jaundice.

Hereditary benign intraepithelial dyskeratosis s., a syndrome characterized by plaques of of bulbar conjunctiva and oral mucosal thickening. Clinically similar to white-folded hypertrophy (white sponge nevus of Cannon); it is inherited as an autosomal dominant trait with a high degree of penetrance.

Hermansky-Pudlak s., an autosomal recessive form of tyrosinase-positive oculocutaneous albinism (ty-pos OCA) with hemorrhagic diathesis secondary to a platelet defect, and accumulation of a ceroid-like substance in the reticuloendothelial system, oral mucosa, and urine.

Hines-Bannick s., intermittent attack of low temperature and disabling sweating.

Hoffmann-Werdnig s., see Werdnig-Hoffmann paralysis.

Holiday heart s., paroxysms of arrhythmias, most commonly atrial fibrillation, in alcoholic patients without overt cardiomyopathy after a weekend bout of alcoholic consumption, especially during the year-end holiday season.

Holmes-Adie s., see Adie's s.

Holt-Oram s., autosomal heart disease of varying severity, usually an atrial or ventricular septal defect, associated with skeletal malformation (hypoplastic thumb and short forearm). Called also heart-hand s.

Homen's s., a genetically determined disease of the nervous system with prominent abnormalities in the lenticular nucleus, marked by vertigo, ataxia, dysarthria, gradually increasing dementia, with rigidity of the body, especially the legs.

Horner's s., Horner-Bernard s., sinking of the eyeball, ptosis of the upper eyelid, slight elevation of the lower lid, constriction of the pupil, narrowing of the palpebral fissure, anhidrosis and flushing of the affected side of the face; caused by paralysis of the cervical sympathetic nerves. Called also Bernard's s; Bernard-Homer s., and Horner's ptosis.

Horton's s., 1. Migrainous neuralgia—a migrant variant characterized by attacks of unilateral excruciating pain over the eye and forehead, with temperature elevation, lacrimation, and rhinorrhea; attacks last 15 to 30 min and tend to occur in clusters. Because attacks identical to the spontaneous attacks may be induced in sufferers by subcutaneous injection of histamine diphosphate, it is also known as histamine cephalgia or headache syndrome 2. Temporal arteritis—a chronic vascular disease of unknown origin, most common in carotid arterial system but also occurring in other large and small systemic arteries, characterized by proliferative inflammation, often with giant cells and granulomas, and by headache, difficulty in chewing, weakness, weight loss, fever, and symptoms of sepsis, with a markedly increase erythrocyte sedimentation rate and leukocytosis. Ocular involvement, ranging from diplopia to complete blindness, occurs in about half the subjects. The disease occurs exclusively in older persons, and is often associated with polymyalgia rheumatica.

Howel-Evan's s., diffuse palmoplantar keratoderma (see Unna-Thost disease) occurring between the ages of 5 and 15 and associated with the development of esophageal cancer later in life.

Hunt's s., see Ramsay Hunt s.

Hunter's s., Hunter-Hurler s., a mucopolysaccharidosis caused by deficient iduronate sulfatase, characterized biochemically by excretion of dermatan sulfate and heparan sulfate in the urine, and differing clinically from the Hurler syndrome by (i) X-linked inheritence; (ii) slower progession, lesser severity, and longer survival (thus resembling the Hurler-Scheie syndrome); and (iii) absence of corneal clouding. Two clinical forms exist. Mucopolysaccharidosis II-XR, severe or

MPS IIA has Hurler-Scheie-like symptoms with death before 15, usually from heart disease; mucopolysaccharidosis II-XR, mild or MPS IIB has onset in first decade, dwarfism, dysostosis multiplex, joint stiffness, visceromegaly, cardiac disease, nerve entrapment, and normal or nearly normal intelligence and lifespan.

Hurler s., the prototype of the mucopolysaccharidoses, and the gravest of the three allelic disorders of mucopolysaccharidosis I, specifically marked by corneal clouding and death by 10 years old. Onset is after the first year with progressive physical and mental deterioration. Further symptoms include gargoyle-like facies with hypertelorism, depressed nasal bridge, large tongue, and widely spaced teeth; dwarfism; severe somatic and skeletal changes, including short neck and trunk, scaphocephaly, and kyphosis with gibbus; short broad hands with short fingers; progressive opacities of the cornea; deafness; cardiovascular defects; hepatosplenomegaly; and joint contractures. Death is usually caused by respiratory infection and heart failure. Called als α-L-iduronidase deficiency, Hurler type, and mucopolysaccharidosis IH.

Hurler-Scheie s., one of the three allelic disorders of mucopolysaccharidosis I, with clinical features intermediate between the Hurler and the Scheie syndromes, specifically characterized by receding chin (micrognathism). Symptoms include mental retardation, dwarfism, dysostosis multiplex, corneal clouding, deafness, hernia, stiff joints (claw hand), and valvular heart disease. Patients survive till their late teens or twenties. Called also mucopolysaccharidosis I H/S, Hurler-Scheie compound, α-L-iduronidase deficiency. Hurler-Scheie type.

Hutchinson's s., diffuse interstitial keratitis, labrynthine disease, and Hutchinson teeth, seen in inherited syphilis.

Hutchinson-Gliford s., see Hutchinson-Gilford disease

Hutchinson s., neuroblastoma with cranial metastasis.

Hyaline membrane s., see Respiratory distress s. of newborn

17-hydroxylase deficiency s., congenital adrenal hyperplasia resulting from a deficiency of the enzyme 17-α-hydroxylase, leading to a deficiency of estrogen and androgen and consequent sexual infantilism; the compensatory increase in secretion of deoxycorticosterone and corticosterone result in hypokalemic alkalosis and hypertension.

Hyperabduction s., thoracic outlet syndrome due to compression of the brachial plexus trunk roots and axillary vessels by the pectoralis minor muscle and the coracoid process when the arms are stretched above the head, as during sleep.

Hyperactive child s., see Attention-deficit hyperactivity disorder.

Hypercalcemia s., see Milk-alkali s.

Hypereosinophilic s., a massive increase in the number of eosinophils in the blood, mimicking leukemia, and characterized by eosinophilic infiltration of the heart, brain, liver, and lungs and by a progressively fatal course.

Hyperimmuno-globulinemia E s., a primary immunodeficiency disorder characterized by recurrent staphylococcal abscesses of skin, lungs, joints, and other sites, pruritic dermatitis very high serum IgE levels, normal levels of IgG, IgA, and IgM, blood and sputum eosinophilia, low anamnestic antibody responses to booster immunization, and poor antibody and cell-mediated responses to neoantigens. Called also Buckley's s.

Hyperkinetic s., see Attention-deficit hyperactivity disorder.

Hyperkinetic heart s., increased cardiac output of unknown cause associated with slightly elevated systolic and pulse pressures, normal mean arterial pressure, and low systemic vascular resistance.

Hyperlucent lung s., a syndrome simulating localized emphysema, but due to congenital absence or hypoplasia of pulmonary arteries; there may be lobar or segmental agenesis; and accessory lungs, lobes, or segments are not unusual.

Hypersomnia-bulimia s., see Kleine-Levin s.

Hypertelorism-hypospadias s., a congenital condition consisting of hypertelorism associated with hypospadias and a neuromuscular abnormality of the esophagus and swallowing mechanism. Called also G s.

Hyperventilation s., a complex of symptoms that accompany hypocapnia caused by hyperventilation, including palitations, a feeling of shortness of breath or air hunger, lightheadeness or giddiness, profuse perspiration, and tingling sensations in the fingertips, face, or toes; prolonged overbreathing may result in vasomotor collapse and loss of consciousness. Hyperventilation unrecognized by the patient is a common cause of the subjective somatic symptoms associated with chronic anxiety or panic attacks.

Hyperviscosity s., any syndrome associated with increased viscosity of the blood. In the syndrome of serum hyperviscosity, there is spontaneous bleeding and neurologic and ocular disorders. The syndrome of polycythemic hyperviscosity, in which increased viscosity is due to large numbers of red cells, is marked by retarded blood flow, organ congestion, reduced capillary perfusion, and increased cardiac effort. Syndromes of sclerocythemic hyperviscosity comprise those in which the deformability of erythrocytes is impaired, as in sickle cell anemia.

Hypoglossia-hypodactyly s., partial to complete absence of the tongue associated with partial to complete absence of the digits or limbs affecting one or more limbs; it occurs sporadically. Called also aglossia-adactylia s.

Hypoplastic left-heart s., a congenital malformation consisting of hypoplasia or atresia of the left ventricle and of the aorta or mitral valve or both, and characterized by respiratory distress and extreme cyanosis, with cardiac failure and death in early infancy.

Idiopathic post-prandial s., the repeated occurrence of the clinical manifestations of hypoglycemia after meals; a controversial disease entity.

Imerslund s., Imerslund-Graesbeck s., familial megaloblastic anemia—a rare familial form of anemia observed in Norwegian and Finnish children, characterized by selective malabsorption of vitamin B_{12} uninfluenced by intrinsic factor, and associated with proteinuria and structural genitourinary tract anomalies.

Immotile-cilia s., a hereditary syndrome of delayed or absent mucociliary clearance from airways and lack of motion of sperm; Kartagener's syndrome is one variety.

Immunodeficiency s., see under disease

S. of inappropriate antidiuretic hormone (SIADH), persistent hyponatremia, an inappropriately elevated urine osmolality, and no discernible stimulus for ADH release; it may occur with neoplasm's (especially oat cell carcinoma of the lung or pancreatic carcinoma, with ectopic production of ADH by the tumor), pulmonary disorders, and central nervous system diseases, including head trauma.

Inferior s. of red nucleus, see Claude's s.

Inhibitory s., the manifestations produced by a somatostatinoma, including diabetes mellitus, cholecystolithiasis, stetorrhea, indigestion, hypochlorhydria, and occasionally anemia.

Inspissated bile s., biliary obstruction caused by plugging of the outflow tract.

Intrauterine parabiotic s., see Placental transfusion s.

Irritable bowel s., irritable colon s., a chronic noninflammatory disease characterized by abdominal pain, altered bowel habits consisting of diarrhea or constipation or both, and no detectable pathologic change; a variant form is characterized by painless diarrhea. It is a common disorder with a psychophysiologic basis. Called also Spastic or irritable colon.

Ivemark's s., congenital splenic agenesis, cardiac defects, and partial situs inversus viscerum. Called also asplenia s and Polhemus-Schafer-Ivemark s.

Jaccoud's s., chronic arthritis occurring after rheumatic fever, usually after repeated attacks, and characterized by fibrous changes in the joint capsules and tendons, leading to deformities that may resemble rheumatoid arthritis (especially ulnar deviation of fingers); the joints may be painful and rheumatic nodules are often present.

Jackson's s., paralysis of the tenth, eleventh, and twelfth cranial nerves, with paralysis of the soft palate, larynx, and one-half of the tongue, associated with paralysis of the sternomastoid and trapezius muscles.

Jadassohn-Lewandowsky s., pachyonychia congenita—an autosomal dominant syndrome characterized by increased thickness of nails that progresses to produce onychogryposis, hyperkeratosis involving the palms, soles, knees, and elbows, widespread tiny cutaneous horns, leukoplakia of the mucous membranes, and usually hyperhidrosis of hands and feet, and sometimes associated with development of bullae on the palms and soles following trauma.

Jaffe-Lichtenstein s., fibrous dysplasia, see Aibright's s.

Jahnke's s., a variant of the Sturge-Weber syndrome in which glaucoma is absent.

Jaw-Winking s., see Gunn's s.

Jejunal s., see Dumping s.

Jervell and Lange-Nielsen s., a syndrome characterized by attacks of syncope and by sudden death in patients with congenital deafness and electrocardiographic anomalies, especially a prolonged Q-T interval.

Jeune's s., asphyxiating thoracic dystrophy—a congenital hereditary syndrome transmitted as an autosomal recessive trait, in which chondrodystrophy of the rib-cage, usually causing asphyxia early in the newborn period, occurs in association with defects of the phalanges and pelvis.

Job s., an autosomal recessive disorder of neutrophils, characterized by the presence of abnormal or absent chemotactic responses, which leads to repeated development of cold staphylococcal abscesses and eczema, and by hyperimmunoglobulinemia E. It is usually associated with red hair and fair skin. Most cases reported have been in girls.

Jugular foramen s., see Vernet's s.

Kallmann's s., hypogonadotropic eunuchoidism—that due to lack of gonadotropin secretion; either luteinizing hormone or follicle stimulating hormone or both may be deficient, and anosmia or hyposmia may be associated.

Kanner's s., see Autistic disorder.

Karroo s., a condition observed in youth among Afrikaners in the Karroo region, consisting of high fever, alimentary tract disturbance, and tenderness in the lymph glands of the neck.

Kartagener's s., a hereditary disorder involving a combination of dextrocardia (situs inversus), bronchiectasis, and sinusitis, transmitted as an autosomal recessive trait.

Kasabach-Merritt s., a syndrome usually occurring in the first few months of life in which severe thrombocytopenia and other evidence of intravascular coagulation occur in infants with rapidly expanding hemangiomas of the trunk, extremities, and abdominal viscera, and may be associated with bleeding and anemia. Bleeding is thought to be due to trapping and destruction of platelets within the tumor and depletion of circulating clotting factors. Called also hemangioma-thrombocytopenia s.

Kast's s., see Maffucci's s.

Kawasaki s., see Mucocutaneous lymph node s.

Kearns-Sayre s., progressive ophthalmoplegia, pigmentary degeneration of the retina, myopathy, ataxia, and cardiac conduction defect; inherited as an autosomal dominant trait, with onset before age 15.

Kennedy's s., retrobulbar optic neuritis, central scotoma, optic atrophy on the side of the lesion and papilledema on the opposite side, occurring in tumors of the frontal lobe of the brain which press downward.

Kiloh-Nevin s., ocular myopathy in patients with ptosis and progressive external ophthalmoplegia.

Kimmelstiel-Wilson s., intercapillary glomerulosclerosis—a degenerative complication of diabetes, manifested as albuminuria, nephrotic edema, hypertension, renal insufficiency, and retinopathy.

Kinky-hair s., see Menkes' s.

Kinsbourne s., myoclonic encephalopathy of childhood—a neurologic disorder of unknown etiology with onset between ages one and three, characterized by myoclonus of trunk and limbs and by opsoclonous, with ataxia of gait and intention tremor, some cases have been associated with occult neuroblastoma.

Kleeblattschadel (cloverleaf skull) s., a congenital disorder, characterized by synostosis of multiple or all cranial sutures, hydrocephalus, and in some cases facial dysostosis and long bone anomalies.

Klein-Waardenburg s., see Waardenburg s., def. 2.

Kleine-Levin s., episodic periods of excessive sleep and overeating lasting for several weeks, usually in adolescent boys.

Klinefelter's s., a condition characterized by small testes with hyalinization of the seminiferous tubules, variable degrees of masculinization, azoospermia and infertility, and increased urinary excretion of gonadotropin; patients tend to be tall, with long legs, and about half have gynecomastia. It is associated typically with an XXY chromosome complement, although variants include XXYY, XXXY, XXXXY, and several mosaic patterns (XY/XXY, XXY. XXXY, etc.).

Klippel-Feil s., a condition characterized by shortness of the neck resulting from reduction in the number of cervical vertebrae or the fusion of multiple hemivertebrae into one osseous mass; the hairline is low and motion of the neck is limited.

Klippel-Trenaunay s., Klippel-Trenaunay-Weber s., a rare condition usually affecting one extremity, characterized by hypertrophy of the bone and related soft tissues, large cutaneous hemangiomas, persistent nevus flammeus (port-wine stain), and skin varices.

Klümpke-Dejerine s., see Klumpke's paralysis.

Kluver-Bucy s., bizarre behavior disturbances following bilateral temporal lobectomy which destroys important limbic structures; it is characterized by a tendency to examine objects orally, depression of drive and emotional reactions, hypermetamorphosis, and lack of sexual inhibitions.

Kocher-Debré-Sémélaigne s., see Debré-Sémélaigne s.

Koerber-Salus-Elschnig s., see Sylvian s

Künig's s., constipation alternating with diarrhea and attended with abdominal pain, meteorism, and gurgling sounds in the right iliac fossa.

Korsakoff's s., a syndrome of anterograde and retrograde amnesia with confabulation associated with alcoholic or nonalcoholic polyneuritis described as "cerebropathia psychica toxemica" by Korsakoff; currently used synonymously with "amnestic syndrome" or, more narrowly, to refer to the amnestic component of the Wernicke-Korsakoff syndrome, i.e., an amnestic syndrome resulting from thiamine deficiency. Called also Korsakoffs psychosis. See also amnestic s. and Wernicke-Korsakoff s.

Kostmann's s., infantile genetic agranulocytosis—an autosomal recessive disorder characterized by early onset of recurrent, severe pyogenic infections, especially of the skins and the lung, total absence of neutrophils in the blood or presence in reduced numbers, absolute monocytosis and eosinophilia, markedly decreased numbers of mature neutrophilic precursors in the bone marrow, and early death.

Krause's s., a retinal and cerebral dysplasia found in premature infants several months after birth, characterized by malformations of the choroid, retina, and optic nerve, and possible blindness, cataract, coloboma, glaucoma, and microphthalmos. Cerebral symptoms include aplasia, hyperplasia, and hypertrophy of the brain, hydrocephaly, microcephaly, and mental retardation. Called also Encephalo-ophthalmic dysplasia.

Kunkel's s; lupoid hepatitis, see Bearn-Kunkel s.,

Ladd's s., congenital obstruction of the duodenum due to peritoneal bands resulting from a malrotated cecum.

Lambert-Eaton s; see Eaton-Lambert s.

Landry's s., acute febrile polyneuritis, see Barre-Guillian s.,

Larsen's s., cleft palate, flattened facies, multiple congenital dislocations, and foot deformities.

Laubry-Soulle s., abnormal localized collections of gas in the colon (splenic flexure) and stomach following acute myocardial infarction.

Launois' s., gigantism due to excessive pituitary secretion, occurring before puberty and: before the epiphyses close; it is most often caused by eosinophilic cell hyperplasia or an eosinophilic adenoma, but sometimes results from a chromophobe adenoma. Called also Hyperpituitary or pituitary gigantism.

Laurence-Moon s., an autosomal recessive disorder characterized by mental retardation pigmentary retinopathy, hypogonadism, and spastic paraplegia; CF: Bardet-Biedl s. and Biemond s., II.

Läwen-Roth s., dwarfism with stippled epiphyses and thyroid deficiency; congenital hypothyroidism or cretinism.

Lawford's s., a variant of the Sturge-Weber syndrome in which there is glaucoma but without an increase in the size of the eye.

Lawrence-Seip s., total lipodystrophy—an autosomal recessive disorder occurring mainly in females, characterized by a generalized loss of subcutaneous fat and extracutaneous adipose tissue, presenting at birth or appearing later in life, and associated with hepatomegaly, hypoglycemia and insulin resistant nonketotic diabetes, hyperlipemia, marked elevation of basal metabolic rate, accelerated somatic growth, advanced bone age, acanthosis nigricans and hirsutism.

Lazy leukocyte s., a syndrome occurring in children, marked by recurrent low-grade infections, associated with a defect in neutrophil chemotaxis and deficient random mobility of neutrophils.

Legg-Calvé-Perthes's., osteochondrosis of the capitular epiphysis, see Legg-Calvé-Perthes' disease.

Leigh s., subacute necrotizing encephalomyelopathy, see Leigh disease.

Lennox s., a childhood epileptic encephalopathy characterized electroencephalographically by diffuse slow spike waves.

Lenz's s., a hereditary syndrome, transmitted as an X-linked trait, consisting of microphthalmia or anophthalmos, unilateral or bilateral, and digital anomalies; narrow shoulders, double thumbs, and other skeletal abnormalities; dental, urogenital, and cardiovascular defects may also occur.

Leopard s., a hereditary syndrome transmitted as an autosomal dominant trait, consisting of multiple lentigines, asymptomatic cardiac defects, and typical coarse facies; it may also be associated with pulmonary stenosis, sensorineural deafness, skeletal changes, ocular hypertelorism, and abnormalities of the genitalia. Called also Multiple lentigines s.

Leredde's s., severe dyspnea on exertion dating from early life, combined with advanced emphysema, recurrent attacks of acute febrile bronchitis; it is a remote sequel of syphilis, usually congenital.

Leriche's s., a syndrome caused by obstruction of the terminal aorta, usually occurring in males and characterized by fatigue in the hips, thighs, or calves on exercising, absence of pulsation in the femoral arteries, and impotence, and often pallor and coldness of the lower extremities.

Lermoyez's s., tinnitus and hearing loss preceding an attack of vertigo and then subsiding after the vertigo has become established.

Lesch-Nyhan s., a rare X-linked disorder of purine metabolism due to deficient hypoxanthine-guanine phosphoribosyltransferase, characterized by physical and mental retardation, compulsive self-mutilation of the fingers and lips by biting, choreoathetosis, spastic cerebral palsy, impaired renal function; and by excessive purine synthesis and consequent hyperuricemia and uricaciduria. Called also Hypoxanthine-guanine phosphoribosyltransferase (HGPRT, HPRT) deficiency.

Levator s., episodic pain and a sensation of fullness and pressure in the rectum and sacrococcygeal area; attributed to spasm of the levator ani muscle.

Levy-Roussy s., see Roussy-Levy s.

Leyden-Moöbius s., limb-girdle muscular dystrophy—a slowly progressive form of muscular dystrophy affecting either sex and usually beginning in childhood, sometimes in maturity or later; it is characterized by weakness and wasting in the shoulder or pelvic girdle.

Lhermitte and McAlpine s., combined pyramidal and extrapyramidal system disease.

Libman-Sacks s., atypical verrucous endocarditis, see Libman-Sacks disease.

Lichtheim's s., subacute combined degeneration of the spinal cord; see Lichtheim's disease.

Lightwood's s., renal tubular acidosis—a variety of metabolic acidosis resulting from impairment of renal function.

Lignac's s., Lignac-Fanconi s., cystinosis—lysosomal storage disorder of unknown molecular defect, characterized by widespread deposition of cystine crystals in reticuloendothelial cells. There are three clinical types:the early onset or infantile nephropathic type, is marked by vitamin D resistant rickets, chronic acidosis, polyuria, and dehydration, all resulting from proximal renal tubular dysfunction, and by corneal opacities, growth failure, uremia, and death before ten. The beningn or adult nephropathic type does not affect kidney or shorten lifespan, is marked, by deposition of cysteine in bone marrow, leukocytes, and corneas, and is diagnosed by ophthalmic examination. The late onset juvenile or adolescent nephropathic type falls within the two extremes: there are ocular and renal manifestations, but the kidney lesion does not always lead to renal insufficiency.

Liver-kidney s., see Hepatorenal s.

Lobstein's s., see osteogenesis imperferta, see Vrolik disease.

"Locked-in" s., a condition of complete paralysis, except for some form of voluntary eye movement, due to bilateral lesions of motor pathways of the lower cranial nerves and limbs.

Loculation s., see Froin's s.

Loffler's s., a condition characterized by transient infiltrations of the lungs, accompanied by cough, fever, dyspnea, and eosinophilia.

Looser-Milkman s., see Milkman s.

Louis-Bar s., see Ataxia-telangiectasia s.

Lowe s., Lowe-Terrey-MacLachlan s., see Oculocerebrorenal s.

Lower radicular s., see Klumpke's paralysis.

Lown-Ganong-Levine s; an electrocardiographic abnormality characterized by a short P-R interval with a normal QRS complex, accompanied by atrial tachycardia.

Lucey-Driscoll s., a syndrome of retention jaundice due to defective bilirubin conjugation, occurring in infants; apparently the result of an unidentified factor, presumably a steroid in maternal blood, transmitted to the infant.

Lupus-like s., a chronic, remitting, relapsing, inflammatory, and often febrile multisystemic disorder of connective tissue, acute or insidious in onset, characterised principally by involvement of skin, joints, kidneys, and serosal membranes. It is of unknown etiology, but it is thought to represent failure of the regulatory mechanisms of the autoimmune system that sustains self-tolerance and preventing body from attacking its own cells, cell constituents, and proteins, suggested by high level of a wide variety of autoantibodies against nuclear and cytoplasmic cellular components seen in affected individuals. The disorder is marked by wide variety of abnormalities, including arthritis and arthralgias, nephritis, central nervous system manifestations, pleurisy, pericarditis, leukopenia or thrombocytopenia, hemolytic anemia, elevated ESR rate, and positive LE-cell preparations. Drug induced lupus, caused, e.g., hydralazine, procainamide, esoniazide, D-penicillamine, and chlorpromazine, is characterized by production of systemic lupus erythematosus-like syndrome that usually resolves following withdrawal of offending drug.

Lutembacher's s., atrial septal defect associated with mitral stenosis. Called also Lutembacher's disease or complex.

Lyell's s., toxic epidermal necrolysis, see Lyell's disease.

Lymphadenopathy s. a condition occurring in a large number of male—homosexuals, characterized by the presence of unexplained lympha-denopathy for three more months involving extrainguinal sites, which on biopsy reveal nonspecific lymphoid hyperplasia; considered by some authorities to be a prodrome of acquired immuno deficiency syndrome.

Lymphoproliferative s., see lymphoproliferative disease.

Lymphoreticulars' s., see lymphoreticular disease.

McArdle s., see glycogen storage disease (type V).

McCune-Albright s., see Albright's s.

Mackenzie's s., associated paralysis of the tongue, soft palate, and vocal cord on the same side.

Macleod's s., see Swyer-James s.

Maffucci's s., enchondromatosis associated with multiple cutaneous or visceral hemangiomas. Called also Kast's s.

Malabsorption s., a group of disorders in which there is subnormal absorption of dietary constituents, and thus excessive loss of nonabsorbed substances in the stool; the malabsorption may be due to an intraluminal (digestive) defect (e.g. pancreatic insufficiency), a mucosal abnormality (celiac disease or disaccharidase deficiency), or a lymphatic obstruction (intestinal lymphangiectasia). Unless there is a specific enzyme transport defect, steatorrhea is usually present.

Deficiency syndromes may result from excessive loss of vitamins, electrolytes, iron, calcium, etc.

Malarial hyper-reactive spleen s., see tropical splenomegaly s.

Malin's s., anemia in which the red cells are ingested by the leukocytes; called also autoerythrophagocytosis.

Mallory-Weiss s., hematemesis or melena that follows typically upon many hours or days of severe vomiting and retching, traceable to one or several slitlike lacerations of the gastric mucosa, longitudinally placed at or slightly below the esophagogastric junction.

Manic s., [DSM III-R], a period of predominantly elevated, expansive, or irritable mood accompanied by some of the associated symptoms of the manic syndrome: inflated self esteem or grandiosity, decreased need for sleep, talkativeness, flight of ideas, distractiblity, hyperactivity or psychomotor agitation, hypersexuality, and reckless behavior.

Marchesani's s., see Weill-Marchesani s.

Marchiafava-Bignami s., see under disease.

Marchiafava-Micheli s., see Marchiafava-Micheli disease.

Marcus Gunn's s., see Gunn's s.

Marfan's s., a congenital disorder of connective tissue characterized by abnormal length the extremities, especially of fingers and toes, subluxation of the lens, cardiovascular abnormalities (commonly dilatation of the ascending aorta), and other deformities. It is autosomal dominant with variable degree of expression.

Marie s., see Marie disease.

Marie-Bamberger s., see Marie disease.

Marie-Robinson s., melancholia, insomnia, and impotence in a form of levulosuria.

Marinesco-Sjögren's s., a hereditary syndrome transmitted as an autosomal recessive trait, consisting of cerebellar ataxia, mental and somatic growth retardation, congenital cataracts, inability to chew, thin brittle fingernails, and sparse, incompletely keratinized hair.

Maroteaux-Lamny s., a mucopolysaccharidosis caused by deficient N-acetygalactosamine 4-sulfatase (arylsulfatase B), and characterized biochemically by the predominance of dermatan sulfate in the urine and the presence of coarse metachromatic granules in the leuckocytes, and clinically by Hurler-like signs with normal intelligence. There are three clinical forms: the severe or classic form shows Hurler like symptoms; the intermediate form has the same phenotype as mucolipidosis III (pseudo-Hurler polydystrophy: the mild form is difficult to distinguish from the Scheie syndrome. Called also mucopolysaccharidosis VI. N-acetylgalactosamine-4-sulfatase and arylsulfatase B (ARSB) deficiency.

Martorell's s., see pulseless disease.

Mastocytosis s., an episodic syndrome occurring in certain patients with systemic mastocytosis, usually those with skin lesions, bone lesions, and hepatosplenomegaly, presumably associated with histamine release from degranulation of mast cells, and characterized mainly in intense pruritus, flushing, headache, tachycardia, hypotension, and syncope.

Maternal deprivation s., growth failure, autistic behavior, and retarded mental development resulting from loss or absence of the mother or lack of proper mothering.

Mauriac s., dwarfism, hepatomegaly, obesity, and retarded sexual maturation, in association with diabetes mellitus.

Mayer-Rokitansky-Kuster-Hauser s., lack of mullerian development, congenital absence of the vagina and rudimentary uterus (typically bicornate remnants), with normal uterine tubes, ovaries, and secondary female sex characteristics and normal growth. Called also Rokitansky-Kuster-Hauser s.

Meckel's s. Meckel-Gruber s., a hereditary syndrome, transmitted as an autosomal recessive trait, most frequently characterized by sloping forehead, posterior meningoencephalocele, polydactyly, and polycystic kidneys, with death occurring in the perinatal period. Called also Gruber's s and dysencephalia splanchnocystica.

Meconium plug s., a syndrome of intestinal obstruction caused by unusually thick or hard meconium in which neither enzymatic nor ganglion cell deficiency can be demonstrated.

Megacystismegaureter s., chronic ureteral dilatation (megaureter) associated with hypotonia and dilatation of the bladder (megacystis) and gaping of ureteral orifices, permitting vesicoureteral reflux of urine, and resulting in chronic pyelonephritis.

Meigs's s., ascites and hydrothorax associated with ovarian fibroma or other pelvic tumor.

Melkersson's s., Melkersson-Rosenthal s., a hereditary syndrome transmitted as an autosomal dominant trait, most often beginning and childhood or adolescence, and characterized chiefly by chronic noninflammatory facial swelling (usually confined to the lips), recurrent peripheral facial palsy, and sometimes fissured tongue. Associated ophthalmic symptoms may include lagophthalmos, burning sensation of the eyes, blepharochalasis, swelling of the eyelids, corneal opacities, retrobulbar neuritis, and bolateral recurrent exophthalmos.

Mendelson's s., see pulmonary acid aspiration syndrome.

Mengert's shock s., a condition resembling shock that sometimes occurs when pregnant women in the late antepartum period lie in the supine position; it is due to the pressure of the uterus on the vena cava.

Meniere's s., see under disease.

Menkes' s., a hereditary abnormality in copper absorption marked by severe cerebral degeneration and arterial changes resulting in death in infancy and by sparse, brittle scalp hair with a twisted appearance microscopically. It is transmitted as an X-linked recessive trait. Called also Menkes' disease and kinky- or steely-hair s.

Metameric s., see Segmentary s.

Methionine malabsorption s., an autosomal recessive disorder of methionine absorption in which the urine has a characteristic odor resembling that of the interior of an oasthouse, due to alpha-hydroxybutyric acid formed by bacterial action on the unabsorbed methionine; it is characterized by white hair, mental retardation, convulsions, and attacks of hyperpnea. Called also Oasthouse urine disease and Smith-Strong disease.

Meyer-Schwickerath and Weyers s., see Dysplasia oculodentodigitalis s.

Middle lobe s., atelectasis of the right middle pulmonary lobe, with chronic pneumonitis called also Brock's s.

Mikulicz's s., a chronic bilateral hypertrophy of the lacrimal, parotid, and salivary glands, associated with decreased or absent lacrimation and xerostomia, and often accompanied by chronic lymphocytic infiltration. It may be associated with other diseases, such as sjogren syndrome, sarcoidosis, lupus erythematosus, leukemia, lymphoma, and tuber-culosis. See also under disease.

Milk-alkali s., a syndrome characterized by hypercalcemia without hypercalciuria or hypophosphatemia, with only mild alkalosis, normal serum phosphatase, severe renal insufficiency with hyperazotemia, and calcinosis, attributed to ingestion of milk and absorbable alkali- for long periods of time; called also Burnett's s. and hypercalcemia s.

Milkman's s., a generalized bone disease marked by multiple transparent stripes of absorption in the long and flat bones, called also Looser-Milkman s.

Millard-Gubler s., crossed paralysis, affecting the limbs on one side of the body and the face on the opposite side, together with paralysis of outward movement of the eye; it is due to infarction of the pons, involving the sixth and seventh cranial nerves and the fibers of the corticospinal tract. Called also Millard-Gubler paralysis. Cf. Foville's s.

Minkowski-Chauffard s., a congenital, familial form of hemolytic anemia characterized by spherocytosis, abnormal fragility of erythrocytes, jaundice and splenomegaly.

Minot-von Willebrand s., see von Willebrand's disease.

Mitral valve prolapse s., prolapse of the mitral valve, often with regurgitation, associated with myxomatous proliferation of the leaflets of the mitral valve, a common, usually benign, often asymptomatic condition characterized by midsystolic clicks and late systolic murmurs on auscultation. Palpitations and chest discomfort may occur, and in some cases progressive mitral regurgitation necessitates valve replacement. Called also Barlow s. and floppy value s.

Moebius's., agenesis or aplasia of the motor nuclei of the cranial nerves characterized by congenital bilateral facial palsy in various combinations, with unilateral or bilateral paralysis of the abductors of the eye, sometimes associated with involvement of the cranial nerves, particularly the oculomotor, trigeminal. and hypoglossal, and anomalies of the extremities. Called also Akinesia algera, congenital facial diplegia, nuclear agenesis or aplasia, congenital abducens-facial paralysis, and congenital oculofacial paralysis.

Mohr s., an autosomal recessive disorder characterized by brachydactyly, clinodactyly, polydactyly, syndactyly, and bilateral hallucal polysyndactyly; by cranial, facial, lingual, palatal, and mandibular anomalies; and by episodic neuromuscular disturbances. Called also oral-facial-digital (OFD) s., type II, orodigitofacial dysostosis, orofaciodigital (OFD) s., type II. See also oral-facial-digital type I.

Monakow's s., hemiplegia on the side opposite the lesion in occlusion of the anterior choroidal artery, sometimes with hemianesthesia and hemianopia.

Moore's s., abdominal epilepsy-paroxysmal pain, the expression of an abnormal neuronal discharge from the brain.

Morel's s., hyperostosis frontalis interna—thickening of the inner table of the frontal bone, which may be associated with hypertrichosis and obesity. It most commonly affects women near menopause.

Morgagni s s., hyperostosis frontalis interna, see Morel's s.

Morgagni-Adams-Stokes s., see Adams-Stokes disease.

Morgagni-Stewart-Morel s., hyperostosis frontalis interna, see Morel's s.

Morning glory s., a coloboma in which there is a funnel-shaped optic nerve head with a dot of whitish, fluffy material in the center, an elevated ring of pigment around the disk, and vessels radiating from the ring like spokes. Vision is severely affected.

Morquio s., two biochemically distinct, but clinically nearly indistinguishable, forms off mucopolysaccharidosis characterized by excretion of keratan sulfate in the urine. Clinical features, affecting primarily the skeletal and secondarily the nervous system, include genu; valgum, pectus carinatum, progressive platyspondyly, short neck and trunk, normal but broad-mouthed facies with spacing between the teeth, progressive deafness, and very mild comeal clouding. Intelligence is normal. The two enzymatic types are: type A, the severe form, caused by N-acetylgalactosamine-6-sulfatase deficiency (patients do not survive their thirties); and type B, caused by β-galactosidase deficiency (patients may live into their sixties). Called mucopolysaccharidosis IV and keratansulfaturia.

Morquio-Ullrich s., see Morquio's s.

Morton's s, a congenital insufficiency of the first metatarsal segment of the foot, characterized by metatarsalgia due to shortening or relaxation of the part.

Morvan's s., 1. Syringomyelia. 2. Manifestation of syringomyelia marked by thickening of the subcutaneous tissues of the hands, which become edematous, soft, swollen, cyanotic, and cold (main succulents, or Marinesco's succulent hand) associated with analgesic ulceration of the tips of the fingers and paresthesia and atrophy of the hands and forearms. Called also analgesic panaris and Morvan's disease.

Mosse's s., polycythemia vera with cirrhosis of the liver.

Moynahan s., 1. Multiple symmetric lentigines, congenital mitral valve stenosis, dwarfism, genital hypoplasia, and mental retardation. Called also progressive cardiomyopathic lentiginosis. 2. A familial congenital syndrome consisting of delayed hair growth on the scalp, epilepsy, mental retardation, and unusual electroencephalogram.

Muckle-Wells s., an autosomal dominant syndrome characterized by amyloidosis involving the kidneys and causing nephritis, recurrent urticaria, deafness, and pain in the extremities.

Mucocutaneous lymph node s. (MLNS), a syndrome of unknown etiology affecting most commonly infants and young children, and marked by fever, conjunctival injection, reddening of the lips and oral cavity, ulcerative gingivitis, enlarged cervical lymph nodes, and maculoerythematous skin eruption that becomes confluent and bright red in a glove-and-sock distribution, the skin becoming indurated and edematous and desquamating from the fingers and toes. It has been observed in Japan since 1967, but has recently been reported in the US with some frequency. Called also Kawasaki disease.

Mucosal neuroma s., multiple endocrine neoplasia. Type III-characterized by medullary carcinoma of thyroid, pheochromocytoma, often bilateral and multiple. The mean survival time is shorter, a marfanoid body habitus may occur and there may be disfiguring neuromas of the lips, buccal mucosa and tongue, ganglioneuromas of the gastrointestinal tract, thickened corneal nerves, and cafe-au-lait spots, neuromas and neurofibromas of the skin. All forms are transmitted as autosomal dominant traits with varying penetrance.

Multiple glandular deficiency s., primary failure of any combination of endocrine glands, including adrenals, thyroid, gonads, parathyroids, and endocrine pancreas, often accompanied by nonendocrine autoimmune abnormalities.

Multiple hamartoma s., see Cowden's disease,

Multiple lentigines s., see Leopard s.

Munchausen s., a condition characterized by habitual presentation for hospital treatment of an apparent acute illness, the patient giving a plausible and dramatic history, all of which is false: called chronic factitious disorder with physical symptoms in DSM III.

Murchison-Sanderson s., see Hodgkin's disease.

Myasthenia gravis s., see Erb's s.

Myasthenic s., see Eaton-Lambert s.

Myelofibrosis-osteosclerosis s., a form of myeloproliferative disease characterized by fibrosis of the bone marrow, splenomegaly, extramedullary hematopoiesis and leukoerythroblastosis.

Myeloproliferative s., pertaining to, or characterized by medullary and extramedullary proliferation of bone marrow constituents including erythroblasts, granulocytes, megakaryocytes and fibrinoblasts. The myeloproliferative disorder comprises group of usally neoplastic diseases, which may be related histogenetically by a common multipotential stem cells, that includes among others acute and chronic granulocytic leukemias, acute and chronic myelomonocytic leukemias, polycythemia vera, myelofibrosis, myeloid metaplasia essential thrombocythemia, and erythroleukemia, an interrelationship with lymphoproliferative disorders is thought to exist.

Naegeli s., see Franceschetti-Jadassohn s.

Naffziger's s., see Scalenus s.

Nail-patella s., onycho-osteodysplasia—a hereditary syndrome with dystrophy of the nails, absence or hypoplasia of the patella, hypoplasia of the lateral side of the elbow joint, and bilateral iliac horns.

Nelson's s., the development of an ACTH-producing pituitary tumor after bilateral adrenalectomy in Cushing's syndrome; it is characterized by aggressive growth of the tumor and hyperpigmentation of the skin.

Neostriatal s., see Hunt's striatal s., def. 2.

Nephrotic s., a condition characterized by massive edema, heavy proteinuria, hypoalbuminemia, and peculiar susceptibility to intercurrent infections; called also Epstein's s.

Netherton's s., a congenital syndrome consisting of lamellar ichthyosis or ichthyosis linearis circumflexa, hair shaft defects, atopic diathesis, and sometimes mental retardation and aminoaciduria. It is believed to be autosomal recessive.

Neurocutaneous s., phakomatosis—any of a group of congenital and hereditary developmental anomalies having in common selective involvement of tissues of ectodermal origin (i.e., central nervous system, eye, and skin) and the development of disseminated glial; hamartomas (phakomas) in these tissues.

Neuroleptic malignant s., a rare, sometimes fatal reaction to neuroleptic drugs, characterized by hyperthermia, rigidity, and coma.

Nevoid basal cell carcinoma s., nevoid basalioma s., see Basal cell nevus s.

Nezelof s., a heterogeneous group of immunodeficiency disorders characterized by profoundly deficient cellular immunity and varying degrees of humeral immunodeficiency. Immunoglobulin levels may be normal or increased, but antibody response to immunization may be absent. Patients are highly susceptible to life threatening infections with low-grade or opportunistic pathogens, such as *Candida albicans*, *Pneumocystis carinii*, and cytomegalovirus. Both autosomal recessive and X-linked inheritance have been described. Called also cellular immunodeficiency with immunoglobulins.

Nitritoid s., a group of symptoms sometimes following the injection of arsphenamine, consisting of redness of the face, dyspnea, feeling of distress, cough, and precordial pain. The condition is named from its resemblance to the symptoms of amyl nitrite poisoning.

Noack s., acrocephalopolysyndactyly.(type 1)—craniostenosis characterized by acrocephaly and syndactyly, probably occurring as an autosomal dominant trait and usually as a new mutation.

Nonne's s., hereditary cerebellar ataxia.

Nonne-Milroy-Meige s., see Milroy's disease.

Nonsense s., see Ganser s.

Noonan's s., webbed neck, ptosis, hypogonadism, congenital heart disease, and short; stature, that is, the phenotype of Turner's syndrome without gonadal dysgenesis; formerly called male Turner's syndrome until the female counterpart was identified. Called also Ullrich-Turner s.

Nothna-Gel's s., unilateral oculomotor paralysis combined with cerebellar ataxia, in lesions of the cerebral peduncles.

OAV **s.**, oculoauriculovertebral dysplasia, see Goldenhar's s.,

Oculocerebral-hypopigmentation s., see Cross s.

Oculocerebrorenal s., an X-linked disorder characterized by vitamin D-refractory rickets, hydrophthalmia, congenital glaucoma and cataracts, mental retardation, and tubule reabsorption dysfunction as evidenced by hypophosphatemia, acidosis, and aminoaciduria. Called also Lowe disease and Lowe-Terrey-Maclachlan s.

Oculodento-osseous s., oculodentodigital dysplasia, see Dysplasia occulodentodigital s.

Oculomandibulofacial s., a syndrome principally characterized by dyscephaly (usually brachycephaly), parrot nose, mandibular hypoplasia, proportionate nanism, hypotrichosis, bilateral congenital cataracts, and microphthalmia; called also Hallermann-Streiff s; Hallermann-Streiff-Francois s., Francois' s., and mandibulo-oculofacial dyscephaly.

OFD s., see Oral-facial-digital s.

Ogilvie's s., a condition simulating colonic obstruction, with persistent contraction of intestinal musculature, but without evidence of organic disease of the colon, occurring as a result of a defect in the sympathetic nerve supply. Called also False colonic obstruction.

Oldfield's s., familial polyposis of the colon associated with extensive sebaceous cysts.

OMM s., ophthalmomandibulomelic dysplasia—a hereditary syndrome transmitted as an autosomal dominant trait, consisting of blindness caused by corneal opacities, temperomandibular fusion, absent coronoid process, obtuse mandibular angle, radiohumeral and radioulnar dislocations, and aplasia of lateral condyle of humerus, radial head and distal ulnar.

Oppenheim's s., see under disease.

Oral- facial-digital (OFD) s., type 1 a male lethal X-linked dominant disorder characterized by camptodactyly, polydactyly, and syndactyly; by cranial, facial, lingual, and dental anomalies; and by mental retardation, familial trembling, alopecia, and seborrhea of the face and milia. Called also orodigitofacial dysostosis, orofaciodigital s. type I. See also Mohr s.

Oral-facial-digital (OFD) s., type II, see Mohr

Oral-facial-digital (OFD) s., type III, an autosomal recessive disorder characterized by postaxial hexadactyly of the hands and feet, by ocular, lingual, and dental anomalies, and by profound mental retardation. Called also orodigitofacial dysostosis, orofaciodigital s., type III.

Organic anxiety s. (DSM III-R), an organic mental syndrome characterized by prominent, recurrent panic attacks or generalized anxiety caused by a specific organic factor and not associated with delirium. Causes include such endocrine disorders as hyperthyroidism, hypothyroidism, pheochromocytoma, fasting hypoglycemia. and hypercortisolism or the use of psychoactive substances.

Organic brain s., see Organic mental s.

Organic delusional s. (DSM III-R), an organic brain syndrome characterized by the presence of delusions caused by a specific organic factor and not associated with delirium. Causes include substances such as amphetamines, cannabis, and hallucinogens and other organic diseases such as temporal lobe epilepsy, head trauma or cerebral lesions, and Huntington's chorea. The substance-induced syndromes are named as "disorders," e.g., "cannabis delusional disorder."

Organic mental s. (DSM III-R), a constellation of psychological or behavioral signs and symptoms associated with one or more specific organic etiologic factors. DSM III-R includes six specific organic brain syndromes, delirium and dementia; amnestic syndrome or organic hallucinosis: organic delusional syndrome, organic mood syndrome, and organic anxiety syndrome; organic personality syndrome: intoxication and withdrawal; and a residual category, organic mental syndrome not otherwise specified. When the etiologic factor is a psychoactive substance, the name of the substance is given, the word "organic" is dropped, and "syndrome" is changed to "disorder," e.g., "alcohol amnestic disorder" or "cannabis delusional disorder." Previous nomenclature classified all organic brain syndromes as "psychotic" or "nonpsychotic" and as "acute" (reversible) or "chronic" (irreversible), the latter pair of terms being used with meanings not in accord with general medical usage.

Organic mood s., (DSM III-R), an organic brain syndrome characterized by the presence of manic or depressive mood disturbance caused by a specific organic factor and not associated with delirium. Common causes are drugs and other psychoactive substances, notably reserpine, methyldopa, and certain hallucinogens; endocrine disorders, notably Cushing's syndrome, Addison's disease, hypothyroidism, and hyperparathyroidism; and viral infections. The substance-induced syndromes are named as "disorders," e.g. hallucinogen mood disorder.

Organic personality s. (DSM Ill-R), an organic brain syndrome characterized by a marked change in behavior or personality, e.g., emotional lability, marked apathy, impaired impulse control, or paranoid ideation, caused by a specific organic factor and not associated with delirium or dementia. The most common causes are space-occupying lesions of the brain, head trauma, and cerebrovascular disease.

Orofaciodigital (OFD) s., type I, see oral-facial-digital s. type I.

Orofaciodigital s., type II, see Mohr s.

Ostrum-Furst s., congenital synostosis of the neck, platybasi (a developmental deformity of the occipital bone and upper end of cervical spine, in which latter appears to have pushed the floor of the occipital bone upward), and Sprengel's deformity (congenital elevation of the scapula, due to failure of desent of the scapula to its normal thoracic position during fetal life).

Outlet s., see Brachial s.

Ovarian-remnant s., pelvic pain, sometimes cyclic, typically occurring several weeks or months after oophorectomy, usually associated with a pelvic mass, most frequently a corpus-luteum cyst, which sometimes leads to unilateral ureteral obstruction. It is due to survival of an ovarian fragment after the operation.

Ovarian vein s., obstruction of the ureter due to compression by an enlarged or varicose ovarian vein; typically the vein becomes enlarged during pregnancy, the symptoms being those of obstruction or infection of the upper urinary tract. The right side is usually affected.

Pain **dysfunction s.**, see Temporomandibular joint s.

Painful arc s., shoulder pain occurring at a particular portion of the arc described when the arm is abducted from the side to the fully raised position, as in inflammation of the tendons of the supraspinatus muscle.

Painful bruising s., a purpuric reaction almost always seen in young to middle-aged women in which spontaneous, chronic recurring painful ecchymoses, single or multiple, occur on the body without antecedent trauma or after insufficient trauma, and may be precipitated by emotional stress. Based on studies that show that certain patients exhibit autoerythrocyte sensitization in which intradermal injection of their own erythrocytes produces a painful ecchymosis, the etiology of the condition has been ascribed by some to an autosensitivity to a component of the erythrocyte membrane; others consider it to be of psychosomatic or factitious origin. Called also autoerythrocyte sensitization s, erythrocyte autosensitization s., and Gardner-Diamond s. Cf; psychogenic purpura.

Paleostriatal s., juvenile paralysis agitans (of Hunt), see Ramsay-Hunt s., (2).

Pallidal s., juvenile paralysis agitans (of Hunt).see Ramsay-Hunt s.,(2).

Pallidomesencephalic s., a syndrome made up of rigidity, poverty of movement, and bradykinesia, amounting to a parkinsonian state.

Pancoast's s., Roentgenographic shadow at apex of lung, neuritic pain in the arm, atrophy of the muscles of the arm and hand, and Homer's syndrome, observed in tumor near the apex of the lung and due to involvement of the brachial plexus. 2. Osteolysis in the posterior part of one or more ribs and sometimes also involving the corresponding vertebra.

Pancreaticohepatic s., extensive destruction of pancreatic tissue and fatty metamorphosis of the liver.

Pancytopenia-dysmelia s., see Fanconi's s. def. 1.

Papillon-Lefevre s., an autosomal recessive disorder occurring between the first and fifth years of life, characterized by psoriasiform palmoplantar keratoderma, which may also involve the elbows, knees, tibias, external malleoli, and other areas; ectopic calcifications of the skull; and periodontitis and premature shedding of both the deciduous and permanent teeth.

Paraneoplastic s., a symptom-complex arising in a cancer-bearing patient that cannot be explained by local or distant spread of the tumor.

Paratrigeminal s., paroxysmal neuralgic pain in the face associated with sympathetic palsy (Homer's syndrome).

Parinaud's s., paralysis of conjugate upward movement of the eyes without paralysis of convergence, associated with lesions of the midbrain, such as a tumor of the pineal gland.

Parinaud's oculoglandular s., a general term applied to conjunctivitis, most often unilateral, usually of the follicular type, followed by tenderness and enlargement of the preauricular lymph nodes; it is often caused by infection with a leptothrix, or may be associated with other infections, such as cat-scratch fever, lymphogranuloma venereum, and tularemia.

Parkinsonian s., a form of parkinsonism due to idiopathic degeneration of the corpus striatum or substantia nigra, frequently occurring as a sequel of lethargic encephalitis, although cerebral arteriosclerosis, toxins, neurosyphilis, and trauma have also been implicated. It is characterized by muscular rigidity, immobile facies (Parkinson's facies), slow involuntary tremor (present at rest but tending to disappear during sleep and on volitional movement), abolition of associated automatic movements, festinating gait, stooped posture, and salivation. Called also postencephalitic parkinsonism.

Parry-Romberg s., facial hemiatrophy, atrophy of one-half of the face which is sometimes progressive, and is of unknown cause.

Patau's s., see trisomy 13s.

Paterson's s., Paterson-Brown-Kelly s., Paterson-Kelly s., see Plummer-Vinson s.

Pellegrini-Stieda s., calcification of the medial collateral ligament of the knee.

Pellizzi's s., see Epiphyseal s.

Pendred's s., a hereditary syndrome of congenital bilateral nerve deafness associated with development of goiter without hypothyroidism in middle childhood; the main biochemical feature is a partial defect in thyroxine biosynthesis.

Pericolic-membrane s., symptoms resembling those of chronic appendicitis due to the pressure of pericolic membranes.

Persistent mullerian duct s., the persistence, in otherwise normal males, of mullerian structures as well as male genital ducts, with undescended testes and bilateral uterine tubes, a uterus, and an upper vagina. There may be unilateral cryptorchidism with contralateral inguinal hernia containing a testis, uterus, and uterine tube (hernia uteri inguinale). The disorder is heritable; fertility has been described.

Pertussis s., 1. see Pertussis-like s. 2. Pertussis—an acute, highly contagious infection of the respiratory tract, most frequently affecting the young children usually caused by *Bordetella pertusis*; It is characterized by catarrhal stage begining after an incubation period of about two weeks, with slight fever, sneezing, running at the nose, and a dry cough. In a week or two the paroxysmal stage begins with the characteristic paroxysmal cough,consisting of deep inspiration, followed by a series of short quick, coughs, continuing until the air is expelled from the lungs; the close of paroxysms is marked by a long drawn, shrill, whooping inspiration, due to spasmodic closure of the glottis. This stage last for 3 to 4 weeks, after which the convalescent stage begins, in which the paroxysms grow less frequent and less violent, and finally ceases.

Pertussis-like s., a syndrome clinically indistinguishable from pertussis but in which there is no evidence of infection with *Bordetella pertussis or B.parapertussis*, although evidence of other infectious agents, such as adenoviruses types 1, 2, 3, 5, and 6, can be demonstrated. Called also pertussis s. Cf parapertussis*.

Peutz s., hereditary intestinal polyposis.

Peutz-Jeghers s., a hereditary syndrome characterized by gastrointestinal polyposis (usually hamartomas of the small bowel) associated with excessive melanin pigmentation of the skin and mucous membranes; gastrointestinal bleeding and intussusception are common complications. It is transmitted as an autosomal dominant trait.

Pfeiffer's s., an autosomal dominant disorder characterized by acrocephalosyndactyly associated with broad short thumbs and big toes. Called also Acrocephalosyndaclyty type V.

Pharyngeal pouch s., see DiGeorge s.

PHC s., an autosomal dominant syndrome consisting of premolar aplasia, hyperhidrosis, and premature canities. Called also Book s.

Picchini's s., inflammation of the three serous membranes connected with the diaphragm, sometimes involving the meninges, synovial sheaths, and tunica vaginalis of the testicle; caused by a trypanosome.

Pick's s., 1. Pick's disease (def. 2). 2 Palpitation of the heart: a feeling of oppression on the chest, dyspnea, cyanosis, and dropsical phenomena; seen in certain heart diseases.

Pickwickian s., the complex of obesity, somnolence, hypoventilation, and erythrocytosis.

Pierre Robin s., an autosomal recessive disorder characterized by brachygnathia and cleft palate, often associated with glossoptosis, backward and upward displacement of the larynx, and angulation of

---

* See Appendix

the manubrium sterni; cleft palate makes sucking and swallowing difficult, permitting easy access of fluids into the larynx. It may appear in several syndromes or as an isolated hypoplasia. Called also Robin's s. and Robin's anomalad.

Pineal s., see Epiphyseal s.

Placental dysfunction s., malnutrition and hypoxia of the fetus due to degenerative changes in the placenta; in the full-blown condition the nails, skin, and vernix are stained a bright yellow and the umbilical cord a yellow-green. Called also yellow vernix s.

Placental transfusion s., the birth of one anemic and one plethoric twin due to the forcing of blood of one fetal twin into the circulation of the other via interconnections between their blood vessels; called also intrauterine parabiotic s.

Plummer-Vinson s., a syndrome usually occurring in middle-aged women with hypochromic anemia, chiefly characterized by cracks or fissures at the corners of the mouth, painful tongue with atrophy of the filiform and later the fungiform papulae, and dysphagia due to esophageal stenosis or webs. Called also Paterson's s., Paterson-Brown Kelly s., Paterson-Brown Kelly s., sideropenic dysphagia, and Vinson's s.

Poland's s., unilateral absence of the sternocostal head of the pectoralis major muscle and ipsilateral syndactyly. Called also Poland's anomaly.

Polhemus-Schafer-lvemark s., see Ivemark's s.

Polycystic ovary s., see Stein-Leventhal s.

Pontine s., see Raymond-Cestan s.

Popliteal pterygium s., 1.see Popliteal web s. 2.see Fevre-Languepin s.

Popliteal web s., a congenital syndrome consisting chiefly of popliteal webs, cleft palate, lower lip pits, and dysplasia of the toenails; a wide-variety of other abnormalities may be associated. Called also popliteal pterygium s.

Postcardiotomy psychosis s., anxiety, confusion, and perceptual disturbances occurring 2 to 5 days after an operation using cardio-pulmonary bypass.

Postcholecystectomy s., the persistence or recurrence of abdominal pain or jaundice following cholecystectomy; it may be due to an incorrect preoperative diagnosis, a retained stone in the common bile duct, or to other physical or psychic abnormalities which are not apparent.

Postcommissurotomy s., see Postpericardiotomy s.

Postconcussional s., amnesia, headache, dizziness, tinnitus, irritability, fatigability, sweating, palpitations of the heart, insomnia and difficulty in concentrating, occurring after concussion of the brain.

Posterior cord s., sensory and ataxic phenomena derived from a lesion of the posterior columns of the spinal cord, as in locomotor ataxia.

Posterolateral s. an ataxic and spasmodic condition due to lesions of the posterolateral elements of the spinal cord.

Postgastrectomy s., see Dumping s.

Postirradiation s., a symptom complex caused by massive irradiation, with hemorrhage, anemia, and malnutrition.

Post-lumbar puncture s., headache in the erect posture, sometimes with nuchal pain, nausea, vomiting, diaphoresis, and malaise, all relieved by recumbency, occurring several hours after lumbar puncture and lasting a few days; it is due to lowering of intracrania pressure by leakage of cerebrospinal fluid through the needle tract.

Postmaturity s., placental dysfunction syndrome occurring in postmature fetuses.

Postmyocardial infarction s., pericarditis with fever, leukocytosis, pleurisy and pneumonia occurring after myocardial infarction; called also Dressler's s.

Postperfusion s., cytomegalovirus mononucleosis occurring about 3 to 6 weeks after extracorporeal circulation or multiple blood transfusion and post-transfusion mononucleosus.

Postpericardiotomy s., delayed pericardial or pleural reaction following opening of the pericardium, characterized by fever, chest pain, and signs of pleural and/or pericardial inflammation.

Postphlebitic s., the various complications associated with deep vein thrombosis which are caused by greatly increased in the deep and communicating veins, resulting in chronic venous insufficiency, and principally characterized by persistent edema, pain, purpura and increased cutaneous pigmentation, eczematoid dermatitis, pruritus, ulceration, and indurated cellulitis. Called also Post-thrombotic s.

Post-thrombotic s., see Post perfusion s.

Post-traumatic brain s., a general term denoting all the symptoms occurring after a head injury; concussion, of the brain, confusion of the brain, and see postconcussional s.

Potter's s., a rare condition combining a characteristic facial appearance with renal agenesis or hypoplasia and other defects. The face is flattened and features may include widely spaced eyes, epicanthal folds, a crease below the lower lids, large, low-set, floppy ears, micrognathia, and skin crease on the lower chin; skeletal abnormalities, such as clubbed feet and contracted joints, are frequent. Infants die shortly after birth.

Prader-Willi s., a congenital disorder characterized by rounded face, almond-shaped eyes, strabismus, low forehead, hypogonadism, hypotonia, insatiable appetite, and mental retardation.

Pre-excitation s., see Wolff-Parkinson-White s.

Premenstrual s., a syndrome of unknown cause sometimes marked by bloating, edema, emotional lability, headache, changes in appetite or cravings for selected foods, breast swelling and tenderness, constipation, and decreased ability to concentrate; called also premenstrual tension.

Premotor s., the association of spastic hemiplegia with increased reflexes, disturbances of skilled movements, forced grasping and transient vasomotor disturbance; occurring in lesion of the premotor cortex.

Profichet's s., a gradual growth of calcareous nodules in the subcutaneous tissues (skin stones) especially about the larger joints, with a tendency to ulceration or cicatrization and attended by atrophic and nervous symptoms.

Prune-belly s., a syndrome in which the lower part of the rectus abdominis muscle and the lower and medial parts of the oblique muscles are absent, the bladder and ureters are usually greatly dilated, the kidneys are small and dysplastic, with hydronephrosis, and the testes are undescended. The abdomen is protruding and thin-walled, with wrinkled skin, giving the syndrome its name.

Pseudoclaudication s., a condition in which symptoms similar to those of intermittent claudication result from compression of the cauda equina owing to hypertrophic ridging or a herniated lumbar disk.

Pulmonary acid aspiration s., the disorder produced, as a complication of anaesthesia, by inhalation of gastric content with a pH of less than 2.5, including bronchoconstriction and destruction of tracheal mucosa, progressing to a syndrome resembling acute respiratory distress syndrome. Called also Mendelson's s.

Pulmonary dysmaturity s., see Wilson-Mikity s.

Putnam-Dana s., subacute combined degeneration of spinal cord, see Lichtheims disease.

Qt s., a combination of prolonged QT interval and torsades de pointes (an atypical rapid ventricular tachycardia with periodic waxing and waning of amplitude of the QRS complexes on the electrocardiogram; it may be self limited or progress to ventricular fibrillation); it may be congenital or acquired, the latter usually the result of drug administration.

Radicular s., a syndrome due to lesion of the roots of the spinal nerves, consisting of restricted mobility of the spine and root pain.

Ramsay Hunt s., 1. Herpes zoster involving the facial and auditory nerves associated with ipsilateral facial paralysis, usually transitory, and herpetic vesicles of the external ear or tympanic membrane, which also may or may not be associated with tinnitus, vertigo, and hearing disorders. Called also geniculate neuralgia, herpes zoster auricularis or oticus and Hunt's disease or neuralgia. 2. Juvenile paralysis agitans (of Hunt). 3. Dyssynergia cerebellaris progressiva.

Raymond-Céstan s., a syndrome due to obstruction of twigs of the basilar artery causing lesions of the pontine region; it is characterized by quadriplegia, anesthesia, and nystagmus.

Refsum's s., see under disease.

Reichmann's s., gastrosuccorrhea—excessive and continous secretion of gastric juice.

Reifenstein's s., a syndrome of male hypergonadotropic hypogonadism, due to an inherited defect of androgen receptors and consequent insensitivity to testosterone, with hypospadias gynecomastia, primary hypogonadism, and postpubertal testicular atrophy and azoospermia.

Reiter's s., a triad of symptoms of unknown etiology comprising urethritis, conjunctivitis, and arthritis (the dominant feature), appearing concomitantly or sequentially associated with mucocutaneous manifestation of keratoderma blennorrhagicum, circinate balanitis and stomatitis, chiefly affecting young men, and usually running a self-limited but relapsing course. Most affected patients have increased levels of the histocompatibilty antigen HLA-B 27. It possibly represents an abnormal immune response to certain infections, perhaps related to hereditary susceptibility. Epidemiologic studies reveal that there are venereal, or postvenereal and dysenteric, or postdysenteric forms. The former occurs mainly in the United States and Great Britain, possibly related to infection with *Chlamydia* or *Ureaplasma urealyticum*; and the latter in Asia, continental Europe, and North Africa, possibly related to *Shigella, Salmonella, Yersinia*, Or *Campylobacter* fetus infection. Called also Fiessinger Leroy-Reiter's disease.

Rendu-Osler-Weber s., hereditary hemorrhagic telangiectasia, see Osler's disease.

Respiratory distress s., of newborn, a condition of the newborn marked by dyspnea with cyanosis, heralded by such prodromal signs as dilatation of the alae nasi, expiratory grunt and retraction of the suprasternal notch or costal margins, most frequently occurring in premature infants, children of diabetic mothers, and infants delivered by cesarean section and sometimes with no apparent predisposing cause. The syndrome includes two patterns: (a) hyaline membrane disease or syndrome, in which affected infant frequently die of respiratory distress in the first few days of life and at autopsy have eosinophilic hyaline material lining the alveoli, alveolar ducts, and bronchioles, and (b) idiopathic respiratory distress of newborn in which the affected infants may live, but in those that die, only resorption atelectasis is seen and there is no formation of a hyaline membrane. Called also Congenital alveolar dysplasia and Congenital aspiration pneumonia.

Restless legs s., unpleasant deep discomfort inside the calves when sitting or lying down, especially just before sleep, producing an irresistible urge to move the legs.

Retraction s., See Duane's s.

S of retroparotid space See Villarets's s.

Rett s., a progressive disorder affecting the gray matter of the brain, occurring exclusively in females and present from birth; it is characterized by autistic behavior, ataxia, dementia, seizures, and loss of purposeful use of the hands, with cerebral atrophy, mild hyperammonemia, and decreased levels of biogenic amines. Called also Cerebroatrophic hyperammonemia.

Reye's s., a rare, acute, and sometimes fatal diseases of childhood, most often occurring as a sequel of varicella or a viral upper respiratory infection. It is marked by recurrent vomiting and elevated serum transaminase levels, with distinctive changes in the liver and other viscera; an encephalopathic phase with acute brain swelling, disturbances of consciousness, and seizures may follow.

Rh-null s., chronic hemolytic anemia affecting individuals who lack all Rh factors (Rh_{null}); it is marked by spherocytosis, stomatocytosis, and increased osmotic fragility.

Richards-Rundle s., a congenital syndrome consisting of ketoaciduria, mental retardation, underdevelopment of secondary sex characteristics, deafness, ataxia, and peripheral muscular wasting which progresses during childhood but eventually becomes static.

Richter's s., chronic lymphocytic leukemia with diffuse histiocytic lymphoma.

Rieger's s., Rieger's anomaly appearing with hypodontia, anal stenosis, hypertelorism, mental deficiency, and agenesis of the facial bones. See also anterior chamber cleavage syndrome.

Riley-Day s., dysautonomia—an autosomal recessive disease of childhood characterized by defective lacrimation, skin blotching, emotional instability, motor incordination, total absence of pain sensation, and hyporeflexia; seen exclusively in Jews.

Riley-Smith s., macrocephaly without hydrocephalus, multiple hemangiomas, and pseudoapilledema; presumed to be transmitted as an autosomal dominant trait.

Robert's s., a hereditary syndrome, transmitted as an autosomal recessive trait, consisting of imperfect development of the long bones of the limbs associated with cleft palate and lip and other anomalies.

Robin s., see Pierre Robin s.

Robinow's s., dwarfism associated with increased interorbital distance, malaligned teeth, bulging forehead, depressed nasal bridge, and short limbs. Called also Robinow's dwarfism and Fetal face s.

Roger's s., a continuous excessive secretion of saliva as the result of cancer in the esophagus, or other esophageal irritation.

Rokitansky-Kuster-Hauser s., see Mayer-Rokitansky-Kuster-Hauser s.

Rolandic vein s., hemiplegia resulting from interference with the cerebral venous circulation.

Romano-Ward s., prolonged Q-t interval and syncope, sometimes with ventricular fibrillation and sudden death; inherited as an autosomal dominant trait.

Rosenbach's s., paroxysmal tachycardia with gastric and respiratory complication.

Rosenthal s., a hereditary hemorrhagic diathesis clinically similar to hemophilia but due to deficiency of coagulation Factor XI.

Rosenthal-Kloepfer s., corneal leukomata, acromegaloid appearance, and cutis verticis gyrata (thickening of the skin of the scalp, most often involving the vertex, and forming fold and furrows resembling sulci and gyri of the brain. It may occur alone or it may be characteristic of another condition, such as pachydermoperiostosis.

Rosewater's s., a mild form of familial primary hypogonadism in the male of unknown pathogenesis, marked only by sterility and gynecomastia.

Rot's s., Rot-Bernhardt s., meralgia paresthetica, see Bernhardt's disease.

Rothmann-Makai s., idiopathic circumscribed panniculitis with fat cell necrosis, lipophagic granuloma, and cyst formation; it usually subsides spontaneously.

Rothmund-Thomson s., an autosomal recessive syndrome occurring principally in females, characterized by the presence of reticulated, atrophic, hyperpigmented, telangiectatic cutaneous plaques, often accompanied by juvenile cataracts, saddle nose, congenital bone defects, disturbances in the growth of hair, nails, and teeth, and hypogonadism. Called also poikiloderma congenitale Cf: Thomson disease.

Rotor's s., chronic familial nonhemolytic jaundice differing from Dubin-Johnson syndrome in the lack of liver pigmentation.

Roussy-Dejerrine s., see Thalamic s.

Roussy-Levy s., a slowly progressive hereditary disorder, transmitted as an autosomal dominant trait, in which sensory ataxia is associated with areflexia, atrophy of the muscles of the distal extremities, especially the peroneal muscles, static tremor of the hands, pes cavus or clawfoot, and sometimes kyphoscoliosis. Called also hereditary areflexic dystasia. Roussy Levy disease and Roussy-Levy hereditery areflex lystasia.

Rovsing s., horseshoe kidney with nausea, abdominal discomfort, and pain on hyperextension.

Rubella s., see Congenital rubella s.

Rubinstein's s., Rubinstein-Taybi s., a congenital condition characterized by mental and motor retardation, broad thumbs and great toes, short stature, characteristic facies, including high-arched palate and straight or beaked nose, various eye abnormalities, pulmonary stenosis, keloid formation in surgical scars, large foramen magnum, and abnormalities of the vertebra and sternum.

Rubrospinal cerebellar peduncle s., see Claude's s.

Rud's s., congenital syndrome consisting of ichthyosis simplex, mental deficiency, epilepsy, and infantilism.

Rudimentary testis s., see Vanishing testis s.

Runting s., graft-vs-host reaction characterized by diarrhea, dermatitis hepatosplenomegaly, hemolytic anemia, and pancytopenia.

Russell's s., see Silver's s.

Rust's s., stiff neck, stiff carriage of the head, with the necessity of grasping the head with both hands in lying down or rising up from a horizontal posture, occurring in tuberculosis, cancer, fracture of the spine, rheumatic or arthritic processes, or syphilitic periostitis.

Sabin-Feldman s., chorioretinitis and cerebral calcifications, similar to the manifestation of toxoplasmosis, but having all tests for toxoplasmosis negative.

Saethre-Chotzen s., see Chotzen's s.

Sakati-Nyhan s., acrocephalopolysyndactyly, type III—autosomal dominant, with hypoplastic tibias and deformed, displaced fibulas.

Salt-depletion s., see Salt-losing s.

Salt-losing s., vomiting, dehydration, hypotension, and, sudden death due to very large sodium losses from the body. It may be seen in abnormal losses of sodium into the urine (as in congenital adrenal hyperplasia, adrenocortical insufficiency, or one of the forms of salt-losing nephritis) or in large extrarenal sodium losses, usually from the gastrointestinal tract. Called also salt-depletion crisis, salt-depletion syndrome, salt-losing crisis, and salt-losing defect.

Sanfilippo's s., four heterogeneous, biochemically distinct, but clinically indistinguishable, forms of mucopolysaccharidosis characterized biochemically by excretion of heparan sulfate in the urine and clinically by severe, rapid mental deterioration and relatively mild somatic symptoms. Onset is from 2 to 6 years of age; the head is large, height normal; Hurler-like features (dysostosis multiplex, hepatomegaly) are mild; hirsutism is generalized; death usually occurs before 20 years of age. The four enzymatic types are: type A, the severest, due to defective heparan N-sulfatase; type B due to defective N-acetyl-α-D-glucosaminidase; type C due to defective acetyl CoA: α-glucosaminide-N-acetyltransferase; and type D, due to defective

N-acetyl-α-D-glucosaminidie-β-sulfatase. Called also Mucopolysaccharidosis III.

Scalded skin s., non-staphylococcal, toxic epidermal necrolysis*, see Lyell's s.

Scalded skin s., staphylococcal, an infectious disease of infants and young children and rarely of older children and adults occurring following infection with certain strains of *Staphylococcus aureus* (phage group II), which elaborate exfoliatin (q.v.), an epidermolytic, erythrogen endotoxin that causes a clinical spectrum ranging from a localized bullous eruption to widespred development of easily ruptured fine vesicles and bullae resulting in exfoliation of large sheets of skin, leaving raw, denuded areas that make the skin surface looked scalded. Called also dermatitis exfoliation neonatorum and Ritter's disease.

Scalenils s., Scalenus anticus s., pain over the shoulder, often extending down the arm (cervicobrachial s.) or radiating up the back of the neck due to compression of the nerves and vessels between a cervical rib and the scalenus anticus muscle; called also Naffziger's s. and cervical rib s.

Scapulocostal s., pain in the superior or posterior aspect of the shoulder girdle, radiating to contiguous regions, as a result of long-standing alteration of the relationship of the scapula and posterior thoracic wall.

Schafer's s., pachyonychia congenital associated with retardation of physical and mental development.

Schanz's s., a series of symptoms indicating spinal weakness, consisting of a sense of fatigue, pain on pressure over the spinous processes, pain on lying prone, and indications of spinal curvature.

Schaumann's s., sarcoidosis, see Boeck and Schaumanns disease.

Scheie's s., a relatively mild allelic variant of the Hurler syndrome and the mildest of the three allelic disorders mucopolysaccharidosis 1, characterized by corneal clouding, claw hand, involvement of the aortic valve, somewhat coarse facies with a broad mouth, genu valgum, and pes cavus. Stature, intelligence, and lifespan are normal. Called also α-L-iduronidase deficiency. Scheie type, and mucopolysaccharidosis IS; formerly called mucopolysaccharidosis V.

---
* See Appendix

Schirmer's s., a variant of the Sturge-Weber syndrome in which glaucoma occurs early in the course of the disease.

Schmidt's s., [1. A. Schmidt] paralysis on one side, affecting the vocal cord, the velum palati, the trapezius muscle, and the sternocleidomastoid muscle, due to a lesion of the nucleus ambiguus and nucleus accessorius. 2. [MB Schmidt] hypofunction of more than one endocrine gland, including the thyroid, adrenal, gonads, parathyroids, and endocrine pancreas, in any combination, along with nonendocrine abnormalities of presumed autoimmune origin, such as vitiligo, alopecia, and pernicious anemia; it occurs primarily in adult females. Originally, primary failure of the adrenals and thyroid only. Called also Polyendocrine autoimmune disease, type II.

Schonlein-Henoch s., see Schonlein-Henoch disease.

Schuller's s., Schuller-Christian s., see Hand Schuller-Christian disease.

Schultz s., agranulocytosis, see Schultz's disease.

Scimitar s., complete or partial venous drainage of the right lung into the inferior vena cava usually with hypoplasia of the right lung; the name is derived from the convex shadow of the anomalous vein to the right of the lower border of the heart in the chest roentgenogram.

S. of sea-blue histiocyte, a rare disorder characterized by the presence of morphologically distinct, sea-blue, granulated histiocyte and by splenomegaly. Clinically, the disorder may range from a relatively benign course with mild purpura secondary to thrombocytopenia, to progressive hepatic cirrhosis, hepatic failure, and death.

Seabright bantam s., pseudohypoparathyrodism—a hereditary condition clinically resembling hypoparathyrodism, but caused by failure to response rather than deficiency of parathyroid hormone. It is characterized by hypocalcemia and hyperphosphatemia, and is commonly associated with short stature, obesity, short metacarpets, and ectopic calcifications.

Seckel's s., a dwarf with proportionately small head, narrow birdlike face with a beaklike protrusion of the nose, large eyes, antimongoloid slant of the palperbral fissures, and recending lower jaw.

Segmentary s., a syndrome produced by a lesion of the gray matter of the spinal cord, and marked by weakness and wasting in the affected segment; called also Metameric s.

Selye s., see General adaptation s.

Senear-Usher s., pemphigus erythematosus—a variant of pemphigus foliaceus, with which it is histologically identical, characterized clinically by the development of lupus erythematosus like rash on the nose, cheeks, ears and seborrhea like lesions elswhere on the body; and immunologically by granular deposition of immunoglobulin and complement along the dermoepidermal junction. These finding suggests the coexistence of lupus erythematosus and pemphigus in the same individual.

S. of sensory dissociation with brachial amyotrophy, see Morvan's disease and syndrome.

Sertoli-cell-only s., congenital absence of the germinal epithelium of the testes, the seminiferous tubules containing only Sertoli cells, characterized by testes which are slightly smaller than normal, azoospermia, and elevated titers of follicle-stimulating hormone and sometimes of luterinizing hormone.

Serum sickness-like s., a hypersensitivity reaction to the administration of foreign serum or serum proteins characterized by fever, urticaria, arthralgia, edema, and lymphadenopathy. It is formed by circulating antigen-antibody complexes that are deposited in tissue and trigger tissue injury mediated by complement anf polymorphonuclear leukocytes. Serum sickness is classed with the Arthur's reaction and immune complex disease as type III in the Gell and Coomb's classification of immune reactions. An identical illness can be produced by hypersensitivity reaction to penicillin and other drugs.

Sezary s., a form of cutaneous T-cell lymphoma manifested by generalized exfoliative erythroderma, intense pruritus, peripheral lymphadenopathy, and abnormal hyperchromatic mononuclear cells in the skin, lymph nodes, and peripheral blood (sezary cells). Called also Sezary erythroderma.

Sheehan's s., postpartum pituitary necrosis.

Short-bowel s., short-gut s., any of the malabsorption conditions resulting from massive resection of the small bowel, the degree and kind of malabsorption depending on the site and extent of the resection; it is characterized by diarrhea, steatorrhea, and malnutrition.

Shoulder-hand s., a clinical disorder of the upper extremity, characterized by pain and stiffness in the shoulder, with puffy swelling and pain in the ipsilateral hand, sometimes occurring after myocardial infarction but also produced by other known or unknown causes.

Shwachman s., Shwachman-Diamond s., primary pancreatic insufficiency and bone marrow failure, characterized by normal sweat chloride values, pancreatic insufficiency and neutropenia; it may be associated with dwarfism and metaphyseal dysostosis of the hips.

Shy-Drager s., a progressive disorder of unknown cause that results in severe disability or death, beginning with symptoms of autonomic insufficiency including impotence (in males), constipation, urinary urgency or retention anhidrosis, and the hallmark of the disorder, orthostatic hypotension, followed by signs of generalized neurologic dysfunction, such as parkinsonian-like disturbances, cerebellar incoordination, muscle wasting and fasciculations, and coarse tremors of the legs.

Sicard's s., see Collet's s.

Sicca s., keratoconjunctivitis and xerostomia without connective tissue disease; Cf. Sjögren's s.

Sick sinus s., a complex cardiac arrhythmia manifested as severe sinus bradycardia alone, sinus bradycardia alternating with tachycardia, or sinus bradycardia with atrioventricular block.

Silver's s., a congenital syndrome consisting of low birth weight despite normal duration of gestation, short stature, lateral asymmetry, slight to moderate increase in excretion of gonadotropins, which may be associated with incurved fifth fingers, cafe-au-lait spots, syndactyly, triangular face, turned down corners of the mouth, and precocious puberty. Cf. Russell's s.

Silverskiold's s., a form of eccentro-osteochondrodysplasia in which the skeletal changes are chiefly in the extremities and which is inherited as a dominant character.

Silvestrini-Corda s., eunuchoid body type, absence of body hair, deficient libido, atrophy of the testes, sterility, and gynecomastia: a syndrome indicative of abnormally high estrogenic activity, due to failure of the liver to inactivate the circulating estrogens.

Simmonds' s., generalised hypopituitarism due to absence of or damage to the pituiary gland, which, in its complete form, leads to absence of gonadal function and insufficiency of thyroid and adrenal cortical function. Dwarfism, regression secondary sex characters and loss of libido, weight loss, fatiguability, bradycardia, hypotension, pallor, depression, and many other manifestations can occur. When cachexia is a prominent feature it is called Simmond's disease.

Sipple's s., multiple endocrine neoplasia, type IIA characterized by medullary carcinoma of thyroid, pheochromocytoma, often bilateral and multiple, and parathyroid hyperplasia.

Sjögren's s., a symptom complex of unknown etiology, usually occurring in middle-aged or older women, marked by the triad of keratoconjunctivitis sicca with or without lacrimal gland-enlargement, xerostomia with or without salivary gland enlargement, and the presence of a connective tissue disease, usually rehumatoid arthritis but sometimes systemic lupus erythematosus, scleroderma, or polymyositis. An abnormal immune response has been implicated. See also sicca s. Called also Sjögren's disease.

Sjögren-Larsson s., congenital oligophrenia, ichthyosis and spastic pyramidal symptoms.

Sleep apnea s., episodes of cessation of breathin occurring at the transition from NREM to REM sleep, with repeated wakening and excessive day time sleepiness; it occurs most frequently in middle-aged obese males and is thought to have several causes, one being collapse or obstruction of the airway with the inhibition of muscle tone that characterizes REM sleep.

SLE-like s., see Lupus like s.

Sluder's s., neuralgia of the sphenopalatine ganglion, causing burning and boring pain in the area of the superior maxilla and radiation of the pain into the neck and shoulder.

Sly s., a mucopolysaccharidosis caused by deficient β-glucuronidase and characterized biochemically by excretion of dermatan sulfate and heparan sulfate in the urine and by granular inclusions in granulocytes. Onset is between 1 and 2 years with mild to moderate Hurler-like features including dysostosis multiplex, pectus carinatum, visceromegaly, cardiac murmurs, short stature, and moderate mental retardation. Milder forms exist. Called also mucopolysaccharidosis VII, β-glucuronidase (GUSB) deficiency.

Smith-Lemli-Opitzs., a hereditary syndrome, transmitted as an autosomal recessive trait, characterized by multiple congenital anomalies, including microcephaly, mental retardation, hypotonia, incomplete development of male genitalia, short nose with anteverted nostrils, syndactyly of second and third toes, etc.

Social breakdown s., symptoms of a mental patient that are due to the effects of long-term institutionalization, rather than the primary illness; they include excessive passivity, assumption of the chronic sick role, and atrophy of work and social skills.

Sohval-Soffer s., a congenital syndrome consisting of male hypogonadism associated with multiple skeletal abnormalities of the cervical spine and ribs and mental retardation.

Somnolence s., a transient condition of drowsiness, lethargy, anorexia, and irritability with electroencephalographic changes, occurring in children after irradiation of the head in acute leukemia or non-Hodgkin's lymphpoma.

Sorsby's s., a congenital condition consisting of bilateral macular coloboma associated with apical dystrophy of the hands and feet, usually brachydactyly confined to the distal two phalanges.

Sotos's s., Sotos's s. of cerebral gigantism, cerebral gigantism—gigantism in the absence of increased level of growth hormone, attributed to cerebral defect; infants are large and acceleratd growth continues for the first four to five years, the rate being normal thereafter. The hands and feet are large, the head large and dolicocephalic, the eyes have a antimongoloid slant, with hypertelorism. The child is clumsy, and mental retardation of varying degree is usually present.

Space adaptation s., a form of motion skickness occurring in a weightless environment during space flight, with nausea, vomiting, anorexia, headache, malaise, drowsiness, and lethargy. It is probably caused by conflicting signals concerning motion from the otolith (whose proper function depends on the presence of gravity) and the visual systems (which affects in the autonomic nervous system). Called also space sickness.

Spens' s., see Adams-Stokes disease.

Spherophakia-brachymorphia s., see Weill-Marchesani s.

Splenic flexure s., discomfort in the left upper abdominal quadrant, which may give rise to pain in the precordium and left shoulder and arm, simulating angina.

Split-brain s. an association of symptoms produced by disruption of or interference with the connection between the hemispheres of the brain.

Sprinz-Dubin s., Sprinz-Nelson s., see Dubin-Johnson s.

Spurway s., osteogenesis imperfecta associated with blue sclerae.

Steele-Richardson-Olszewski s., a progressive neurological disorder, having onset during the sixth decade, characterized by supranuclear ophthalmoplegia, especially paralysis of the downward gaze, pseudo-bulbar palsy, dysarthria, dystonic rigidity of the neck and trunk, and dementia.

Steely-hair s., see Menkes's.

Stein-Leventhal s., a clinical symptom complex characterized by oligomenorrhea or amenorrhea, anovulation (hence infertility), and hirsutism, and regularly associated with bilateral polycystic ovaries; excretion of follicle-stimulating hormone and 17-ketosteroids is essentially normal. Called also polycystic ovary disease or syndrome.

Stein-brocker's s., see Shoulder-hand s.

Steiner's s., see Curtisu's.

Stevens-Johnson s., a sometimes fatal form of erythema multiforme presenting with a flu like prodrome, and chracterized by systemic as well as more severe mucocutaneous lesions. The oronasal and anogenital mucous membranes may become involved with a characteristic gray or white pseudomemebrane; hemorrhagic crusts often occur on the lips; ocular lesions vary from injected conjunctivitis, ititis, uveitis, corneal vesicles, erosions, and perforaton which may result in corneal opacities and blindness; and pulmonary, gastrointestinal, cardiac, and renal involvement occur. Called also ectodermosis erosiva pluriorificialis, erythema multiforme exudativum, erythema multiforme major, and Johnson-Stevens disease.

Stewart-Morel s., hyperostosis frontalis interna, see Morgagni-Stewart-Morel s.

Stewart-Treves s., lymphangiosarcoma which occurs as a late complication of severe lymphedema of the arm following excision of lymph nodes, usually associated with radical mastectomy.

"Stiff heart" s., any cardiac disease characterized by restrictive hemodynamics; it may result from any pathologic process that renders the myocardial fibers anomally rigid or that extremelly applies a constricting pressure and as a consequence impedes flow of blood into the ventricular cavities.

Stiffman s., a condition of unknown etiology characterized by progressive fluctuating rigidity of axial and limb muscles in the absence of signs of cerebral and spinal cord disease but with continuous electromyographic activity.

Still-Chauffard s., see Chauffard's s.

Stilling s., Stilling-Turk-Duane s., see Duane s.

Strokes' s., Stokes-Adams., see Adams-Stokes disease.

Stokvis-Talma s., enterogenous cyanosis—a syndrome due to absorption of nitrites and sulfides from the intestine, principally marked by metemoglobinemia and/or sulfhemoglobinemia associated with cyanosis. It is accompanied by severe enteritis, abdominal pain, constipation or diarrhea, headache, dyspnea, dizziness, syncope, anemia, and occassionally, digital clubbing and indicanuria.

Straight back s., a skeletal deformity characterized by loss of the anterior concavity of the vertebral column in the upper thoracic region, with consequent reduction in the anteroposterior diameter of the thorax and compression of the heart between the dorsal spine and the sternum.

Stroke s., a condition with sudden onset caused by acute vascular lesions of the brain, such as hemorrhage, embolism, thrombosis, or rupturing aneurysm, which may be marked by hemiplegia or hemiparesis, vertigo, numbness, aphasia and dysarthria; it is often followed by permanent neurologic damage. Called also Cerebrovascular accident and stroke.

Sturge's s., Sturge-Kalischer-Weber s., see Sturge-Weber s.

Sturge-Weber s., a congenital syndrome of unknown etiology consisting of a portwine stain type of nevus flammeus distributed over the trigeminal nerve accompanied by a similar vascular disorder of the underlying meninges and cerebral cortex; it usually occurs unilaterally. Called also encephalofacial or encephalotrigeminal angiomatosis. Sturge's or Sturge-Kalischer-Weber s., and Sturge's or Weber's disease.

Subclavian steal s., cerebral or brainstem ischemia resulting from diversion of blood flow from the basilar artery to the subclavian artery, in the presence of occlusive disease of the proximal portion of the subclavian artery.

Sudden infant death s., the sudden and unexpected death of an apparently healthy infant, typically occurring between the ages of three weeks and five months, and not explained by careful postmortem studies; called also crib or cot death. Abbreviated as SIDS.

Sudden unexplained death s., death for which no underlying cause can be found of a person, 2 years old or older of South-East Asian origin; abbreviated as SUDS.

Sudeck-Leriche s., post-traumatic osteoporosis associated with vasospasm.

Sulzberger-Carbe s., exudative discoid and lichenoid dermatitis, see Oid-Oid disease.

Superior mesenteric artery s., compression of the third, or transverse, portion of the duodenum against the aorta by the superior mesenteric artery, resulting in complete or partial obstruction that may be chronic, intermittent, or acute; symptoms range from mild to severe, including nausea and vomiting, pain, and extreme distention of the stomach and duodenum.

Superior orbital fissure s., deep orbital and unilateral frontal headache with progressive sixth, third, and fourth cranial nerve palsies, occurring as a rare complication of sphenoid sinusitis and caused by extension of the infection to the structures of the superior orbital fissure.

Superior sulcus tumor s., see Pancoast's s., def. 1.

Superior vena cava s., suffusion and brawny edema of the face, neck, or upper arms due to increased venous pressure incident to compression of the superior vena cava, most commonly caused by primary bronchial tumors or metastatic mediastinal lymph nodes in lung cancer.

Supraspinatus s., tenderness over the supraspinatus tendon, a painful arc on movement of the arm, and a reversal of scapulohumeral rhythm.

Sweat retention s., 1. A dermatologic condition due to occlusion of sweat ducts, which may result in symptoms ranging from pruritus, scratch dermatitis, and miliaria to very persistent infalmmatory changes depending upon the extent of the blockage, environmental temperature, and duration of sweating stimulus. 2. Tropical anhidrotic asthenia—a rare condition occurring under conditions of heat stress, in which miliaria profunda causes extensive occlusion of the sweat ducts, producing anhidrosis and heat retention that may lead to weakness, dyspnea, tachycardia, elevation of the body temperature, and collapse.

Sweet's s., acute febrile neutrophilic dermatosis—a condition usually seen on the upper body of the middle aged women characterized by the presence of one or more large, rapidly expanding, erythematous, tender or painful plaques, and occurring in association with fever and dense infiltration of the neutrophilic leukocytes in the upper and mid dermis.

Swyer-James s., acquired unilateral hyperlucent lung, the severe airway obstruction during expiration, oligemia, and a small hilum; called also Macleod s.

Sylvian s., Sylvian aqueduct s., impairment of vertical gaze, retraction nystagmus, convergence nystagmus, convergence spasms, and poor or absent reaction of the pupils (which are usually of normal size) to light or near vision. It is caused by a neoplasm, inflammation, or vascular lesion adjacent to the periductal gray matter of the aqueduct of Sylvius. Called also Koerber-Salus-Elschnig s. and nystagmus refractorius.

Syringomelic s., syringomelia.

Takayasu's s., see Pulseless disease.

Tapia's s., unilateral paralysis of the tongue and larynx, the velum palati being unaffected.

Tarsal tunnel s., a complex of symptoms resulting from compression of the posterior tibial nerve of the plantar nerves in the tarsal tunnel, with pain, numbness, and tingling paresthesia of the sole of the foot.

Taussig-Bing s., a rare congenital malformation of the heart characterized by transposition of the great vessels and a ventricular septal defect straddled by a large pulmonary artery hemodynamically it is characterized by pulmonary hypertension, pulmonary plethora cyanosis, and greater O_2 saturation of blood in the pulmonary artery than in the aorta.

Tegmental s., hemiplegia, alternating with disordered eye movements, indicative of lesions of the tegmentum.

Temporomandibular dysfunction s., Temporomandibular Joint s., a symptom complex described as consisting of partial deafness, stuffy sensation in the ears; tinnitus, clicking and snapping in the temporomandibular joint, dizziness, headache, and burning pain in the ear throat, tongue, and nose. Numerous causes have been proposed, such as mandibular overclosure, lesions of the temporo-mandibular joint, and stress, but some researches feel that the anatomical and physiological evidence to justify this syndrome is lacking. Called also Costen's s. and myofascial pain dysfunction.

Terry's s., retrolental fibroplasia—a bilateral retinopathy occurring in premature infants treated with excessively high concentrations of oxygen, characterized by vascular dilatation, proliferation, and tortuosity, edema, and retinal detatchment, with ultimate conversions of the retina into fibrous mass that can be seen as a dense retrolental membrane; usually growth of the eye is arrested and may result in microphthalmia, and blindness may occur.

Terson's s. hemorrhage into the vitreous.

Testicular feminization s., an extreme form of male pseudohermaphroditism, with female external development, including secondary sex characteristics, but with presence of testes and absence of uterus and tubes; it is due to end-organ resistance to the action of 5α-testosterone.

Tethered cord s., an abnormally low conus medullaris tethered by one or more forms of intradural abnormality such as a short, thickened filum terminale, fibrous bands or adhesions, or an intradural lipoma.

Thalamic s., a combination of the following symptoms (i) superficial persistent hemianesthesia (ii) mild hemiplegia; (iii) mild hemiataxia and more or less complete astereognosis; (iv) severe and persistent pains in the hemiplegic side; (vi) choreoathetoid movements in the members of the paralyzed side. Called also Dejerine-Roussy s. and thalamic hyperesthetic anesthesia.

Thibierge-Weissenbach s., calcinosis—a condition marked by deposition of calcium salts in various tissues of the body.

Thiele s., tenderness and pain in the region of the lower portion of the sacrum and coccyx, or in contiguous soft tissues and muscles.

Thiemann's s., see under disease.

Thoracic outlet s., compression of the brachial plexus nerve trunks, characterized by pain in arms, paresthesia of fingers, vasomotor symptoms (pallor, acrocyanosis, secondary Raynaud's phenomenon, etc.) and weakness and wasting of the small muscles of the hand; it may be caused by drooping shoulder girdle, a cervical rib or fibrous band, an abnormal first rib, continual hyperabduction of the arm (see hyperabduction s), or (rarely) compression of the edge of the scalenus anterior muscle.

Thorn's s., see Salt losing s.

Thrombocytopenia-absent radius (TAR) s., an autosomal recessive syndrome consisting of thrombocytopenia associated with absence or hypoplasia of the radius and sometimes congenital heart disease and renal anomalies.

Thromboembolic s., the association between the formation of thrombi in the deep veins of the leg and pulmonary embolism.

Tietze's s., 1. (Alexander Tietze) idiopathic painful nonsuppurative swellings of one or more costal cartilages, especially of the second rib; the anterior chest pain may mimic that of coronary artery disease. Called also costal chondritis and Tietze's disease. 2. albinism, except for normal eye pigment, deaf-mutism, and hypoplasia of the eyebrows.

Tirea housewife s., a form of mild hypothyroidism manifested in symptoms such as mild lassitude, fatigue, slight anemia, constipation, apathy, slight cold intolerance, menstrual irregularities, inability to conceive, dry skin, some loss of hair,, and slight to moderate weight gain.

Tolosa-Hunt s., unilateral ophthalmoplegia associated with pain behind the orbit and in the area supplied by the first division of the trigeminal nerve; it is thought to be due to nonspecific inflammation and granulation tissue in the superior orbital fissure or cavernous sinus.

Tommaselli's s., see under disease.

Torres s., multiple carcinomas, primarily of the gastrointestinal tract, in association with a large number of sebaceous gland neoplasms.

Touraine-Solente-Gole s., pachydermoperiostosis—a condition believed to be inherited as an autosomal dominant trait, chiefly characterized by 1 thickening of the skin of the head and distal extremities deep folds and furrows of the skin of the forehead, cheeks, and scalp, seborrhea, hyperhidrosis, periostosis of the long bones, digital clubbing, and spade like enlargement of the hands and feet. It is more prevalent in the male, and usually first evident during adolescence.

Toxic fat s., a condition occurring in 3 to 10 weeks old chickens that have been fed fat supplemented diets marked by edema of the pericardium and abdomen, waddling gait, and sudden death; called also water belly.

Toxic shock s., a severe illness characterized by high fever of sudden onset, vomiting diarrhea, and myalgia, followed by hypotension and, in severe cases, shock; a sunburn-like rash with peeling of the skin, especially of the palms and soles, occurs during the acute phase. The syndrome affects almost exclusively menstruating women using tampons, although a few women who do not use tampons and a few males have been affected. It is thought to be caused by infection with *Staphylococcus aureus*.

Transfusion s., see Placental transfusion s.

Translocation Down s., Down syndrome in which the excess chromosomal material (the long arm of chromosome 21) is translocated to another acrocentric chromosome (in standard trisomy 21 there is an additional chromosome 21). A carrier of the translocation chromosome has 45 chromosomes including the translocation chromosome and may be at increased risk of having a child with Down syndrome.

Treacher Collins s., Treacher Collins-Franceschetti s., mandibulofacial dysostosis, see Franceschetti s.

Trichorhinophalangeal s., an autosomal recessive syndrome consisting of sparse, slowly growing hair, pear-shaped nose with high philtrum, and brachyphalangia with deformity of the fingers and wedge-shaped epiphyses.

Triparanol s., alopecia, poliosis, ichthyosis, irreversible cataracts, and impotence, due to the use of triparanol, a drug formerly used to depress the synthesis of cholesterol.

Trisomy C s., see trisomy 8 s.

Trisomy D s., see trisomy 13s.

Trisomy E s., see trisomy 18s.

Trisomy 8 s., a syndrome associated with an extrachromosome 8, usually mosaic (trisomy 8/normal), characterized by mild to severe mental retardation, prominent forehead, deep-set eyes, thick lips, prominent ears, and camptodactyly.

Trisomy 13s., a chromosome aberration in which an extrachromosome 13 causes central nervous system defects and mental retardation, together with cleft palate ,and lip, polydactyly, dermal pattern anomalies, and abnormalities of the heart, viscera, and genitalia.Called also Patau s.

Trisomy 18 s., a condition characterized by mental retardation scaphocephaly or other skull abnormality micrognathia, blepharoptosis, low-set ears, corhealopacities deafness, webbed neck, short digits, ventricular septal defects, Meckel's diverticulum, and other deformities. It is due to the presence of an extra chromosome 18. Called also Edwards' s. and trisomy E s.

Trisomy 21 s., see Down's s.

Trisomy 22 s., a syndrome due to an extrachromosome 22, characterized typically by mental and growth retardation, microcephaly, low-set or malformed ears, micrognathia, long philtrum, preauricular skin tag or sinus, and congenital heart disease. In males, there is small penis and/or undescended testes.

Troisier's s., bronzed cachexia occurring in the diabetes associated with hemochromatosis.

Tropical splenomegaly s., a condition seen in endemic malarious areas that is said to be due to an aberrant immunological response to malaria, characterized by massive splenomegaly, hepatomegaly, anemia with increased reticulocyte count, and lymphocytic infiltration of the hepatic sinusoids. Patients often have elevated malaria antibody titers anserum IgM levels. Malaria prophylaxis usually causes the condition to improve. Called also Malarial hyperreactive spleen s.

Trousseau's s., spontaneous venous thrombosis of upper and lower extremities occurring in association with visceral carcinoma.

Tumor lysis s., severe hyperphosphatemia, hyperkalemia, hyperuricemia, and hypocalcemia occurring after effective induction chemotherapy of rapidly growing malignant neoplasms, thought to be due to release of intracellular products after cell lysis.

Turcot s, familial polyposis of the colon associated with malignant tumors (gliomas) of the central nervous system.

Turner's s., a disorder of gonadal differentiation, marked by short stature, undifferentiated (streak) gonads, and variable abnormalities that may include webbing of the neck, low posterior hair line, increased carrying angle of the elbow, cubitus valgus, and cardiac defects; it is typically associated with absence of the second sex chromosome (XO, or 45, X), although structural abnormality of one X chromosome or mosaicism (e.g. XX/XX or X/XXX) may also be responsible. The phenotype is female; patients are usually sterile. Called also Gonadal dysgenesis.

Turner's s' male, see Noonan's s.

Ullrich-Feichtiger s., a condition of micrognathia, hexadactyly, and genital abnormalities with depressed nose, small eyes, hypertelorism, and protuberant ears, along with other defects.

Ullrich-Turner s., see Noonan's s.

Unilateral nevoid telangiectasia s., generalized essential telangiectasia representing latent vascular nevus that becomes manifest under the possible influence of estrogen (pregnancy, menarche) or increased venous pressure (liver disease). Called also unilateral nevoid telangiectasia.

Unna-Thost s., diffuse palmoplantar keratoderma, see Unna-Thost disease.

Unverricht's s., myoclonus epilepsy, see Lafora's disease.

Urethral s., suprapubic aching and cramping, urinary frequency, and such bladder complaints as dysuria, urinary tenesmus, and low back pain, without evidence of urinary infection.

V**agoaccessory s.**, see Schmidt's s.

van Buchem's s., hyperostosis corticalis generalista—a hereditary disorder, transmitted as an autosomal recessive trait, characterized principally by osteosclerosis of the skull, mandible, clavicles, ribs, and diaphyses of long bones, associated with elevated blood alkaline phosphatase; beginning during puberty, it sometimes lead to optic atrophy and perceptive deafness due to nerve pressure exerted by thickening of base of the skull.

van der Hoeve's s., a hereditary syndrome consisting of blue scleras, osteogenesis imperfecta, and otosclerotic deafness, usually transmitted as an autosomal dominant trait. Called also Adair-Dighton s. and Dighton-Adair s.

van der Woude's s., a hereditary syndrome, transmitted as an autosomal dominant trait consisting of cleft lip and/or cleft palate occurring in association with cysts of the lower lip.

Vanishing testes s., a disorder characterized by the absence of gonadal tissue, a small penis, and no adolescent virilization; the testes are thought to have been present in the embryo but to have "vanished" before completion of male sexual differentiation. The chromosome pattern is XY (male).

Vascular s., any syndrome due to occlusion or stenosis of vessels supplying the nervous system.

Verner-Morrison s., a rare syndrome of profuse watery diarrhea, hypokalemia, and achlorhydria, usually due to a beta cell neoplasm of pancreatic islets and associated with excess levels of vasoactive intestinal polypeptide; called also pancreatic cholera and WDHA syndrome.

Vernet's s., paralysis of the ninth, tenth, and eleventh cranial nerves due to a lesion in the region of the jugular foramen, and marked by paralysis of the superior constriction of the pharynx and difficulty in swallowing solids; paralysis of the soft palate and fauces with anesthesia of these parts and of the pharynx, and loss of taste in the posterior third of the tongue; paralysis of the vocal cords and anesthesia of the larynx; paralysis of the sternocleidomastoid and trapezius muscles. Called also Jugular foramen s.

Villaret's s., unilateral paralysis of the ninth, tenth, eleventh, and twelfth cranial nerves and sometimes the seventh, due to a lesion in the retroparotid space, and characterized by paralysis of the superior constriction of the pharynx and difficulty in swallowing solids; paralysis of soft palate and fauces with anesthesia of these parts and of the pharynx; loss of taste in the posterior third of the tongue; paralysis of the vocal cords and anesthesia of the larynx; paralysis of the sternocleidomastoid and trapezius; and paralysis of the cervical sympathetic nerves (Horner's syndrome). Called also s. of retroparotid space.

Vinsons s., see Plummer-Vinson s.

Vogt's s., a syndrome frequently associated with birth trauma, characterized by bilateral athetosis, walking difficulties, spasmodic outbursts of laughing or crying, speech disorders, excessive myelination of the nerve fibers of the corpus striatum giving it a marbled appearance (status marmoratus), and sometimes mental deficiency. Called also Vogt's disease and s. of corpus striatum.

Vogt-Koyanagi s., uveomeningitis characterized by exudative iridocyclitis and choroiditis associated with patchy depigmentation of the skin and hair: the lashes and eyebrows a become whitened, and there may also be retinal detachment and associated deafness tinnitus. Cf: Harada s.

Vohwinkel's s., keratoma hereditarium mutilans—an autosomal dominant, progressive dystrophic form of palmoplantar keratoderma, begning in the childhood, characterized by stellate pattern of hyperkeratosis on the backs of the hands and feet, linear keratoses on elbows and knees, and annular ainhum-like constriction of the digits, and sometimes associated with scarring alopecia and deafness.

Volkmann's s., post-traumatic muscular hypertonia and degenerative neuritis; Volkmann's contracture.

Waardenburg's s., 1. An autosomal dominant disorder characterized by wide bridge of the nose due to lateral displacement of the inner canthi and puncta, pigmentary disturbances, including white forelock, heterochromia irides, white eyelashes, leukoderma, and sometimes cochlear deafness. 2. An autosomal dominant disorder characterized by acrocephaly, orbital and facial deformities, and brachydactyly with mild soft tissue syndactyly; cleft palate, hydrophthalmos, cardiac malformation, and contractures of the elbows and knees may also be present. Called also acrocephalosyndactyly type IV and Klein-Waardenburg s.

Wallenberg's s., a syndrome due to occlusion of the posterior inferior cerebellar artery, marked by ipsilateral loss of temperature and pain sensations of the face and contralateral loss of these sensations of the extremities and trunk, ipsilateral ataxia, dysphagia, dysarthria, and nystagmus.

Ward-Romano s., see Romano-Ward s.

Waterhouse-Friderichsen s., the malignant or fulminating form of epidemic cerebrospinal meningitis, marked by sudden onset and short course, fever, coma, and collapse, cyanosis, petechial hemorrhages of the skin and mucous membranes, and bilateral adrenal hemorrhage.

WDHA s. watery diarrhea, hypokalemia, achlorhydria, see Verner-Morrison s.

S. of Weber, paralysis of the oculomotor nerve on the same side as the lesion, producing ptosis, strabismus, and loss of light reflex and of accommodation; also spastic hemiplegia on the side opposite the lesion with increased reflexes and loss of superficial reflexes. Called also alternating oculomotor hemiplegia and Weber's paralysis.

Weber-Christian s., relapsing febrile nodular nonsuppurative panniculitis, see Weber-Christian disease.

Weber-Cockayne s., localized epidermolysis bullosa simplex—a form of epidermolysis bullosa primarily confined to the hands and feet, especially the palms and soles, appearing in infancy or later life, and often associated with hyperhidrosis. It may be exacerbated by unusual trauma such as prolonged walking.

Weber-Dubler s., see S. of Weber.

Wegener's s., a multisystem disease chiefly affecting males, characterized by necrotizing granulomatous vasculitis involving the upper and lower respiratory tracts, glomerulonephritis, and variable degrees of systemic, small vessel vasculitis, which is generally considered to represent an aberrant hypersensitivity reaction to an unknown antigen.

Weils s., a severe form of leptospirosis (qv) characterized by jaundice usually accompanied by azotemia, hemorrhages, anemia, disturbances of consciousness, and continued fever. It is usually caused by *Leptospira interrogans* serogroup icterohemorrhagica but may be caused by other serogroups such as bataviae. The disease has been known by various eponymous and clinically descriptive names, including Fiedler's Lancereaux-Mathieu-Weil, Landouzy's, and Weil's disease; infectious, infective, leptospiral and spirochetal jaundice; and leptospirosis icterohemorrhagica.

Weill-Marchesard s., a congenital disorder of connective tissue transmitted as autosomal dominant or recessive trait, characterized by brachycephaly brachydactyly, stature with a broad chest and heavy musculature, reduced joint mobility, spherophakia ectopia lentis, myopia, and glaucoma; called also dystrophia mesodermalis congenita hyperplastica, Marchesani's s., and spherophakia-brachymorphia s.

Weingarten's s., tropical eosinophilia—a subacute or chronic form of occult filariasis, usually involving *Brugia malayi* or *Wuchereria bancrofti* occurring in the tropics and chiefly affecting Asiatic Indians, in whom it may represent genetic predisposition. It is characterized episodic nocturnal wheezing and coughing, strikingly elevated eosinophilia, and diffuse reticulonodular infiltrations of the lungs. Microfilariae are seldom detected in peripheral blood films since the parasites are confined primarily to the lungs.

Wermer's s., multiple endocrine neoplasia, type tumors of the pituitary, parathyroid glands, and pancreatic islet cells in association with high incidence of peptic ulcer the Zollinger-Ellison syndrome can occur in affected families.

Werner s., premature aging in the adult, transmitted as an autosomal recessive trait, and characterized principally by scleroderma-like skin changes, involving especially the extremities, cataracts, subcutaneous calcification, muscular atrophy, a tendency to diabetes mellitus, aged appearance of the face, canities (diffuse grayness or whiteness of the scalp hair, especially as associated with aging) and baldness, and a high incidence of neoplasm.

Wernicke's s., encephalopathy, see Wernicke's disease.

Wernicke-Korsakoff s., the neuropsychiatric disorder caused by thiamine deficiency, most commonly due to chronic alcohol abuse and associated with other nutritional polyneuropathies. Wernicke's encephalopathy (confusion, ataxia of gait, nystagmus, and ophthalmoplegia) occurs as an acute attack and is reversible, except for some residual ataxia or nystagmus, by administration of thiamine; Korsakoffs syndrome (severe anterograde and retrograde amnesia) may occur in conjunction with Wernicke's encephalopathy or may become apparent later; only about 20 percent of patients recover completely from the amnesia.

Weyers' oligodactyly s., a congenital syndrome consisting of deficiency of the ulna and' ulnar rays, antecubital pterygia, reduced sternal segments, malformations of the kidney and spleen, and cleft lip and palate.

Whiplash shake s., a constellation of injuries to the brain and eye that may occur when a child less than 3 years old, usually less than 1 year old, is shaken vigorously while being held by the trunk or limbs with the head unsupported. This causes stretching and tearing of the cerebral vessels and brain substance, commonly leading to subdural hematomas and retinal hemorrhages, and sometimes associated with cerebral contusion. It may result in paralysis, blindness and other visual disturbances, convulsions, and death.

Whistling face s., whistling face windmill vane hand s., craniocarpotarsal dystrophy, see Freeman-Sheldon s.

Widal s., icteroanemia—a disease marked by the development of icterus and anemia, with splenic enlargement, urobilinuria, and a hemolysis associated with fragility of the red blood corpuscles.

Willebrand's s., see von Willebrand's disease.

Williams s., supravalvular aortic stenosis, mental retardation, elfin facies, and transient hypercalcemia in infancy. Called also elfin facies s.

Williams-Campbell s., congenital bronchomalacia due to absence of annular cartilage distal to the first division of the peripheral bronchi; it is marked by bronchiectasis.

Wilson's s., see under disease.

Wilson-Mikity s., a rare form of pulmonary insufficiency in low-birth-weight infants, marked by hyperpnea and cyanosis of insidious onset during the first month of life and often resulting in death. Radiographically, there are multiple cyst like foci of hyperaeration throughout the lung with coarse thickening of the interstitial supporting structures. The disorder has been attributed to disparity of maturation of parenchymal elements, especially of alveoli proliferation, and hence has been called pulmonary dysmaturity.

Winter's s., a congenital syndrome consisting of renal hypoplasia or aplasia, anomalies of the internal genitalia, especially vaginal atresia, and anomaly of the ossicles of the middle ear.

Wiskott-Aldrich s., an X-linked immunodeficiency syndrome characterized by eczema, thrombocytopenia, and recurrent pyogenic infection. There is an inability to produce antibodies to polysaccharide antigens and increased susceptibility to infection with encapsulated bacteria (*Haemophilus influezae, Meningocoocus, Pneumococcus*). Typically IgM is low and IgA and IgE are elevated; cutaneous anergy is common. There is also a high incidence of lymphoreticular malignant disease. Called also Aldrich syndrome and mmunodeficiency with thrombocytopenia and eczema.

Withdrawal s., see Abstinence s.

Wolf-Hirschhorn s., a syndrome associated with partial deletion of the short arm of chromosome 4, characterized by microcephaly, ocular hypertelorism, epicanthus, cleft palate, micrognathia, low-set ears simplified in form, cryptorchidism and hypospadias.

Wolff-Parkinson-White s., the association of paroxysmal tachycardia (or atrial fibrillation) and pre-excitation, in which the electrocardiogram displays a short P-R interval and a wide QRS complex which characteristically shows an early QRS vector (delta wave); called also anomalous atrioventricular excitation.

Wolfram s., a hereditary association of diabetes mellitus, diabetes insipidus, optic atrophy and neural deafness.

Woringer-Kolopp s., pagetoid reticulosis, see Woringer-kolopp disease.

Wright's s., 1. (Irving S. Wright) A neurovascular syndrome caused by hyperabduction of the arm. Such hyperabduction may cause occlusion of the subclavian artery, leading to gangrene, or may produce sensory symptoms due to stretching of the brachial plexus. 2. A condition marked by multifocal areas of osteitis fibrosa, patchy cutaneous pigmentation, and precocious puberty.X

X-inked lymphoproliferative s., an immunodeficiency disorder characterized by defective cellular or humoral immune response to Epstein-Barr virus (EBV). Fulminant infectious mononucleosis, fatal B cell malignancies, or hypogammaglobulinemia can result from EBV fection. Called also X-linked lymphoproliferative disease and Duncan's disease or Syndrome.

XXY s., see Klinefelter's s.

Yellow nail s., a syndrome associated with lymphedema, especially of the legs, consisting a yellowish to greenish discoloration of the nails, which may be smooth, thickened, excessively curved on the long axis, and slow growing, and may become loose and be shed.

Yellow vernix s., see Placental dysfunction s.

Young's s., obstructive azoospermia and chronic sinopulmonary infections.

Zellweger s., see Cerebrohepatorenal s.

Zieve s., hypercholesterolemia, hepatosplenomegaly, fatty infiltration of the liver, hemolyticanemia, and hypertriglyceridemia following the ingestion of large amounts of ethanol.

Zinsser Cole-Engman s., dyskeratosis congenita—an X-linked syndrome with onset in childhood, and characterized by nail dystrophy, reticular cutaneous hyperpigmentation, mucosal leukokeratosis, and pancytopenia.

Zollinger-Ellison s., a triad comprising (i) intractable, sometimes fulminating, and in many atypical peptic ulcers; (ii) extreme gastric hyperacidity; and (iii) gastrin-secreting, non-β islet cell tumors of the pancreas, which may be single or multiple, small or large, benign malignant. The gastrinoma sometimes occurs in sites (e.g., the duodenum) other than the pancreas.

2
Diseases

Disease: Any deviation from or interruption of the normal structure or function of any part, organ, or system (or combination thereof) of the body that is manifested by a characteristic set of symptoms and signs and whose etiology, pathology, and prognosis may be known or unknown.

Accumulation d., thesaurismosis*.

Acosta's d., acute mountain sickness.

Adams, Adams-Stokes d., a condition caused by heart block and characterized by sudden attacks of unconsciousness, with or without convulsions: also called Adams-Stokes syndrome or syncope, Stokes-Adams d., syndrome, or syncope. Morgagni-Adams-Stokes syndrome, and Stokes' syndrome.

D's of adaptation, a concept introduced by Hans Selye that certain diseases are byproducts of physiologic adaptations to chronic stress; he included in this category rheumatoid arthritis, peptic ulcer, essential hypertension, and possibly atherosclerosis.

Addison's d., a disease characterized by hypotension, weight loss, anorexia, weakness, and sometimes a bronzelike melanotic hyperpigmentation of the skin; it is due to tuberculosis or autoimmune-induced disease (hypofunction) of the adrenal glands that results in deficiency of aldosterone and cortisol and, in the absence of replacement therapy, is usually fatal.

Adult celiac d., the adult form of celiac disease, or nontropical sprue.

---

* See Appendix

Airsac d., infectious sinusitis of turkeys.

Akamushi d., scrub typhus.

Akureyri d., epidemic neuromyasthenia; named for a town in Northern Iceland where more than 1000 cases occurred in 1948.

Aland eye d., see Forsius-Eriksson syndrome.

Albers-Schönberg d., osteopetrosis—a rare genetic disease characterized by abnormally dense bone, due to defective resorption of immature bone; in this, the proliferation of bone obliterates the marrow cavity, causing anemia and hepato-splenomegaly, and the nerve foramina of the skull, causing compression of cranial nerves, which may result in deafness and blindness.

Aleutian mink d., a chronic, progressive disease of mink, perhaps of viral origin, marked by inappetance, weight loss, lethargy, polydipsia, and hemorrhages.

Alexander's d., an infantile form of leukodystrophy, characterized histologically by the presence of eosinophilic material at the surface of the brain and around its blood vessels, resulting in brain enlargement.

Alkali d., 1. Botulism in ducks. 2. A disease of livestock; a form of poisoning of livestock of the North central great plains region of the United States due to feeding on plants which have absorbed selenium from the soil and characterized by cirrhosis of the liver, anemia, loss of hair, erosions of long bones, emaciation.

Allogeneic d., graft' versus-host reaction occurring in immunosuppressed animals receiving injections of allogeneic lymphocytes.

Almeida's d., paracoccidioidomycosis*.

Alpers' d., poliodystrophia cerebri—a rare disease of young children, characterized by neuronal degeneration of the cerebral cortex and elsewhere, accompanied by progressive mental deterioration, motor disturbances, and early death.

Alpha chain d., the most common heavy chain disease, occurring predominantly in young adults in the Mediterranean area, and

---

* See Appendix

characterized by plasma cell infiltration of the lamina propria of the small intestine resulting in malabsorption with diarrhea, abdominal pain, and weight loss, or, exceedingly rarely, by pulmonary involvement. The gastrointestinal form called is also immunoproliferative small intestine disease.

Altitude d., high-altitude sickness—the condition resulting from difficulty in adjusting to diminised oxygen pressure at high altitudes. It may take the form of mountain sickness, high-altitude pulmonary edema, or cerebral edema.

Alzheimer's d., a progressive degenerative disease of the brain of unknown etiology characterized by diffuse atrophy throughout the cerebral cortex with distinctive histopathologic changes termed "senile plaques" (microscopic lesions composed of fragmented axon terminals and dendrites surrounding a core of amyloid) and "neurofibrillary tangles" (intracellular knots or clumps of neurofibrils). There is a loss of choline acetyltransferase activity in the cortex, and it appears that many of the degenerating neurons are cholinergic neurons projecting from the substantia innominata to the cortex. The first signs of the disease are slight memory disturbance or subtle changes in personality; there is progressive deterioration resulting in profound dementia over a course of 5 to 10 years. Onset may occur at any age; the disease was originally described as presenile dementia, occurring in persons under 65 as opposed to senile dementia, which was supposed to be a consequence of the aging process, but there is no clinical or pathophysiological distinction between the two classes of patients. Women are affected twice as frequently as men.

Anders' d., adiposis tuberosa simplex—a disorder resembling adiposa dolorosa, marked by development in the subcutaneous tissue of fatty masses which are sometimes painful to pressure.

Andersen's d., see glycogen storage d. (type IV).

Andes d., chronic mountain sickness—is characterized by loss of tolerance to hypoxia in a previously acclimatized person, and by secondary polycythemia. It occurs in two types: an emphysematous type, in which dyspnea is the dominant symptom and bronchitis and laryngitis are common and cyanosis is present and in an erythremic type, in which the prominent symptoms include an erythremic color that turns to cyanosis on mild exertion, fatigue, headache, episodic stupor, paresthesias, anorexia, nausea, vomiting, and diminution of visual acuity.

Antiglomerular basement membrane (anti-GBM) antibody d., glomerulonephritis, usually of a generalized proliferative crescent-forming histologic type with a rapidly progressive course, marked by circulating anti-GBM antibodies and linear deposits of immunoglobulin and complement along the glomerular basement membrane. When associated with pulmonary hemorrhage, the condition is called Goodpasture's syndrome.

Aperts d., acrocephalosyndactyly-craniostenosis characterized by acrocephaly (a condition in which the top of the head is pointed or conical owing to premature closure of the coronal and lambdoid sutures) and syndactyly (congenital anomaly of the hand or foot, marked by persistence of the webbing between adjacent digits) probably occurring as an autosomal dominant trait and usually as a new mutation.

Apert-Crouzon d., an autosomal dominant disorder, consisting of the hand and foot malformations associated with Apert's syndrome, together with the facial characteristics of Crouzon's disease. Also called acrocephalosyndactyly type and Vogt's cephalodactyly.

Aran-Duchenne d., spinal muscular atrophy—a progressive degenerative disease of the motor cells of the spinal cord. Begining usually in the small muscles of the hands, but in some cases (scapulohumeral type) in those of the upper arm and shoulder, the atrophy progresses slowly to muscles of the lower extremity.

Arc-welders' d., siderosis-pneumoconiosis due to the inhalation of iron particles.

Armstrong's d., lymphocytic choriomeningitis.

Atopic d., atopy—a genetic predisposition toward the development of immediate (type I) hypersensitivity reactions against common environmental antigens (atopic allergy), occurring in 10 percent of general population, 50 percent of those with one affected parent, and 75 percent of those with two affected parents. The most common clinical manifestation is allergic rhinitis, bronchial asthma, atopic dermatitis, and food allergy occur less frequently. The form exhibited may vary over time and may differ from that exhibited by the parents.

Aujeszky's d., pseudorabies.

Australian X d., an acute epidemic encephalitis of viral origin observed in Australia during the summer months between 1917 and 1926, which resembled Japanese B encephalitis both symptomatically and pathologically; the virus appeared to be a variant of Japanese B encephalitis virus, but the culture was lost before it could be identified.

Autoimmune d., a disorder caused by an immune response directed against self-antigens. Ideally, there should be not only demonstrable circulating autoantibodies or cell-mediated immunity against auto-antigens in conjunction with inflammatory lesions caused by immunologically competent cells or immune complexes in tissues containing the autoantigens but also clinical or experimental evidence that the autoimmune process is pathogenic not secondary to other tissue damage. In practice, many diseases, such as systemic lupus erythematosus (SLE) and rheumatoid arthritis are often classified as autoimmune diseases although their pathogenesis is unclear.

Aviators' d., high-altitude sickness—see altitude disease.

Ayerza's d., a form of polycythemia vera marked by chronic cyanosis, chronic dyspnea, chronic bronchitis, bronchiectasis, enlargement of liver and spleen, hyperplasia of bone marrow, and associated with sclerosis of the pulmonary artery.

Azorean d., a progressive degenerative disease of the central nervous system occurring in families of Portuguese-Azorean descent, having a variety of forms and inherited as an autosomal dominant trait. There are four major types: Type I, with pyramidal and extrapyramidal deficits; Type II, with cerebellar, pyramidal, and extrapyramidal deficits; Type III, with cerebellar deficits and distal sensorimotor neuropathy; Type IV, with parkinsonism and distal sensory neuropathy. Also called Joseph's d., Machado-Joseph d., and Portuguese-Azorean d.

Azorean d. of nervous system, see Machado-Joseph d.

Baastrup's d., kissing spine—a condition in which the spinous processes of adjacent vertebrae are in contact.

Baelz's d., a rare disease in which the lower lip becomes enlarged, firm, and finally everted, exposing the openings of accessory salivary glands, which are inflamed and; dilated, appearing as pinhead-sized red macules on the mucosa. The glands themselves are enlarged and sometimes nodular. The condition may be associated with carcinoma of the lip. It occurs in three basic types: the simple type is characterized by multiple painless, pinhead-sized lesions, with central depressions and dilated canals, and may develop into either of the other two types. The superficial suppurative type is characterized by painless swelling, induration, crusting and superficial and deep ulcerations of the lip. The deep suppurative type is basically a deep-seated infection, with abscesses and fistulous tracts that eventually form scars.

Baló's d., an atypical form of Schilder's disease in which the demyelination is arranged in concentric rings around a central circle; also called encephalitis periaxialis concentrica and leukoencephalitis periaxialis concentrica.

Bamberger's d., 1. Saltatory spasm or tic of the lower extremities. 2. See Concato's d.

Bamberger-Marie d., hypertrophic pulmonary osteoarthropathy—symmetrical osteitis of the four limbs, chiefly localized to the phalanges and the terminal epiphyses of the long bones of the forearm and leg, sometimes extending to the proximal ends of the limbs and the flat bones, and accompanied by a dorsal kyphosis and some affection of the joints. It is often secondary to chronic conditions of the lungs and heart.

Bang's d., infectious abortion in cattle caused by *Brucella abortus*.

Bannister's d., angioneurotic edema—a vascular reaction involving deep dermis or subcutaneous or submucosal tissues, representing localized edema caused by dilatation and increased permeability of the capillaries, and characterized by development of giant wheals. Hereditary angioedema, transmitted as an autosomal dominant trait, tends to involve more visceral lesions than the sporadic form and is caused by a deficiency or functional impairment of complement component C1 esterase inhibitor (C1INH), resulting in increased levels of several vasoactive mediators of anaphylaxis.

Banti's d., originally described as a primary disease of the spleen associated with splenomegaly and pancytopenia, but later considered secondary to portal hypertension; also called congestive splenomegaly, Klemperer's d. and splenic anemia.

Barcoo d., desert sore—a phagedenic ulcer occurring in South Africa and Australia characterized initially by the development of papulovesicular lesions on the extremities, especially on the back of hands, forearm, knees, and shins that rupture and form painful, crusted purulent ulcers. The condition probably represents an infected ulcer from some secondarily antecedent neglected lesion.

Barlow's d., infantile scurvy—nutritional disease of infants characterized by the same symptoms as scurvy in adults.

Barometer-maker's d., chronic mercurial poisoning in makers of barometers, due to the inhalation of the fumes of mercury.

Barraquer's d., partial lipodystrophy—a condition occurring especially in females in the first olacade of life, characterized by a symmetrical loss of subcutaneous fat, usually beginning on the face and gradually extending to the chest, neck, back, and upper extremities, giving the lower part of the body an apparent, and possibly real, adiposity of the buttocks, thighs, and legs, some affected patients develop insulin-resistant diabetes mellitus, triglyceridemia and renal disease.

Basedow's d., see Graves' d.

Batten d., a term for several lipidoses differing biochemically in clinical manifestation. The juvenile type is a neuronal ceroid lipofuscinosis with onset between 5 to 10 years, a prolonged course, and death during adolescence; is relatively common among Scandinavians and show a "salt and pepper" pigmentary degeneration (atypical retinitis pigmentosa), then cerebellar ataxia, polymyoclonia, and dementia.

Bauxite workers' d., bauxite pneumoconiosis—rapidly progressive pneumoconiosis leading to extreme pulmonary emphysema, frequently accompanied by pneumothorax, caused by inhalation of bauxite fumes containing fine particles of alumina and silica.

Bayle's d., general paresis-parenchymatous neurosyphilis in which chronic meningoencephalitis causes gradual loss of cortical function, resulting in progressive dementia and generalised paralysis, which generally occurs 10 to 20 years after the initial infection of syphilis.

Bazin's d., a type of panniculitis characterized histologically by the presence of granulomas vasculitis, and caseation necrosis, traditionally considered to be the tuberculous conterpart of nodular vasculitis but now known often to occur without tuberculous causation, although of uncertain etiology. It is seen most commonly in adolescent and menopausal women, is initiated or exacerbated by cold weather, and typically presents as one or more recurrent erythrocyanotic nodules or plaques on the calves, which may progress to form deep-seated indurations, ulcerations, and scars.

Beard's d., neurasthenia—a syndrome of chronic mental and physical weakness and fatigue, which was supposed to be caused by exhaustion of the nervous system.

Beau's d., cardiac insufficiency.

Beauvais' d., rheumatoid arthritis—a chronic systemic disease primarily of the joints, usually polyarticular, marked by inflammatory changes in the synovial membranes and articular structures and by atrophy and rarefaction of the bones. In late stages deformity and ankylosis develop. The cause is unknown, but autoimmune mechanisms and virus infection have been postulated.

Beck's d., a disease affecting young people in Siberia and marked by fatigue and swelling of the phalanges; later all the joints of the body become enlarged and normal growth is retarded.

Béguez César d., see Chediak-Higashi syndrome.

Behçet's d., see under syndrome.

Behr's d., degeneration of the macula retinae in adult life.

Beigel's d., piedra—a fungal infection of the hair shaft characterized by presence of dark or pale, firm, irregular nodules composed of fungal elements.

Bekhterev's d., rheumatoid spondylitis—the form of rheumatoid arthritis that affects the spine. It is a systemic illness of unknown etiology, affecting young males predominantly, and producing pain and stiffness as a result of inflammation of the sacroiliac intervertebral, and costovertebral joints; paraspinal calcification, with ossification and ankylosis of the spinal joints, may cause complete rigidity of spine and thorax.

Benson's d., asteroid hyalosis—a usually unilateral condition of the eye, most frequently seen in older men, characterized by the presence of spherical or star-shaped, calcium-containing opacities in the vitreous humor, which, when illuminated under an examining light, appear to sparkle; vision is usually unaffected.

Berger's d., IgA glomerulonephritis—a chronic form marked by hematuria and proteinuria and by deposits of IgA immunoglobin in the mesangial areas of the renal glomeruli with subsequent reactive hyperplasia of mesangial cells.

Bergeron's d., electric chorea of childhood, characterized by violent rhythmic spasms, but running a benign course.

Berlin's d., commotio retinae—edema around the macular region of the retina, caused by a severe blow to the eyeball, and producing a permanent central scotoma as a result of destruction of the delicate cones in the fovea.

Bernard-Soulier d., an autosomal recessive disorder characterized by platelets with a wide range in size and morphology. The platelet membranes lack glycoprotein Ib, the probable receptor for plasma von Willebrand's factor (vWF); this deficiency keeps the platelets from binding the vWF necessary for their adhesion to the subendothelial surfaces of blood vessels. The clinical signs are variable and include mucocutaneous and visceral hemorrhaging, purpura, and prolonged bleeding time. See also von Willebrand's disease, under disease. Also called Bernard-Soulier syndrome and giant platelet d. or syndrome.

Bernhardt's d., Bernhardt-Roth d., meralgia paresthetica—a disease marked by paresthesia, pain, and numbness in the outer surface of the thigh, in the region supplied by the lateral femoral cutaneous nerve, due to entrapment of the nerve at the inguinal ligament.

Besnier-Boeck d., sarcoidosis—a chronic, progressive, systemic granulomatous reticulosis of unknown etiology, involving almost any organ or tissue, including the skin, lungs, lymph nodes, liver, spleen, eyes, and small bones of the hands and feet. It is characterized histologically by the presence in all affected organs or tissues of noncaseating epitheloid cell tubercles (naked or hard tubercles). Laboratory findings may include hypercalcemia and hypergammaglobulinemia; there is usually diminised or absent reactivity to tuberculin and in most active cases, a positive Kveim reaction. The acute form has an abrupt onset and a high spontaneous remission rate, whereas the chronic form, insidious in onset, is progressive.

Best's d., congenital macular degeneration—an autosomal dominant form of macular degeneration characterized by the presence of a cyst like lesion that in the early stages resembles egg yolk.

Bettlach May d., a fatal disease affecting adult honeybees, principally in Switzerland, marked by paralysis with inability to fly, caused by ingestion of the pollens of certain buttercups, which contain a poisonous substance.

Biedl's d., see Bardet-Biedel syndrome, under syndrome.

Bielschowsky-Jansky d., see Jansky-Biel-Schowsky d.

Biermer's d., pernicious anemia—a megaloblastic anemia occurring in children but more commonly in later life, characterized by histamine-fast achlorhydria, in which the laboratory and clinical manifestations are based on malabsorption of vitamin B_{12} due to a failure of the gastric mucosa to secrete adequate and potent intrinsic factor.

Bilderbeck's d., acrodynia—a disease of infancy and early childhood characterized by pain and swelling in, and pink coloration of the fingers and toes, and by listlessness, irritability, failure to thrive, generalized inconstant rashes, profuse perspiration, photophobia, loss of teeth, and sometimes scarlet coloration of cheeks and tip of nose; repeated ingestion of or contact with mercury is the cause of most, if not all, cases, and individual sensitivity may also be a factor.

Billroth's d., 1. Meningocele due to skull fracture and tearing of the arachnoid; Also called cephalhydrocele traumatica and spurious meningocele. 2. Lymphoma.

Binswanger's d., a degenerative dementia of presenile, onset caused by demyelination of the subcortical white matter of the brain accompanying sclerotic changes in the blood vessels supplying it.

Black d., infectious necrotic hepatitis of sheep: a fatal disease of sheep, and occasionally of man, in the United States (in Montana) and in Australia (in New South Wales, Victoria, Tasmania), marked by necrotic areas in the liver; it is caused by *Clostridium novyi*.

Blinding fiiarial d., blindness caused by onchocerciasis.

Blocq's d., astasia-abasia—motor incoordination with an inability to stand or walk despite normal ability to move the legs when sitting or lying down, a form of hysterical ataxia.

Bloodgood's d., see cystic d. of breast.

Blount's d., tibia vara-medial angulation of the tibia in the metaphyseal region, due to a growth disturbance of the medial aspect of the proximal tibial epiphyses; there is an infantile and an adolescent type.

Blue d., 1. An old term for congenital heart disease; 2. Rocky Mountain spotted fever—an acute infections sometimes fatal disease caused by *Rickettsia rickettsii*, usually transmitted by the bites of several species of infected ixodid ticks, the two most important vectors being *Dermacentor andersoni* (wood tick) and *D. vriabilis* (dog tick) and occurring only in North and South America. It is characterized by sudden onset, with chills; fever lasting about 2 to 3 weeks; cutaneous rash that generally appears between second and sixth days of illness, at first involving the wrists, ankles, palms, soles, and forearms and spreading to the proximal extremities, trunk and face; myalgias; severe headache; and prostration.

Blue nose d., a disease of horses, apparently due to photosensitization following the ingestion of certain meadow plants, in which there is usually a blue discoloration of muzzle, sloughing of nonpigmented skin, and frequently intense excitement.

Boeck's d., see Besnier-Boeck d.,

Border d. of sheep., a disease of unknown etiology and very high mortality that affects sheep on the English-Welsh border; it is manifested by an increase in the amount of hair in the fleece, slow growth, diminished stature, slight abnormality of head shape, and a slightly swaying gait.

Borna d., a fatal enzootic encephalitis of horses, cattle, and sheep, caused by a virus; also called enzootic encephalitis of horses, equine encephalitis, and crazy d.

Bornholm's d., epidemic pleurodynia—an acute, febrile, infectious disease generally occurring in epidemics, most often seen in persons under the age of 20, and usually caused by group B coxsackieviruses and sometimes by group A cocksackieviruses, echoviruses, and other enteroviruses. It is typically characterized by sudden sharp paroxysmal pain located over the rib area of the chest or upper abdomen, relapses occur frequently after asymptomatic periods.

Bostock's d., hay fever—a seasonal variety of allergic rhinitis, marked by acute conjunctivitis with lacrimation and itching, swelling of the nasal mucosa, nasal catarrh, sudden attacks of sneezing, and often with asthmatic symptoms. It is regarded as an anaphylactic or allergic condition excited by a specific allergen (e.g., a pollen) to which the individiual is sensitized.

Bottom d., crotalism—a disease of animals caused by eating leguminous plants of the genus *Crotalaria*, which are in low bottom land. The disease is characterized by congestion and hemorrhage of the liver and spleen, emaciation, weakness, and stupor.

Bouchard's d., dilatation of the stomach from inefficiency of the gastric muscles.

Bouchet-Gsell d., see Swineherd's d.

Bouillaud's d., rheumatic endocarditis.

Bourneville's d., tuberous sclerosis—an autosomal dominant disease characterized principally by the presence of hamartomas of the brain (tubers), retina (phakomas), and viscera, mental retardation, seizures, and adenoma sebaceum, and often associated with other skin lesions including subungual fibromas, vitiliginous patches, shagreen patches, and cafe-au-lait spots.

Bouveret's d., paroxysmal tachycardia—a condition marked by attacks of rapid action of the heart having sudden onset and cessation.

Bowen's d., intraepidermal squamous cell carcinoma, often occurring in multiple primary sites; also called Bowen's precancerous dermatosis and precancerous dermatitis.

Bradley's d., epidemic nausea and vomiting

Brancher glycogen storage d., see glycogen storage d (type IV).

Breda's d., yaws—an endemic, infectious, tropical disease caused by *Treponema pertenue*, usually affecting persons under the age of 15, and spread by direct contact with skin lesions or by contaminated fomites. It is characterized by the appearance at the site of innoculation of the spirochete, which enters the body through abraded or otherwise compromised skin, of a painless papule that grows into a papilloma (mother yaw). This heals, leaving a scar which is followed by crops of generalized secondary granulomatous papule that may relapse repeatedly. Late manifestations include destructive and deforming lesions of the skin, bones and joints.

Breisky's d., kraurosis vulvae—an atrophy affecting the female external genitalia, most often of an older woman, resulting in drying and shriveling of the parts, and marked by leukoplakic patches on the mucosa, itching, dyspareunia, dysuria, and soreness. It occurs most commonly as a result of lichen sclerosus et atrophicus of the vulva, but may be associated with other types of genital atrophy.

Bretonneau's d., diphtheria.

Bright's d., a broad descriptive term once used for kidney disease with proteinuria, usually glomerulonephritis.

Brill's d., see Brill-Zinsser d.

Brill-Symmers d., nodular lymphoma—malignant lymphoma in which the lymphomatous cells are clustered into identifiable nodules within the lymph nodes that somewhat resembles the germinal centers of lymph node follicles. Nodular lymphomas usually occur in older persons, commonly involving many (or all) nodes as well as possibly extranodal sites.

Brill-Zinsser d., a recrudescence of epidemic typhus occurring years after the initial infection, in which the etiologic agent, *Rickettsia prowazekii*, persists in the body tissue in an inactive state (perhaps as long as 70 years), with humans as the reservoir. Compared with epidemic typhus, it is milder, the fever is not as high and is of shorter duration, the rash is less intense and is often absent; and the fatality rate is much lower; also called Brill's d., and latent or recrudescent typhus.

Brinton's d., lintis plastica.

Brion-Kayser d., paratyphoid fever.

Brisket d., a disease resembling mountain sickness in man, affecting young cattle living at altitudes above 7600 feet; it is sometimes seen in sheep and has been produced experimentally in pigs.

Broad-beta d., familial hyperlipoproteinemia (type III); so called because on electrophoresis the lipoproteins show a broadband of beta lipoproteins.

Brodie's d., 1. Chronic synovitis, especially of the knee, with a pulpy degeneration of the parts affected. 2. Hysterical pseudofracture of the spine.

Bronzed d., see Addison's d.

Brooke's d., 1. Keratosis follicularis contagiosa—a widespread, symmetrical eruption of the skin resembling keratosis follicularis, most often involving the back of the neck, shoulders, and extensor surfaces of the extremities, which occur in children, and is apparently an infectious disease. 2. Trichoepithelioma papillosum multiplex—hereditary multiple trichoepithelioma.

Brown-Séquard d., see under syndrome.

Brown-Symmers d., fatal, acute serous encephalitis in children.

Bruck's d., a condition marked by deformity of bones, multiple fractures, ankylosis of joints, and atrophy of muscles.

Brushfield-Wyatt d., see under syndrome.

Bruton's d., X-linked infantile agammaglobulinemia—a primary immunodeficiency disorder with X-linked recessive inheritance characterized by absence of circulating B lymphocytes, absence of plasma cells and germinal centers in lymphoid tissues, and very low levels of circulating immunoglobulins. Infants with the disorder are well during the first 6-9 months of life because of the presence of transplacentally acquired maternal immunoglobulin. They then acquire repeated severe bacterial infections with highly virulent, encapsulated, extracellular organisms, e.g., staphylococci, streptococci, pneumococci, and *Haemophilus influenzae*, which must be controlled by antibiotic prophylaxis and immune globulin replacement therapy. Response to most viral infections and live vaccines is normal; there is increased susceptiblity to hepatitis virus and enterovirus infection, the pathogenic defect appears to be a failure of pre-B cells to differentiate into mature B-cells.

Budd's d. (obs.). Budd's cirrhosis—chronic hepatic enlargement once thought to be caused by intestinal intoxication.

Budd-Chiari d., see under syndrome.

Buerger's d., thromboangiitis obliterans—an inflammatory and obliterative disease of the blood vessels of the extremities, primarily the lower extremities, occurring chiefly in young men and leading to ischemia of the tissues and gangrene.

Buerger-Grütz d., idiopathic hyperlipemia—a group of genetic disorders of lipoprotein metabolism, classified into five major phenotypes based on clinical features, enzymatic abnormalities, and serum lipoprotein electrophoretic patterns. Type 1, a recessive trait, due to lipoprotein lipase deficiency, is manifested by abdominal pain and vomiting, acute pancreatitis, xanthomas, hepatosplenomegaly, and lipemia retinalis.

Buffalo d., buffalo encephalitis—a viral encephalitis of the asiatic water buffalo.

Buhl's d., an acute sepsis affecting newborn infants, marked by hemorrhages into the skin, mucous membranes, and navel attended with cyanosis and jaundice; there are also hemorrhages in the intestinal organs.

Buschke's d., i.e., cryptococcosis.

Bush d., a disease of sheep and cattle in certain parts of New Zealand, marked by progressive anemia; it is due to an iron or an iron and copper deficiency.

Busquet's d., exostoses on the dorsum of the foot due to osteoperiostitis of the metatarsal bones.

Buss d., a viral encephalomyelitis with pleuritis affecting cattle in the United States and Japan, marked by dullness, labored breathing, cough, diarrhea, staggering gait, and, sometimes, drooling of saliva and a discharge from the nose; also called sporadic bovine encephalomyelitis.

Busse-Buschke d., cryptococcosis.

Cacchi-Ricci d., sponge kidney—a rare congenital condition, anatomically characterized by multiple small cystic dilatations of the collecting tubules of the medullary portions of the renal pyramids, giving the organ a spongy, porous feeling and appearance. It is usually asymptomatic, but there may be calculus formation within the cysts, hematuria, renal colic, or recurrent renal infection.

Caffey's d., infantile cortical hyperostosis—a disease of young infants characterized by soft tissue swellings over the affected bones, fever, and irritability, and marked by periods of remission and exacerbation.

Caisson d., decompression sickness—a disorder characterized by joint pains, respiratory manifestations, skin lesions, and neurologic signs, occurring in aviators flying at high altitudes and following rapid reduction of air pressures in persons who have been breathing compressed air in caissons and diving apparatus.

California d., coccidioidomycosis—a fungous disease caused by infection with *Coccidiodes immitis*, occurring in a primary and a secondary form. The primary form is an acute, benign, self-limited respiratory infection due to inhalation of spores, and varying in severity from that of a common cold to symptoms resembling those accompanying influenza, with pneumonia, cavitation, high fever, and, rarely erythema nodosum (bumps). The secondary form (or progressive) is a virulent and severe, chronic, progressive, granulomatous disease resulting in involvement of the cutaneous and subcutaneous tissues, viscera, central nervous system, and lungs, with anemia, phlebitis, and various allergic responses. This form may be caused by a new infection or by reactivation of arrested primary disease.

Caloric d., any disease due to exposure to high temperature.

Calvé-Perthes d., osteochondrosis of the capitular epiphysis of the femur.

Camurati-Engelmann d., diaphyseal dysplasia—a condition characterized by thickening of the cortex of the midshaft area of the long bones, progressing toward the epiphyses, the thickening sometimes occurring also in the flat bones; excessive growth in length of bones of the extremities usually results in abnormal stature.

Canavan's d., Canavan-van Bogaert-Bertrand d., spongy degeneration of the central nervous system; a rare, autosomal recessive form of leukodystrophy, characterized by early onset, widespread demyelination and vacuolation of the cerebral white matter that gives rise to a spongy appearance, severe mental retardation, megalocephaly, atony of the neck muscles, spasticity of arms and legs, and blindness, with death usually occurring at about 18 months of age.

Canine parvovirus d., an acute, often fatal gastroenteritis of dogs caused by a parvovirus related to the virus of feline panleukopenia or of mink enteritis.

Caroli's d, congenital dilatation of the intrahepatic bile ducts.

Carrión's d., bartonellosis—Infection with *Bartonella bacilliformis*, transmitted by sandflies of the genus *Phlebotomus*, especially *P.verrucarum*. The first stage (Oroya fever) is an acute, highly fatal, febrile illness associated with severe hemolytic anemia. The second stage (hemmorhagic pain, Peruvian wart, verruca peruviana, verruga perviana) is manifested by a chronic, benign skin eruption of hemangioma-like macules surrounded by hyperpigmented borders.

Castellani's d., bronchospirochetosis—an infectious disease caused by presence in the bronchi of the *Spirochaeta bronchialis* and marked by chronic bronchitis attended by the spitting of blood.

Cat scratch d., a usually benign, self-limited infectious disease of the regional lymph nodes, chiefly characterized by subacute painful regional lymphadenitis and mild fever of short duration. It is most often associated with close contact with a cat, the primary symptom being an isolated papule or pustule at the site of a cat scratch. Various organisms, including viruses, rickettsiae, and chlamydiae, have been suspected as etiologic agents. Although the disease has traditionally been considered to be nonbacterial in origin (being also called nonbacterial regional lymphadenitis), evidence has implicated a gram-negative, silver-staining bacillus as the causative agent. Also called benign lymphoreticulosis, cat scratch fever, and regional lymphadenitis.

Cavare's d., familial periodic paralysis—an autosomal dominant trait marked by recurring attacks of rapidly progressive flaccid paralysis; there are three types: I, associated with a fall in serum potassium levels (hypokalemic periodic paralysis); II, associated with a rise therein (hyperkalemic periodic p; also called adynamia episodica hereditaria); and III, with normal levels (normokalemic periodic p.).

Celiac d., a malabsorption syndrome affecting both children and adults, precipitated by the ingestion of gluten-containing foods; its etiology is unknown but a hereditary factor has been implicated. Pathologically, the proximal intestinal mucosa loses its villous structure, surface epithelial cells exhibit degenerative changes, and the absorptive function of these cells is severely impaired. It is characterized by diarrhea in which the stools are bulky, frothy, fatty (steatorrhea), and fetid (occasionally, malabsorption may be associated with the passage of a single bulky stool without diarrhea); abdominal distention; flatulence; weight loss; asthenia; deficiency of vitamins B, D, and K; and electrolyte depletion. Also called gluten enteropathy and nontropical sprue. In the infantile form the onset is insidious, and is marked by irritability, loss of appetite, weakness, extreme wasting, growth retardation, and celiac crisis. The adult form is marked by extreme lassitude, fatigue, difficulty in breathing, clubbing of the fingers, bone pain, cramping of the muscles, tetany, abdominal distention during the day, megacolon, tympanitis, and skin pigmentation. Until recently, it was thought that the infantile form and the adult form were different entities, but it is now believed that they are the same.

Central core d. of muscle., a rare hereditary disease, transmitted as an autosomal dominant trait, in which severe hypotonia arrests motor development in infancy, but the course is benign and by school age affected children can walk; histologically, the diagnostic feature is a central core in each muscle fiber.

Chabert's d., blackleg Chagas' d., Chagas-Cruz d., an acute, subacute, or chronic form of trypanosomiasis occurring widely in Central and South America, caused by *Trypanosoma cruzi*, and transmitted by the bites of reduviid bugs of the genera *Triatomo*, *Panstrongylus*, and *Rhodnius*, with various domestic and wild animals, including cats, dogs, rodents, armadillos, bats, foxes, and other mammals, serving as reservoir hosts. The acute form (prevalent in children) is marked initially by an erythematous nodule (chagoma) at the site of inoculation; high fever; unilateral swelling of the face with edema of the eyelid (Romana's sign); regional lymphadenopathy; hepatosplenomegaly; and meningoencephalic irritation. If death does not occur, the disease may resolve completely, or the subacute or chronic form may follow. Subacute Chagas' disease, which may last for several months or years, is characterized by mild fever, severe asthenia, and generalized lymphadenopathy. The chronic form, which may or may not be preceded by an acute episode, is characterized principally by cardiac manifestations (chagasic myocarditis) and gastrointestinal manifestations associated with megaesophagus and megacolon. Also called Cruz-Chagas d., American Cruz, or South American trypanosomiasis. and schizotrypanosomicusis.

Charcot's d., neuropathic arthropathy—a chronic progressive degeneration of the stress-bearing portion of a joint, with bizarre hypertrophic changes at the periphery. It is probably a complication of a variety of neurologic disorders, particularly tabes dorsalis, involving loss of sensation, which leads to relaxation of supporting structures and chronic instability of the joint.

Charcot-Marie-Tooth d., progressive neuropathic (peroneal) muscular atrophy—a hereditary form of muscular atrophy, beginning in muscles supplied by peroneal nerves, progressing slowly to involve muscles of hands and arms.

Charlouis' d., yaws, see Breda's d.

Chédiak-Higashi d., see under syndrome.

Cherchevski's (Cherchewski's) d., ileus of nervous origin.

Chester's d., xanthomatosis of the long bones with spontaneous fractures.

Chiari's d., see Budd-Chiari syndrome.

Chiari-Frommel d., see under syndrome.

Chicago d., North American blastomycosis—an infection usually acquired through the pulmonary route, caused by *Blastomyces dermatidis*, and marked by suppurating tumors in the skin (cutaneous b) or by lesions in the lungs, bones, subcutaneous tissues, liver, spleen, and kidneys.

Cholesteryl ester storage d. (CESD), a relatively mild lysosomal storage disease due to acid lipase deficiency, hepatomegaly may be the only clinical abnormality; hyperbetalipoproteinemia is common, and there is often severe premature atherosclerosis; patients may survive past 40.

Christian's d. see Hand-Schuller-Christina d.

Christian-Weber d., a nodular nonsuppurative panniculitis—a form of panniculitis characterized by recurrent episodes of fever accompanied by crops of single or multiple, erythematous tender or painless subcutaneous nodule on the lower extremities and trunk, which resolves and usually leaves a depression in the skin. The condition is most often seen in women, and it may occur alone or it may be associated with numerous other disorders.

Christmas d., Factor IX deficiency—deficiency of this factor results in a hemorrhagic syndrome called hemophilia B or Christmas disease, which is similar to classical hemophilia (hemophilia A). More than one molecular form has been discovered. A transient form, known as hemophilia B Leyden, is clinically indistinguishable from ordinary hemophilia, but the bleeding tendency abates after puberty.

Chronic granulomatous d. (CGD), chronic granulomatous d. of childhood., a group of immunodeficiencies of X-linked or autosomal recessive inheritance, caused by the failure of the respiratory or metabolic burst, which results in deficient microbicidal ability. Clinically, the picture resembles glucose-6-phosphate dehydrogenase deficiency anemia, and patients usually suffer frequent, severe, and prolonged bacterial and fungal infections affecting the skin, oral and intestinal muscosa, reticuloendothelial system, bones, lungs, and genitourinary tract. The course of the disease varies: symptoms may appear at one week of age, with death during the first decade, or patients may survive well into middle age with no medical intervention. There appear to be no physiologic differences between the X-linked and the autosomal recessive types. Thereapy includes antibiotic prophylaxis and supportive treatment against infection.

Chronic obstructive pulmonary d. (COPD)., any disorder, e.g., asthma, chronic bronchitis, and pulmonary emphysema, marked by persistent obstruction of bronchial air flow.

Chronic respiratory d. of poultry., a common respiratory disease of chicken caused by *Mycoplasma*, and marked by distressed breathing, swelling of the face, and discharge from the nostrils; abbreviated as CRD.

Chylopoietic d. (obs), one which affects the digestive organs.

Circling d., listeriosis—infection caused by *Listeria monocytogenes*. In humans, *in utero* infections occur transplacentally and result in abortion, stillbirth, and premature birth; infections acquired during birth cause cardiorespiratory distress, diarrhea, vomiting, and meningitis. Infection in adults produces meningitis, endocarditis, and disseminated granulomatous lesion. Infection in cattle and sheep causes encephalitis and abortion. Nervous signs are common in ruminants, and necrosis of the liver in monogastric animals.

Climatic d., any disease thought to be produced by a change of climate.

Coast d, a disease of domestic animals similar to enzootic marasmus (qv), occurring in Tasmania.

Coats' d., chronic, progressive exudative retinopathy usually occurring in male children and young adults.

Cogan's d., see under syndrome.

Cold agglutinin d., see under syndrome.

Collagen d., any of a group of diseases that, although clinically distinct and not necessarily related etiologically, have in common widespread pathologic changes in the connective tissue; they include lupus erythematosus, dermatomyositis, scleroderma, polyarteritis nodosa, thrombotic purpura, rheumatic fever, and rheumatoid arthritis. Collagen disease is not to be confused with collagen disorder (qv).

Comb d., favus of fowl—chronic dermatomycosis affecting the comb of fowl, caused by *Trychophyton gallinae*.

Combined immunodeficiency d., deficiency of lymphoid cells that mediate both antibody (B-lymphocytes) and cellular (T-lymphocytes) immunity.

Combined system d., subacute combined degeneration of the spinal cord-degeneration of both the posterior and lateral columns of the spinal cord caused by vitamin B_{12} deficiency; a progressive disease, most often affecting persons over forty years of age, it is usually associated with pernicious anemia. The symptoms include paresthesias, ataxia, unsteadiness of gait, and sometimes emotional disorders.

Communicable d., an infectious disease transmitted from one individual to another, either by direct contact or indirectly by means of a vector or fomites; the terms communicable disease and contagious disease are used synonymously. Cf: infectious d.

Complicating d., one which occurs in the course of some other disease as a complication.

Compressed-air d., decompression sickness—a disorder characterized by joint pains, respiratory manifestations, skin lesions, and neurologic signs, occurring in aviators flying at high altitudes and following rapid reduction of air pressure in persons who have been breathing compressed air in caissons and diving apparatus.

Concato's d., progressive malignant polyserositis with large effusions into the pericardium, pleura, and peritoneum.

Conor and Bruch d., boutonneuse fever—an acute febrile disease caused by *Rickettsia conorii*, transmitted by the bites of various ixodid ticks, with dogs and rodents being the chief hosts, and characterized by a primary lesion (tachenoire) at the site of tick bite, maculopapular or petechial skin rash, headache, arthralgia. myalgia, chills, fever, and photophobia; there are usually no sequelae. The disease is widely distributed along the Mediterranean, Black Sea, and Caspian Sea, Littorals, and apparent variant forms of the infection occur in Africa and on the Indian subcontinent.

Conradi's d., chondrodysplasia punctata—a heterogeneous group of bone dysplasias, the common characteristic of which is stippling of epiphyses in infancy. The group includes a severe autosomal recessive form (rhizomelic dwarfism), an autosomal dominant form (Conradi-Hünermann syndrome), and a milder X-linked form.

Constitutional d., one that involves a system of organs or one characterized by widespread symptoms.

Contagious d., a communicable disease transmitted by contact; the terms contagious disease and communicable disease are used synonymously. Cf: infectious d.

Cooley's d., β-thalassemial—that is caused by diminised synthesis of β-chains of hemoglobin. The homozygous form in which hemoglobin A is completely absent and which appears in the newborn period, is a severe form marked by a hemolytic, hypochromic-microcytic anemia, pronounced hepatomegaly, skeletal deformation, mongloid fades, and cardiac enlargement. The heterozygous form (thalassemia minor), in which hemoglobin A synthesis usually retarded, is asymptomatic, but there are sometimes moderate anemia and splenomegaly.

Cooper's d. (obs)., chronic cystic disease of the breast.

Corbus' d., gangrenous balanitis—a rapidly destructive infection producing erosion of the glans penis and often destruction of the entire external genitalia the infection believed to be due to a spirochete.

Cori's d., glycogen storage d. (type III).

Cornstalk d., toxic encephalomalacia of dietary origin affecting horses,

Corridor d., a tick-borne protozoal disease resembling East Coast fever, due to *Theileria lawrencei*, first reported in the Corridor, a region in South Africa. It is highly pathogenic for cattle, with buffalo serving as a reservoir of infection.

Corrigan's d., aortic insufficiency—the back flow of blood into the heart, or between the chambers of the heart when a valve is incompetent.

Corvisart's d., 1. Chronic hypertrophic myocarditis. 2. Tetralogy of Fallot associated with right aortic arch.

Cotugno's d., sciatica—a syndrome characterized by pain radiating from the back into buttock and into the lower extremity along its posterior or lateral aspect, and most commonly caused by prolapse of the intervertebral disk; the terms also used to refer to the course of the sciatic nerve.

Covering d., dourine—veneral trypanosomiasis affecting horses and asses in Africa, Asia and certain regions of North and South America caused by *Trypanosoma equiperdum* transmitted by coitus, and characterized by edematous swelling of the external genitalia and a mucopurulent discharge from the urethra or vagina, cutaneous plaques, and progressive emaciation and weakness.

Cowden's d., an autosomal dominant disorder comprising a combination of ectodermal, mesodermal, and endodermal anomalies, characterized by the development of a wide variety of multiple hamartomatous lesions, especially in the skin, oral mucosa, breast, thyroid, colon, and intestines, and associated with a high incidence of malignancies in the organs involved. Also called Cowden's syndrome and multiple hamartoma syndrome.

Crazy d., see Borna disease.

Crazy cluck d., 1. Avian encephalomalacia—a disease of young chickens due to vitamin E deficiency, in which there is ataxia, incoordination, paralyses, and severe encephalomalacia in several areas of the brain, especially the cerebellum. 2. Avian encephalomyelitis—a virus disease of chickens under six weeks old, marked by weakness of the legs, trembling of the head and neck, and degeneration of the neurons in the pons, medulla and anterior horns of the spinal cord. Clinically, it resembles avian encephalomalacia and must be differentiated from that condition.

Creeping d., a condition marked by cutaneous lesions similar to those seen in larva migrans, but produced by nematodes of the genus *Gnathostoma.*

Creutzfeldt-Jakob d., a rare, usually fatal, transmissible spongiform encephalopathy, occurring in middle life, in which there is partial degeneration of the pyramidal and extrapyramidal systems accompanied by progressive dementia and sometimes wasting of the muscles, tremor, athetosis, and spastic dysarthria. Also called Creutzfeldt-Jakob syndrome, Jakob's disease, Jakob-Creutzfeldt disease, and spastic pseudoparalysis.

Crigler-Najjar d., see under syndrome.

Crocq's d. (obs.), acrocyanosis—a condition marked by symmetrical cyanosis of the extremities with persistant, uneven mottled blue or red discoloration of the skin of the digits, wrist, and ankles and with profuse sweating and coldness of the digits.

Crohn's d., a chronic granulomatous inflammatory disease of unknown etiology, involving any part of the gastrointestinal tract from mouth to anus, but commonly involving the terminal ileum with scarring and thickening of the bowel wall; it frequently leads to intestinal obstruction and fistula and abscess formation and has a high rate of recurrence after treatment. Also called regional enteritis or ileitis.

Crouzon's d., craniofacial dysostosis—an autosomal dominant disorder characterized by acrocephaly, exophthalmos, hypertelorism, strabismus, parrot-beaked nose, and hypoplastic maxilla with relative mandibular prognathism.

Cruveilhier's d., 1. Spinal muscular atrophy—a progressive degenerative disease of the motor cells of the spinal cord. Beginning usually in the small muscles of the hands, but in some cases (scapulohumeral type) in those of the upper arm and shoulder, the atrophy progresses slowly to the muscles of the lower extremity. 2. Cruveilhier's ulcer—simple gastric ulcer.

Cruz-Chagas d., see Chagas' d.

Csillag's d. (obs.), lichen sclerosus et atrophicus—a chronic atrophic skin disease characterized by white, angular, flat, well defined, indurated papules with an erythematous halo and follicular, black, keratotic plugs. It is the most common cause of kraurosis vulvae in females and balanitis xerotica obliterans in males.

Curschmann's d. (obs.), perihepatitis chronica plastica—a disease in which the peritoneal covering of the liver becomes converted into white mass resembling the icing of a cake.

Cushing's d., Cushing's syndrome in which the hyperadrenocorticism is secondary to excessive anterior pituitary secretion of adrenocorticotropic hormone, with or without a pituitary adenoma.

Cystic d. of breast., a form of mammary dysplasia with formation of cysts of various sizes containing a semitransparent, turbid-fluid that imparts a brown to blue color (blue dome cyst) to the unopened cysts; considered to be due to abnormal hyperplasia of the ductal epithelium and dilatation of the ducts of the mammary gland, occurring as a result of an exaggeration and distortion of the cyclic breast changes that normally occur in the menstrual cycle. Also called chronic cystic mastitis, fibrocystic disease, fibrocystic disease of breast, and Schimmelbusch's disease.

Cystic d. of lung, a condition in which there are abnormally large air spaces in the lung parenchyma; the term is sometimes applied to cystic emphysema. Also called pseudocysts of lung and pulmonary pseudocysts.

Cysticercus d., infection with larval forms (*Cysticercus cellulosae*) of *Taenia solium* (the pork tapeworm)—a larval form of tape-worm, consisting of a single scolex enclosed in a bladder-like cyst.

Cystine d., Cystine storage d., cystinosis—lysosomal storage disorders of unknown molecular defect, characterized by widespread deposition of cystine crystals in reticuloendothelial cells, there are three clinical types. The late onset juvenile or polescent nephropathic type falls within the two extremes; there are ocular and renal manifestations, but the kidney lesion does not always lead to renal insufficiency.

Cytomegalic inclusion d., any of a group of diseases caused by cytomegalovirus infection marked by characteristic inclusion bodies in enlarged infected cells. The classic disease is congenital, being acquired *in utero* from the mother: infection can also be transmitted from mother to infant in passage through the birth canal or from ingestion of the virus present in the mother's milk. Most infected infants are asymptomatic, but in some hepatosplenomegaly, jaundice, chorioretinitis, purpura, microcephaly, cerebral calcifications, and severe central nervous system sequelae resulting in blindness, deafness, quadriplegia, and mental retardation may occur. Acquired disease is transmitted via respiratory droplets or tissue or blood donation, or it may be sexually transmitted. The group also includes an infectious mononucleosis-like syndrome in previously well individuals and in those receiving multiple blood transfusions and a fatal disseminated infection in patients immunosuppressed or otherwise immunocompromised. See postperfusion syndrome, under syndrome.

Czerny's d., periodic hydrarthrosis of the knee.

Daae's d., epidemic pleurodynia—an acute, febrile, infectious disease generally occurring in epidemics, most often seen in persons under the age of 20, and usually caused by group B coxsackieviruses and sometimes by group A coxsackieviruses, echoviruses, and other enteroviruses. It is typically characterized by sudden sharp paroxysmal pain located over the rib area of the chest or upper abdomen; relapses occur frequently after asymptomatic period.

Dalrymple's d., cyclokeratitis—inflammation of the cornea and cilliary body.

Danlos' d., see Ehlers-Danlos syndrome.

Darier's d., keratosis follicularis*.

* See Appendix

Darling's d., histoplasmosis—an infection resulting from inhalation or infrequently, the ingestion of spores of *Histoplasma capsulatum*. Worldwide in distribution, it is particularly in midwestern United States. The infection is asymptomatic in most cases, but in 1 to 5 percent it causes acute pneumonia, or disseminated reticuloendothelial hyperplasia with hepatosplenomegaly and anemia, or an influenza-like illness with joint effusion and erythema nodosum. Reactivated infection involves the lungs, meninges, heart, peritoneum, and adrenals in that order of frequency. It can be diagnosed by culture, or by demonstration of a rise in complement-fixing antibody titers in serum.

David's d., tuberculosis of the spine, see Pott's d.

Debrancher glycogen storage d., see glycogen storage d (type III).

Deficiency d., a condition produced by dietary or metabolic deficiency; the term includes all diseases—e.g., kwashiorkor, beriberi, scurvy, pellagra, calcium deficiency, etc. caused by an insufficient supply of the essential nutrients, i.e., protein (or amino acids), vitamins, and minerals.

Degenerative joint d., osteoarthritis—noninflammatory degenerative joint disease occurring chiefly in older persons, characterized by degeneration of articular cartilage, hypertrophy of bone at the margins, and changes in the synovial membrane. It is accompanied by pain and stiffness, particularly after prolonged activity.

Degos' d., malignant papulosis.

Dejerine's d., Dejerine-Sottas d., progressive hypertrophic interstitial neuropathy—a condition characterized by hyperplasia of the interstitial connective tissue, causing thickening of peripheral nerve trunks and posterior roots, and by sclerosis of posterior columns of the spinal cord. It is a slowly progressive familial disease beginning in early life, marked by atrophy of distal parts of legs, and by diminution of tendon reflexes and of sensation.

Demyelinating d., any condition characterized by destruction of myelin.

Dense deposit d., type II, membranoproliferative glomerulonephritis—marked by heavy dense deposits in the glomerular basement membrane and alternative compliment pathway activation involving

C3 nephritic factor. It occurs in older children young adults and follows a slowly progressive course with irregular remissions ultimately resulting in renal failure.

Deprivation d., see deficiency d.

De Quervain's d., painful tendosynovitis (inflammation of tendon sheath) due to relative narrowness of the common tendon sheath of the abductor pollicis longus and the extensor pollicis brevis.

Dercum's d., adiposis dolorosa—a disease accompanied by painful localized fatty swellings and by various nerve lesions. The disease is usually seen in women, and may cause death from pulmonary complications.

Dermopathic herpesvirus d., a herpesvirus disease of cattle, characterized by ulcerative lesions in the skin. It resembles lumpy skin disease (qv), a poxvirus disease indigenous to African cattle.

Deutschländer's d., 1. Tumor of the metatarsal bones. 2. March foot (fracture)—fracture of bone of the lower extremity, developing after repeated stresses, as seen in soldiers.

Devic's d., neuromyelitis optica—combined demyelination of the optic nerve and the spinal cord; it is marked by diminution of vision and possibly blindness, flaccid paralysis of the extremities, and sensory and genitourinary disturbances.

Diamond-skin d., the urticarial and mildest form of swine erysipelas—a contagious disease of swine of worldwide distribution, caused by *Erysipelothrix rhusiopathiae*, of great economic importance, it occurs in four clinical forms: An acute septicemic form, marked by high fever, lesions of the internal organs and viscera, and a high mortality. An urticarial form, marked by sudden onset, high fever, general debility, formation of reddish to purplish quadrangular or rhomboid blotches on the neck and body and sometimes by involvement of viscera; this is the mildest form and is rarely fatal.

Di Guglieimo d., erythremic myelosis—a malignant blood dyscrasia regarded as one of the myeloproliferative disorders and characterized by progressive anemia hepatoblastic erythroid hyperplasia, myeloid dysplasia, hepatosplenomegaly and hemorrhagic phenomena.

Diverticular d., a general term embracing the prediverticular state, diverticulosis, and diverticulitis.

Döhle's d., syphilitic aortitis—aortitis caused by syphilis; its complications include insufficiency of the aortic valve, stenosis or occlusion of the coronary orifices, and aortic aneurysm.

Down's d., see under syndrome.

Drug d., 1. A morbid condition due to long-continued use of a drug. 2. In homeopathy, the group of symptoms seen after the administration of a drug for the purpose of proving.

Dubin-Sprinz d., see Dubin-Johnson syndrome.

Dubini's d., an acute, fatal form of electric chorea due to acute infection of the central nervous system.

Dubois' d., abscess(es) of the thymus in congenital syphilis.

Duchenne's d., 1. Spinal muscular atrophy—see Cruveilhier's disease. 2. Bulbar paralysis—paralysis due to changes in the motor centers of the medulla oblongata; a chronic, usually fatal disease, most commonly affecting persons over 50 years old but also occurring in the course of amyotrophic lateral sclerosis, syringobulbia, and multiple sclerosis. It is marked by progressive paralysis and atrophy of the muscles of the lips, tongue, mouth, pharynx, and larynx, and is due to degeneration of the nerve nuclei of the floor of the fourth ventricle. 3. Tabesdorsalis—parenchymatous neurosyphilis in which there is slowly progressive degeneration of the posterior columns and posterior roots; and ganglia of the spinal cord, occurring 15 to 20 years after the initial infection of syphilis, characterized by lancinating pains, urinary incontinence, ataxia, impaired position and vibratory sense, optic atrophy, hypotonia, hyperreflexia, and trophic joint degeneration (Charcot's joints).

Duchenne-Aran d., spinal muscular atrophy-see Cruveilhier's disease.

Duchenne-Griesinger d., pseudohypertrophic muscular dystrophy—a chronic progressive disease affecting the shoulder and pelvic girdles, commencing in early childhood. It is characterized by increasing weakness, pseudohypertrophy of the muscles followed by atrophy, lordosis, and a peculiar swaying gait with the legs kept wide apart. The disorder is transmitted as an X-linked trait, and affected individuals, predominantly males, rarely survive to maturity; death is usually due to respiratory weakness or heart failure.

Duhring's d., dermatitis herpetiformis—a chronic, relapsing multisystem disease in which the primary clinical manifestations are cutaneous, presenting as an extremely pruritic eruption consisting of various combinations of grouped, erythematous, symmetrical, papular, papulovesicular, vesicular, eczematous, and bullous lesions, which frequently heal with hyperpigmentation or occasionally hypopigmentation and sometimes scarring. It usually occurs in association with an asymptomatic gluten-sensitive enteropathy. The cause is unknown, but immunogenetic factors are thought to play a role.

Dukes' d., a mild febrile disease of childhood characterized by a bright rosy red, generalized exanthematous eruption, probably a viral exanthem of the coxsackie-ECHO group; it was given the ordinal designation fourth disease to differentiate it from other exanthems. Also called Filatov-oukes d. and scarlatinella.

Duncan's d., X-linked lymphoproliferative syndrome—pertaining to or characterized by proliferation of the cells of the lymphoreticular system. The lymphoproliferative disorders comprise a group of malignant neoplasms arising from cells related to the common multipotential, primitive lympho-reticular cell that includes among others the lymphocytic, histocytic and monocytic leukemias, multiple myeloma, plasmacytoma, Hodgkin's disease, all lymphocytic lymphomas, and immunosecretory disorders associated with monoclonal gammopathy. An interrelationship with the myelo-proliferative disorders is thought to exist.

Duplay's d. (obs.), subacromial or subdeltoid bursitis; inflammation and calcification of subacromial or subdeltoid bursa, resulting in pain, tenderness, and limitation of motion in the shoulder.

Dupre's d., meningism—the symptoms and signs of meningeal irritation associated with acute febrile illness or dehydration without actual infection of the meninges.

Durand-Nicolas-Favre d., lymphogranuloma venereum—a sexually transmitted infection, occurring in warm climates, due to specific strains of *Chlamydia trachomatis*, characterized by a primary cutaneous or mucosal lesion at the site of infection, which may be papular, ulcerative, herpetiform, or erosive lesion or urethritis or endocervicitis that heals spontaneously and may go unnoticed, followed by acute unilateral or bilateral lymphadenopathy. The site of the initial infection or primary lesion determines the subsequent manifestations; in men, the primary lesion is usually found on the prepuce, glans, and shaft of the penis, and is most commonly associated with inguinal lymphadenitis, often with draining buboes (the inguinal syndrome); in women, the primary lesion usually involves the posterior vagina and the cervix and the labia, and is most often associated with hemorrhagic proctocolitis (anogenitorectal syndrome). Late complications in untreated cases chiefly seen in women, include locally destructive ulcerations, rectal strictures, rectovaginal fistulas, and genital elephantiasis.

Durant's d., osteogenesis imperfecta (OI)—a collagen disorder due to defective synthesis of type collagen and generally characterized by brittle, osteoporotic, easily fractured bones. Other defects that may appear include blue sclerae, wormian bones, lax joints, and dentinogenesis imperfecta. OI is variable in manifestation and severity and has great molecular, genetic, and clinical heterogeneity. There are four major types (I-IV) plus variants of OI. Type I, the classic, the most common, mildest type, is autosomal dominant; also called osteogenesis imperfecta with blue sclera and osteogenesis imperfecta tarda. Type II, the perinatal lethal type, has at least three clinical and genetic subtypes and may be an autosomal dominant trait, an autosomal recessive trait, or an autosomal dominant new mutation. The dominant type is also called osteogenesis imperfecta congenita, neonatal lethal form; OI type II, dominant form; and lethal perinatal OI. The recessive form is also called osteogenesis imperfecta congenita; OIC: Vrolik type of osteogenesis imperfecta; OI type II recessive form; and lethal perinatal OI. Type III, the progressive deforming type, may be autosomal recessive or a new mutation; also called osteogenesis imperfecta, progressively deforming, with normal sclerae. Type IV is an autosomal dominant form; called osteogenesis imperfecta with normal sclerae.

Duroziez's d., congenital mitral stenosis.

Eales' d., a condition marked by recurrent hemorrhages into the retina and vitreous, affecting mainly males in the second and third decades of life.

Ebola virus d., a highly fatal, acute hemorrhagic fever, clinically very similar to Marburg virus disease, caused by the Ebola virus, which is morphologically but not antigenically similar to Marburg virus, and occurring in the Sudan and adjacent areas in north western Zaire; the natural reservoir and mode of transmission of the virus are unknown, but secondary infection is by direct contact with infected blood and other body secretions and by airborne particles.

Ebstein's d., 1. Hyaline degeneration and necrosis of the epithelial cells of the renal tubules; seen in diabetes. 2. A malformation of the tricuspid of the septal and posterior leaflets being attatched to walls of right ventricle to a varying degree, and the anterior leaflet being normally attached to the annulus firosus; usually associated with atrial septal defect.

Echinococcus d., see hydatid d.

Economo's d., lethargic encephalitis—a form of epidemic encephalitis, the orignal type described by von Economo, characterized by increasing langour, apathy and drowsiness, passing into lethargy.

Eddowes' d., see under syndrome.

Edsall's d., heat cramp—a form of heat exhaustion in which muscular spasm is attended by pains, dilated pupils, and weak pulse; seen in those who labor in intense (stokers, miners, cane-cutters) and lose much water and salt.

Ehlers-Danlos d., see under syndrome.

Elevator d., respiratory distress affecting persons who work in grain elevators.

Endemic d., one present or usually prevalent in a population or geographical area at all times; such diseases are usually of low morbidity. Also called endemia. See also holoendemic d. and hyperendemic d. Cf: epidemic d.

Engelmann's d., diaphyseal dysplasia—a conditioned characterized by thickening of the cortex of the midshaft area of the long bones, progressing toward the epiphyses, the thickening sometimes occurring also in the flat bones; excessive growth in the length of bones of the extremities usually result in abnormal stature.

Engel-Recklinghausen d., osteitis fibrosa cystica—rarefying osteitis with fibrous degeneration and formation of cysts, and with the presence of fibrous nodules on the affected bones; it is due to marked osteoclastic activity secondary to hyperfunction of the parathyroid gland.

English d., rickets—a condition caused by deficiency of vitamin D, especially in infancy and childhood, with disturbance of normal ossification. The disease is marked by bending and distortion of the bones under muscular action, by the formation of nodular enlargements on the ends and sides of the bones, by delayed closure of the fontanels, pain in the muscles, and sweating of the head. Vitamin D and sunlight together with an adequate diet are curative, provided that the parathyroid glands are functioning properly.

English sweating d., anglicus sudor—a deadly pestilential fever which several time ravaged England during the Middle Ages.

Enzootic d., a disease which is at all times present in a small number of animals in a particular region.

Eosinophilic endomyocardial d., Loffler's endocarditis—endocarditis associated with eosinophilia, marked by fibroplastic thickening of the endocardium, and resulting in congestive heart failure, persistent tachycardia, hepatomegaly, splenomegaly, serous effusions into the pleural cavity, edema of the legs, and edema and ascites of the arms.

Epidemic d., an infectious or other disease that suddenly affects individuals in a population or geographical area clearly in excess of the number of cases normally expected. Cf: endemic d.

Epizootic d., a disease which affects a large number of animals in some particular region within a short period of time.

Epstein's d., pseudodiphtheria—presence of false membranes not due to *Corynebacterium diphtheriae*.

Erb's d., progressive muscular dystrophy.

Erb-Charcot d., Erb's spastic paraplegia—an uncommnon form of meningovascular syphilis marked by progressive spasticity and weakness of the legs, paraplegia, muscular atrophy, paresthesia, increased knee and ankle reflexes, and incontinence.

Erb-Goldflam d., myasthenia gravis—a disorder of neuromuscular function due to the presence of antibodies to acetylcholine receptors at the neuromuscular junction; clinically, there is fatigue and exhaustion of the muscular system with a tendency to fluctuate in severity and without sensory disturbance or atrophy. The disorder may be restricted to a muscle group or become generalized with severe weakness and, in some cases, ventilatory insufficiency. It may affect any muscle of the body, but especially those of the eye, face, lips, tongue, throat, and neck.

Erb-Landouzy d., muscular dystrophy—a group of genetic degenerative myopathies characterized by weakness and atrophy of muscle without involvement of the nervous system. There are three main types: pseudohypertrophic muscular dystrophy, facioscapulohumeral dystrophy, and limb girdle muscular dystrophy. Other forms include distal muscular dystrophy, ocular myopathy, and myotonic dystrophy.

Eulenburg's d., paramyotonia congenita—an autosomal dominant disorder clinically similar to myotonia congenita, except that the precipitating factor is exposure to cold, the myotonia is aggravated by activity, and only the proximal muscles of the limbs, eyelids and tongue are affected.

Extensor process d., buttress foot—a condition of periostitis or ostitis in the region of the pyramidal process of the os pedis of the horse, with fracture of the process, deformity of the hoof, and alteration of the normal angle of the joint.

Extrapyramidal d., any of a group of clinical disorders marked by abnormal involuntary movements, alterations in muscle tone, and postural disturbances and involving lesions of the extrapyramidal tract, it includes parkinsonism, chorea, athetosis, etc.

Fabry's d., an X-linked lysosomal storage disease of glycosphingolipid catabolism resulting from deficient α-galactosidase A and leading to accumulation of globotriaosylceramide in the cardiovascular and renal systems. Clinical manifestations include telangiectases in the "bathing suit area", corneal opacities, burning pain in the palms, soles, and abdomen, chronic paresthesias of the hands and feet, cardiopulmonary involvement, edema of the legs, osteoporosis, retarded growth, and delayed puberty. Patients usually die of renal failure or cardiac or cerebrovascular disease. Detection of female heterozygotes and prenatal testing (amniocentesis) are available. Also called angiokeratoma carports diffusum, diffuse angiokeratoma, α-galactosidase A deficiency, and ceramide trihexosidase deficiency.

Fahr-Volhard d., malignant nephrosclerosis—an uncommon form of arteriolar nephrosclerosis affecting all the vessels of the body, especially the small arteries and arterioles of the kidneys, and frequently associated with malignant hypertension and hyperplastic arteriosclerosis. It may occur in the absence of previous history of hypertension of primary renal disease, especially glomerulonephritis, beningn nephrosclerosis, and pyelonephritis.

Fallot's d., tetralogy of Fallot—a combination of congenital cardiac defects consisting of pulmonary stenosis, interventricular septal defect, dextroposition of the aorta so that it overrides the interventricular septum and receives venous as well as arterial blood, and right ventricular hypertrophy.

Fanconi's d., see under syndrome.

Farber's d., a lysosomal storage disease of ceramide metabolism due to defective ceramidase and marked by hoarseness, aphonia, and a brownish desquamating dermatitis beginning at about three months of age, followed by foam cell infiltration of bones and joints, resulting in deformations; granulomatous reaction in lymph nodes, heart, lungs, and kidneys, and psychomotor retardation. Also called Farber's lipogranu-lomatosis, and ceramidase deficiency.

Fat-deficiency d., a condition characterized by cessation of growth and skin lesions that result when essential fatty acids (arachidonic and linoleic acid) are absent from the diet.

Fauchard's d., marginal periodontitis—a chronic destructive inflammatory periodontal disease that begins as a simple marginal gingivitis and may migrate along the tooth toward the apex producing periodontal pockets, usually with pus formation, and destruction of the periodontal and alveolar structures, causing the teeth to become loose.

Favre-Durand-Nicholas d., see Durand-Nicholas-Favre d.

Feer's d., acrodynia—a disease of infancy and early childhood characterized by pain and coloration of, the fingers and toes, and by listlessness, failure to thrive, irritability, generalized inconstant rashes, profuse perspiration, photophobia, loss of teeth and sometimes scarlet coloration of cheeks and tip of the nose; repeated ingestion of or contact with mercury is the cause of most, if not all, cases, and individiual sensitivity may also be a factor.

Fenwick's d., idiopathic atrophic gastritis (chronic gastritis with atrophy of the mucous membrane and gland), first described by Fenwick in a patient with pernicious anemia.

Fibrocystic d. of breast, see cystic d. of breast.

Fibrocystic d. of the pancreas, cystic fibrosis.

Fiedler's d., see Weil's syndrome.

Fifth d., erythema infectiosum—a moderately contagious, beningn epidemic disease seen mainly in children, probably of viral etiology, and characterized by abrupt onset of rash, which occurs in three stages: livid erythema appears on the cheeks giving them appearance of having being slapped; an erythematous maculopapular rash then involves the trunk extremities; the rash fades with central clearing, leaving a lace-like pattern.

Fifth venereal d., lymphogranuloma venereum—see Durand-Nicholas-Favre d.

Filatov's d., infectious mononucleosis—a common, acute, usually self-limited infectious disease caused by the Epstein-Barr virus, characterized by fever, membranous pharyngitis, lymph node and splenic enlargement, lymphocyte proliferation, and the presence of atypical lymphocytes, and giving rise to various immune reactions, including the development of a transient heterophile and a persistent Epstein-Barr virus antibody response. Potential complications include hepatitis and encephalo-meningitis. It affects adolescents and young adults, being spread by saliva transfer and possibly other modes; in children, the infection is largely subclinical.

Filatov-Dukes d., see Dukes' d.

File-cutters' d., lead poisoning from inhaling particles of lead which arise from the bed of lead used in file cutting.

Fingertoe and toe d., a disease of cabbage and other cruciferous plants due to the protozoan *Plasmodiophora brassicae*, and characterized by knotty enlargement of the affected plant's roots. Also called clubroot.

Fish-slime d., septicemia following a puncture wound made by the spine of a fish.

Flajani's d., see Graves' d.

Flatau-Schilder d., see Schilder's d.

Flax-dresser's d., a pulmonary disorder seen in flax-dressers, and caused by inhaling of flax.

Flegel's d., hyperkeratosis lenticularis perstans—an autosomal dominant skin disorder usually occurring in the third or fourth decade of life, characterized clinically by the presence of pink or reddish or yellowish brown hyperkeratotic scaly papules on the lower leg and dorsum of the foot, sometimes involving the trunk, thigh, arms, and dorsum of the hand, and usually associated with punctate keratoses on the palms and soles; and histologically by a lack of keratinosomes and a reduction of keratohyalin granules in the epidermis underlying the lesions.

Fleischner's d., osteochondritis affecting the middle phalanges of the hand.

Flint d., chalicosis—a disorder of the lungs or bronchioles (chiefly among stone-cutters), due to the inhalation of fine particles of stones; it is a form of pneumoconiosis.

Floating-beta d., see broad-beta d.

Fluke d., infection with flukes—a class of the Platyhelminthes which includes the flukes. The trematodes or flukes are parasitic in man and animals, infection generally resulting from the ingestion of uncooked or insufficiently cooked fish, crustaceans, and vegetation. All flukes require a mollusk as their first intermediate host, in which complex developmental cycle takes place. The larval stage, which escapes from the mollusk, may then enter a second intermediate host (fish—crustacean, or another mollusk), encyst on vegetation, or penetrate directly into the skin of the definitive host.

Focal d., one which is localized at one or more foci.

Folling d., phenylketonuria-hyperphenylalaninemia, type—phenylalanine accumulation resulting in mental retardation, neurologic manifestations (including hyperkinesia, epilepsy, and microcephaly), light pigmentation, eczema and a mousy odor, unless treated by a diet very low in phenylalanine.

Foot-and-mouth d., an acute, naturally occurring, extremely contagious viral disease of wild and domestic animals, chiefly cattle, pigs, sheep, goats, and other ruminants, and very rarely of man. It is marked by an eruption of vesicles on the lips, buccal cavity, pharynx, legs, and feet; sometimes the skin of the udder or teats is involved. Also called hoof-and-mouth d.; aftosa; contagious, epizootic, or malignant aphthae: aphthous fever and aphthobullous, epidemic or epizootic stomatitis.

Forbes' d., see glycogen storage d (type III).

Fordyce's d., 1. Ectopic sebaceous glands found on the lips and gums and in the mucosa of the cheeks, which presents as yellowish white milia. 2. See Fox-Fordyce d.

Forestier d., hyperostosis of the anterolateral vertebral column, especially in the thoracic region.

Förster's d., that which starts around or near the macula lutea and progresses toward the periphery. Unlike other forms of choroiditis, the lesions are pigmented at first and then lose their pigmentation.

Fothergill's d., 1. Scarlatina anginosa—scarlet fever associated with painful pharyngitis, with tonsillar enlargement or peritonsillar abscess. 2. Trigeminal neuralgia—excruciating episodic pain in the area supplied by the trigeminal nerve, often precipitated by stimulation of well-defined trigger points.

Fournier's d., an acute gangrenous infection of the scrotum, penis, or perineum involving gram-positive organisms, enteric bacilli, and anaerobes, which occurs following trauma, operative procedures, an underlying urinary tract disease, or a distant acute inflammatory process.

Fourth d., see Dukes' d.

Fourth venereal d., 1. Specific gangrenous and ulcerative balanoposthilis—an acute inflammatory disease of the glans penis and opposed surface of the prepuce, marked by ulcerations and sometimes by gangrene, with a flow of odorous pus, and caused by spirochete.

2. **Granuloma inguinale**—a chronic, slowly progressive, ulcerative granulomatous disease, assumed to be sexually transmitted, caused by *Calymmatobacterium granulomatis*, and primarily involving the skin and the lymphatics of the anogenital region but sometimes spreading to the perineum and perianal area or inguinal region; it occurs especially in the tropics and is usually seen in dark-skinned people even in the temperate areas, where it is rare.

Fox-Fordyce d., a chronic, usually pruritic disease chiefly seen in women, characterized by the development of small follicular papular eruptions of apocrine gland-bearing areas, especially the axillae and pubes, and caused by obstruction, and rupture of the intraepidermal portion of the ducts of affected apocrine glands, resulting in alteration of the regional ductal epidermis, apocrine secretory tubule, and adjacent dermis. Also called apocrine mitiaria.

Francis' d., tularemia—an infectious plague like, zoonotic disease found primarily in rodents but also affecting humans and many kinds of wildlife, with rabbits, squirrels, and muskrats being the primary source of infection by the etiologic agent, the bacillus *Francisella tularensis*. It is transmitted by bites of deer flies, fleas, and ticks, as a result of handling contaminated animals or their products, by inhalation of aerosolized *F.tularensis*, or by ingestion of contaminated food or water. In addition to a marked reaction at the portal of entry of the pathogen, which has lead to classification of the various forms of tularemia, most cases are characterized by abrupt onset of fever, chills, weakness, headache, backache, and malaise.

Frankl-Hochwart's d., polyneuritis cerebralis menieriformis—symptoms of cochlear vestibular, facial, and trigeminal nerve irritation occurring in the early period of syphilis.

Frei's d., see Durand-Nicolas-Farve d.,

Freiberg's d., oeteochondrosis of the head of the second metatarsal.

Friedländer's d., endarteritis obliterans—endarteritis in which the lumina of the small vessels become narrowed or obliterated as a result of proliferation of the tissue of the intimal layer.

Friedreich's d., 1. Paramyoclonus multiplex—a condition occurring more often in males than in females, characterized by sudden shock like contractions affecting first the proximal muscles of the arms and the shoulder girdle, with any muscles of the limbs and trunk being involved later, and finally involving the face bulbar muscles. 2. Friedreich's ataxia—an autosomal recessive disease, usually beginning in childhood or youth, with sclerosis of lateral and dorsal columns of the spinal cord. It is attended by ataxia, speech impairment, lateral curvature of the spinal column, and peculiar swaying and irregular movements, with paralysis of the muscles, especially of the lower extremities. It is often associated with hypertrophic cardiomyopathy.

Fright d., canine hysteria—psychic disturbance in dogs marked by symptoms of fright and by hysterical barking and running.

Frommel's d., see Chiari-Frommel syndrome.

Functional d., a disease involving functions without tissue damage.

Functional cardiovascular d., neurocirculatory asthenia—a syndrome characterized by palpitations, dyspnea, a sense of fatigue, fear of effort and discomfort brought on by exersice or even slight effort; considered by most authorities to be a particular presentation of anxiety neurosis (anxiety state), the physical symptoms being attributed to autonomic responses to anxiety or to hyperventilation.

Fürstner's d., pseudospastic paralysis with tremor.

Gaisböck's d., stress polycythemia—chronic relative polycythemia usually affecting white, middle-aged, mildly obese who are active, anxiety-prone, and hypertensive, occurring without the characteristic symptoms associated with polycythemia vera, i.e., without leukocytosis, splenomegaly, and thrombocytosis.

Gamma chain d., a heavy chain disease occurring usually in elderly persons that clinically resembles a malignant lymphoma, with symptoms of lymphadenopathy, hepatosplenomegaly, and recurrent infections.

Gamna's d., a form of splenomegaly, with thickening of the splenic capsule and the presence of small brownish areas (Gamna's nodules) which are usually surrounded by hematogenous zone; feruginous pigment is deposited in the splenic pulp.

Gamstorp's d., adynamia episodica hereditaria—an autosomal dominant trait marked by recurring attacks of rapidly progressive flaccid paralysis, associated with rise in serum potassium levels.

Gandy-Nanta d., siderotic splenomegaly—splenomegaly characterized by marked fibrosis with deposit of iron and calcium (Gamna's nodules).

Gannister d., pneumoconiosis due to the inhalation of dust by workers in the manufacture of refractory brick or fire clay.

Garre's d., sclerosing nonsuppurative osteomyelitis—chronic idiopathic osteomyelitis involving the long bones, particularly tibia and femur, characterized by a diffuse inflammatory reaction, increased density and spindle-shaped sclerotic thickening of the cortex, and an absence of suppuration.

Gaucher's d., a lipidosis caused by deficient glucocerebrosidase (glucosylceramidase) with glucocerebroside (glucosylceramide) accumulation in storage cells (Gaucher's cells) in the liver, spleen, lymph nodes, alveolar capillaries, and bone marrow. There are three clinical types: type 1 (chronic non-neuronopathic or "adult") may appear at any age and is associated with hypersplenism, thrombocytopenia, anemia, jaundice, and bone lesions; type 2 (acute neuronopathic or "infantile") is associated with onset in infancy, hepatosplenomegaly, severe CNS impairment, and death usually within the first year; type 3 (subacute neuronopathic or "juvenile") is the most varied, having the same clinical features as types 1 and 2 but a longer course. Also called glucosylceramide lipidosis.

Gee's d., Gee Herter d., Gee-Herter-Heubner d., the infantile form of celiac disease or nontropical sprue—a malabsorption syndrome affecting both children and adults, precipitated by ingestion of gluten-containing food; its etiology is unknown, but a hereditary factor has been implicated. Pathologically, the proximal intestinal mucosa loses its villous structure, surface epithelial cells exhibit degenerative changes, and their absorptive function is severely impaired. It is characterized by diarrhea in which the stools are bulky, frothy, fatty (steatorrhea), and fetid (occasionally, malabsorption may be associated with the passage of a single bulky stool without diarrhea), and by abdominal distention, flatulence, weight loss, asthenia, deficiency of vitamins B, D, and K, and electrolyte depletion; also called celiac disease and gluten enteropathy. In the infantile form onset is insidious, and marked by irritability, loss of appetite, weakness, extreme wasting, growth retardation, and celiac crisis; also called infantile celiac disease.

Gee-Thaysen d., adult celiac disease, the adult form of nontropical sprue—the adult form is marked by extreme lassitude, fatigue, difficulty in breathing, clubbing of the fingers, bone pain, cramping of the muscles, tetany, abdominal distention during the day, megacolon, tympanitis, and skin pigmentation.

Genetic d., a general term for any disorder caused by a genetic mechanism, comprising chromosome aberrations or anomalies, mendelian or monogenic or single-gene disorders and multifactorial disorders.

Gerhardt's d., erythromelagia—a disease affecting chiefly extremities of the body, the feet more often than the hands, and marked by paroxysmal, bilateral vasodilation, particularly of the extremities, with burning pain, and increased skin temperature and redness.

Gerlier's d., a disease of the nerves and nerve centers attacking farm laborers and stablemen, and characterized by pain, paresis, vertigo, ptosis, and muscular contractions; also called endemic paralytic vertigo, paralyzing vertigo and Gerlier's syndrome.

Giant platelet d., see Bernard-Soulier d.

Gibney's d., perispondyhitis—a painful condition of the spinal muscles.

Gierke's d., see glycogen storage d. (type I).

Gilbert's d., see Gilbert's syndrome.

Gilchrist's d., North American blastomycosis—an infection usually acquired through pulmonary route, caused by *Blastomyces dermatitidis*, and marked by suppurating tumors in the skin or by lesions in the lungs, bones, subcutaneous tissues, liver, spleen and kidneys.

Gilles de la Tourette's d., see under syndrome.

Glanzmann's d., thrombosthenia—a platelet abnormality characterized by defective clot retraction, abnormal glass adhesion, impaired aggregation to ADP, collagen, and thrombin, and prolonged bleeding time; it is manifested clinically as Glanzmann's d., with epistaxis, inappropriate bruising, and excessive bleeding, as during surgery.

Glasser's d., a disease mainly affecting pigs 5 to 14 weeks old, in which swelling of the hocks or knee joints, or both is accompanied by fever, lameness, and a disinclination to move: if untreated, death usually results. It is caused by 's' strain of *Haemophilus influenzae*.

Glénard's d., (obs), splanchnoptosis—the prolapse or downward displacement of the viscera; also called visceroptosis.

Glisson's d., see English disease.

Glucose-6-phosphate dehydrogenase (G6PD) d., the most common inborn error of metabolism, affecting over 100 million people with varying degrees of hemolytic anemia. The G6PD locus, Xq28, is very closely linked to the genes for deutanomaly, protanomaly, hemophilia A, and adrenoleukodystrophy, and closely linked to the genes (on Xq27) for the fragile X syndrome and HPRT deficiency (the Lesch-Nyhan syndrome. The G6PD deficiency provides heterozygote advantage against falciparum malaria. The G6PD gene is highly polymorphous, with over 300 variants known. Glucose-6-phosphate dehydrogenase deficiency anemia—a genetically determined anemia caused by a deficiency of this enzyme in erythrocytes which results in hemolysis of the erythrocytes by drugs of certain groups (such as antimalarials, sulfonamides, nitrofurans, antipyretics and analgesics, and sulfones), fava beans, and other agents. Recent studies imply that this predisposition to hemolysis may be expressed in varying degrees and that other biochemical defects, in addition to that involving glucose-6-phosphate dehydrogenase, may also be present in erythrocytes.

Glycogen storage d., any of at least 14 types or subtypes of rare inborn errors of metabolism due to a defect in a specific enzyme involved in glycogen catabolism. In type I, defective glucose-6-phosphatase affects liver and kidneys, causing hepatomegaly, hypoglycemia, hyperuricemia, xanthomas, bleeding, and adiposity; patient may live well into adulthood. Also called Gierke (von Gierke) d., hepatorenal glycogenosis, hepatorenal glycogen storage d, and glucose-6-phosphatase deficiency. In type II, defective α-1, 4-glucosidase (acid maltase) causes generalized glycogen accumulation with CNS involvement and psychomotor retardation, with cardiomegaly and cardiorespiratory failure; most infants die by one year of age. Also called Pompe d., α-1, 4-glucosidase deficiency, acid-maltase deficiency, and generalized glycogenosis. In type III, a defect in the debranching enzyme amylo-1,6 glucosidase affects the heart and liver;

signs include stunted growth, hepatomegaly, hypoglycemia, and acidosis. Six different subgroups (III A through III F) are known. Also called debrancher deficiency, Cori's d., Forbes' d: limit dextrinosis, amylo-1,6 glucosidase deficiency, and debrancher glycogen storage d. In type IV, a defect in the branching enzyme amylo-1:4, 1:6-transglucosidase causes early cirrhosis with liver failure and hepatosplenomegaly; the child dies usually in his second year. Also called amylopectinosis, Andersen's d., brancher deficiency, brancher deficiency glycogenosis, brancher glycogen storage d., amylo 1:4, 1-6-transglucosidase deficiency, and α-1, 4 glucan: α-1,4 glucan 5-glucosyl-transferase deficiency. In type V, a deficiency of muscle phosphorylase affects the skeletal muscles, causing muscle cramps and a depressed blood lactate level during exercise. Also called McArdle's d., McArdle's syndrome, myophosphorylase deficiency glycogenosis, and muscle phosphorylase deficiency. In type VI, a deficiency of liver phosphorylase is manifested in the liver and leukocytes, with hepatomegaly, moderate hypoglycemia, mild acidosis, and growth retardation. Also called Hers' d., hepatic phosphorylase deficiency, and hepatophosphorylase deficiency glycogenosis. In type VII, a deficiency, and hepatophosphorylase deficiency. glycogenosis. In type VII a deficiency in phosphofructokinase affects muscle and erythrocytes, with temporary weakness and skeletal muscle cramping after exercise. Also called muscle phosphofructokinase deficiency and Tarui's d. In type VIII, an X-linked disorder, a defect in hepatic phosphorylase kinase reduces liver and leuckocyte phosphorylase and causes hepatomegaly and increased concentrations of liver glycogen; patients are otherwise asymptomatic. Also called hepatic phosphorylase kinase deficiency.

Goldflam's d., Goldflam-Erb d., myasthenia gravis—a disorder of neuromuscular function due to the presence of antibodies to acetylcholine receptors at the neuromuscular junction; clinically, there is fatigue and exhaustion of the muscular system with a tendency to fluctuate in severity and without sensory disturbance or atrophy. The disorder may be restricted to muscle group or become generalized with severe weakness and, in some cases ventilatory insufficiency. It may affect any muscle of the body, but especially those of the eye, face, lips, tongue, throat, and neck.

Goldstein's d., hereditary hemorrhagic telangiectasia—an autosomal dominant vascular anomaly characterized by presence of multiple small telangiectases of the skin, mucous membranes, gastrointestinal tract, and other organs, associated with recurrent episodes of bleeding from affected sites and gross or occult melena.

Graft-versus-host (GVH) d., disease caused by the immune response of histoincompatible, immunocompetent donor cells against the tissues of immunoincompetent host, which can occur as a complication of bone marrow transplantation or as a result of maternal-fetal blood transfusion or therapeutic blood transfusion in which the recipient has a cellular immunodeficiency disease. Clinical manifestation include skin disease ranging from a maculopapular eruption to epidermal necrosis, intestinal disease marked by diarrhea, malabsorption, and abdnominal pain, and liver dysfunction caused by cholestatic hepatitis or veno-occulsive disease and marked by serum enzyme abnormalities. Also called graft-versus-host reaction.

Grass d., a usually fatal disease of horses occurring after they have been put to graze on grass, usually between May and July; first seen in Scotland, it has spread to Wales, England and Sweden. It is marked by dysphagia, severe diarrhea, dehydration, interrupted peristalsis, and priapism. Also called grass sickness.

Graves' d., a disorder of the thyroid of unknown but probably autoimmune etiology, occurring most often in women, characterized by thyrotoxicosis with diffuse goiter, exophthalmos, or pretibial myxedema, or any combination of the three. Signs and symptoms include fatigability, nervousness, emotional lability and irritability, heat intolerance and increased sweating, weight loss, palpitation, and tremor of the hands and tongue. Some patients have varying degrees of exophthalmos. Most patients have circulation thyroid-stimulating immunoglobulins (TSI) that cause excessive secretion of thyroid hormones by binding to TSH receptors on thyroid cells. Called Basedow's d. in continental Europe. Also called cachexia exopthalmica, diffuse toxic goiter, exophthalmic goiter, Flajani's d., Parry's d., and tachycardia strumosa exophthalmica.

Greasy pig d., seborrhea of piglets, which is thought to be associated with a vitamin B deficiency.

Greenfield's d., metachromatic leukodystrophy—an autosomal recessive form of leukoencephalopathy due to defective aryl sulfatase and characterized by an accumulation of a sphingolipid (sulfatide) in neural and non-neural tissues, with a diffuse loss of myelin in the central nervous system. The infantile form usually begins in the third year of life, most commonly before the thirtieth month, with blindness, motor disturbances, rigidity, mental deterioration, and sometimes convulsions. The adult form begins after 16 years of age, usually with psychiatric disturbances that progress to dementia; the motor and posture disturbances appear late in the course of this form. A juvenile form with an onset between 4 and 10 years of age has also been observed.

Griesinger's d. (obs), see hookworm d.

Grinder's d., pneumoconiosis of grinders.

Gross' d., encysted rectum; saccular dilatation of anal wall with retained inspissated feces.

Guinea worm d., dracunculiasis—the guinea worm or medina worm, a thread-like worm, 30 to 120 cm long, which inhabits the subcutaneous and intermuscular tissues of man and several domestic animals in India, Africa, and Arabia. Its embryos are discharged through an opening in the skin upon contact with water, in which they enter bodies of a small crustacean, cyclops, where they undergo larval development.

Guinon's d., see Gilles de la Tourette's syndrome.

Gull's d., atrophy of the thyroid with myxedema.

Gumboro d., see infectious bursal d.

Gunther's d., congenital erythropoietic porphyria—autosomal recessive porphyria in which increased synthesis of uroporphyrinogen I relative to uroporphyringen III occurs in bone marrow normoblasts; it is characterized by cutaneous photosensitivity, leading to mutilating skin lesions, by hemolytic anemia and splenomegaly, and by greatly increased urinary excretion of uroporphyrin (corproporphyrin I excretion is slightly elevated). Erythrodontia and hypertrychosis are invariably present.

H d., see Hartnup's d.

Habermann's d., acute lichenoid pityriasis—an acute or subacute, sometimes relapsing, widespread macular, papular, or vesicular eruption that tends to crusting, necrosis, and hemorrhage, which heals, leaving pigmented depressed scars, followed by the develop-ment of a new crop of lesions. Occasionally, progression to the chronic lichenoid form may occur.

Haff d., a condition affecting fishermen of the Konigsberg (Frisches) Haff, lagoon joining the Baltic Sea. The men are suddenly seized with severe pain in the limbs great weariness, and myoglobinuria. The disease is said to be the result of poisoning by arsine introduced into the Haff through the waste water of cellulose factories. Several epidemics occurred prior to the World War II.

Haglund's d., bursitis in the region of the Achilles tendon.

Hagner's d., an obscure bone disease somewhat resembling acromegaly (Pierre Marie described this obscure bone disease in the two Hagner brothers).

Hailey-Hailey d., benign familial pemphigus—a benign persistently recurrent bullous and vesicular autosomal dominant dermatitis involving chiefly sides of the neck, axillae, groin and flexural and opposing surfaces of the body, and characterized by crops of lesions, which may remain localized or become generalized, that rupture, undergo erosion, and become thickly crusted. The histopathologic features are suggestive of keratosis follicularis as well as pemphigus.

Hallervorden-Spatz d., see under syndrome.

Hamman's d., pneumomediastinum—the presence of air or gas in the mediastinum, which may interfere with respiration and circulation, and may lead to such conditions as penumothorax or pneumopericardium. It may occur spontaneously or as a result of trauma or a pathological process, or it may be introduced deliberately as a diagnostic procedure.

Hammond's d., athetosis—a derangement marked by ceaseless occurrence of slow, sinuous, twisting movements, especially severe in the hands, and performed involuntarily; it may occur after hemiplegia, and is then as posthemiplegic chorea. Also called mobile spasm.

Hand's d., see Hand-Schüller-Christian d.

Hand-foot-and-mouth d., a usually mild and self-limited exanthematous eruption most often caused by coxsackievirus A 16, primarily seen in preschool children, and characterized by vesicles on the buccal mucosa, tongue, soft palate, gingivae, and hands and feet, including the palms and soles. Also called hand-foot-and-mouth syndrome.

Hand-Schüller-Christian d., a chronic idiopathic form of histiocytosis, sometimes with accumulation of cholesterol, characterized classically by the triad of: defects in the membranous bones, exophthalmos, and diabetes insipidus. In most cases, this triad is not seen, but there is multiple system, soft tissue, and bone involvement. Also called chronic idiopathic xanthomatosis and cholesterol thesaurismosis.

Hanot's d., 1. Primary biliary cirrhosis—a rare form of biliary cirrhosis of unknown etiology in which small interhepatic bile ducts are destroyed while the major intrahepatic and extrahepatic ducts remain patent; 90 percent of patients are female most are middle aged; it is characterized by chronic cholestasis with pruritus, jaundice, hypercholesterolemia and xanthomas, steomalacia, and, in the later stages by portal hypertension and liver failure. Almost all patients have circulating antimitochondrial antibodies. 2. Secondary biliary cirrhosis—cirrhosis of the liver resulting from chronic bile obstruction due to congenital atresia or stricture.

Hansen's d., leprosy—a slowly progressive, chronic infectious disease caused by *Mycobacterium leprae* and characterized by development of granulomatous or neurotrophic lesions in the skin, mucous membranes, nerves, bones, and viscera. It is manifested by a broad spectrum of clinical symptoms, consisting of two principal, or polar types, with the lepromatous type at one end of the spectrum and the tuberculoid type at the other; between these two polar types is the borderline type, with two subtypes., borderline tuberculoid and borderline lepromatous.

Hapsburg's d., hemophilia—a hemorrhagic diathesis occurring in two main forms (i) hemophilia A (classical hemophilia, factor VIII deficiency), an X-linked disorder due to deficiency of coagulation factor VIII; (ii) hemophilia B (factor IX deficiency, Christmas disease), also X-linked, due to deficiency of coagulation factor IX. Both forms are determined by a mutant gene near the telomere of the long arm of X chromosome (Xq), but at different loci, and are characterized by subcutaneous and intramuscular hemorrhages; bleeding from mouth, gums, lips, and tongue; hematuria and hemarthroses.

Harada's d., see under syndrome.

Hard pad d., hyperkeratosis of the footpads of young dogs, occurring in canine distemper.

Hartnup's d., an inborn error of metabolism characterized by cerebellar ataxia, apellagra-like condition of the skin, and massive aminoaciduria involving a group of neutral mono-aminomonocarboxylic amino acids sharing a common renal reabsorption mechanism; patients respond well to prolonged oral administration of nicotinamide.

Hashimoto's d., a progressive autoimmune disease of the thyroid gland, with lymphocytic infiltration of the gland and circulating antithyroid antibodies. Women are most commonly affected, and there is a familial predisposition to the disease. It sometimes occurs after the subsidence of Graves' disease. Patients have goiter and gradually develop hypothyroidism. Also called autoimmune and Hashimoto's thyroiditis and struma lymphomatosa.

Heart d., any organic, mechanical, or functional abnormality of the heart; it may be valvular, myocardial, or neurogenic.

Heartwater d., a fatal disease of cattle, sheep, and goats, marked by fluid accumulation in the pleura, pericardium and pleural cavity. it is caused by *Cowdria ruminantium*, which is transmitted by the ticks *Amblyomma hebraeum* and *A.variegata*.

Heavy-chain d., a group of rare malignant neoplasms of lymphoplasmacytic cells that secrete an M component consisting of monoclonal immunoglobulin heavy chains or heavy chain fragments; they are classified according to heavy chain type. See also alpha chain d., gamma chain d., and muchian d.

Heberden's d., 1. Rheumatism of the smaller joints, accompanied by nodules in or about the distal interphalangeal joints. 2. Angina pectoris.

Hebra's d., erythema multiforme minor—a mild self-limited mucocutaneous form of erythema multiforme that may have a prodrome of fever, cough, and pharyngitis. In addition to the characteristic iris lesions, erythematous macules and papules, purpura, and occasional vessiculobullous lesions may be present, which are usually asymptomatic, but may burn or itch slightly.

Heerfordt's d., see under syndrome.

Heine-Medin d., the major form of poliomyelitis—an acute viral disease, occurring sporadically and in epidemics, and characterized clinically by fever, sore throat, headache, and vomiting, often with stiffness of back and neck. The major form is characterized by involvement of central nervous system, stiff neck, pleocytosis in the spinal fluid, and perhaps paralysis. There may be subsequent atrophy of groups if muscles, ending in contraction and permanent deformity.

Heller-Döhle d., syphilitic aortitis—see Döhle d.

Helminthic d., a disease caused by worms.

Hemoglobin d., any of a group of hereditary molecular diseases, characterized by the presence of various abnormal hemoglobins, e.g., hemoglobins C_2-D, E, H, or S, in the red blood cells, in which the homozygous form is manifested by hemolytic anemia.

Hemoglobin C-thalassemia d., a hereditary disorder involving simultaneous heterozygosity for hemoglobin C and thalassemia, manifested by mild hemolytic anemia and persistent splenomegaly; also called hemoglobin C-thalassemia.

Hemoglobin E-thalassemia d., a hereditary condition involving simultaneous heterozygosity for hemoglobin E and thalassemia, manifested by mild hemolytic anemia and persistent splenomegaly; called als hemoglobin E-thalassemia.

Hemolytic d., of newborn, erthythroblastosis fetalis—hemolytic anemia of the fetus or newborn, usually secondary to an incompatibility between the blood group of the mother and that of her offspring, characterized by accelerated destruction of erythrocytes and consequent jaundice and by increased red cell regeneration (nucleated red cells in the blood) and hepatosplenomegaly. Infants with severe jaundice, kernicterus may result.

Hemorrhagic d., of the newborn, a self-limited hemorrhagic disorder of the first days of life, caused by a deficiency of the vitamin K-dependent blood coagulation factor II, VII, IX, and X.

Henderson-Jones d., osteochondromatosis characterized by the presence of numerous cartilaginous foreign bodies in the joint cavity or in the bursa of a tendon sheath.

Hepatolenticular d., see Wilson's d.

Hepatorenal glycogen storage d., see glycogen storage d (type I).

Hereditary d., one that is transmitted genetically from parents to children.

Heredoconstitutional d., an inherited pathologic condition which does not progress.

Heredodegenerative d., any disease of the central nervous system characterized by specific loss of neural tissue due to hereditary influence.

Herlitz's d., junctional epidermolysis bullosa—an autosomal recessive disorder having onset at birth or during the neonatal period, characterized clinically by severe generalized blistering, particularly in the perioral area, scalp, legs, diaper area and trunk, and extensive denudation that may be associated with secondary infection and death from septicemia, nail dystrophy, and dental dysplasia; growth retardation and refractory anemia are frequent findings in those who survive. On electron microscopy, a cleavage plane between the plasma membranes of the basal cells and the basement membranes is seen.

Hers' d., see glycogen storage d. (type VI).

Herter's d., Herter-Heubner d., the infantile form of nontropical sprue, see Gee-Herter d.

Heubner's d., syphilitic endarteritis of the cerebral vessels; also called Heubner's specific endarteritis.

Hip joint d., tuberculosis of the hip joint.

Hippel's d., see von Hippel's d.

Hippel-Lindau d., see von Hippel-Lindau d.

Hirschsprung's d., congenital megacolon—megacolon due to congenital absence of myenteric ganglionic cells in a distal segment of the large bowel. The resultant loss of motor function in the segment causes massive hypertrophic dilatation of the normal proximal colon; the aganglionic segment usually remains narrowed, but may dilate passively. The condition appears soon after birth, is more common in males, and causes extreme constipation, abdominal distention, sometimes vomiting, and, when severe, growth retardation.

His' d., His-Werner d., trench fever—a self-limited louse-borne, rickettsial disease due to *Rochalimaea quintana*, transmitted by the body louse, *Pediculus humanus*, and characterized by intermittent fever, generalized aches and pains, particularly severe in the shins, chills, sweating, vertigo, malaise, typhus-like rash, and multiple relapses.

Hock d., perosis—a disease of chicks marked by bone deformities and associated with deficiency of certain dietary factory, such as choline and manganese.

Hodgkin's d., a form of malignant lymphoma characterized by painless, progressive enlargement of the lymph nodes, spleen, and general lymphoid tissue; other symptoms may include anorexia, lassitude, weight loss, fever, pruritus, night sweats, and anemia. The characteristic histologic feature is presence of Reed-Sternberg cells. Hodgkin's disease is usually classified as: (i) diffuse, according to the number of lumphocyte and histiocytes (lymphocytes predominant; mixed cellularity; lymphocytes depleted) and (ii) nodular sclerosing (marked by birefringent bands of collagen and the presence of the lacunar cells). The condition, which affects twice as many males as females and usually occurs between the ages of 15 and 34 or after 50 is considered by many to be neoplastic in origin, but neither an infectious origin nor an immune response to the development of Reed-Sternberg cells has been excluded. Also called Hodgkin's lymphoma. Cf. non-Hodgkin's lymphoma.

Hodgson's d., an aneurysmal dilatation of the proximal part of the aorta, often accompanied by dilatation or hypertrophy of the heart.

Hoffa's d., traumatic proliferation of fatty tissue (solitary lipoma) in the knee joint.

Holoendemic d., a disease endemic in most of the children in a population, with the adults in the same population being less often affected.

Hoof-and-mouth d., see foot-and-mouth d.

Hookworm d., a condition due to infection with *Ancylostoma duodenale* or *Necator americanus*, nematode worms that closely resemble each other (In dogs, the disease is usually caused by *Ancylostoma caninum*). The disease occurs in practically all tropical and subtropical countries, including the southern United States and the West Indies. In temperate regions, it may occur in mines and tunnels, where conditions of temperature and moisture resemble the tropics. The larvae of the parasite live in soil and gain entrance to the digestive tract indirectly by way of the skin of the feet or legs or directly with contaminated food or water. The percutaneous infection is followed by a transitory eruption known as "ground itch". From here the parasites are carried by the blood to the lungs, ascend the trachea, are swallowed, and settle in the small intestine, where they attach to the intestinal mucosa and ingest blood. Symptoms, which vary with diet and with severity of infection, may include abdominal pain, diarrhea, and colic or nausea. Anemia is seen only in moderate to severe infections or when other adverse nutritional factors operate in conjunction with the parasite-induced blood loss.

Horton's d., 1. Migrainous neuralgia—a migraine variant characterized by attacks of unilateral excruciating pain over the eye and forehead, with temperature elevation, lacrimation, and rhinorrhea; attacks last 15 to 30 min and tend to occur in clusters. Because attacks identical to the spontaneous attacks may be induced in sufferers by subcutaneous injection of histamine diphosphate. 2. Temporal arteritis—a chronic vascular disease of unknown origin, most common in the carotid arterial system but also occurring in other large and small systemic arteries, characterized by proliferative inflammation, often with giant cells and granulomas, and by headache, difficulty in chewing, weakness, weight loss, fever, and symptoms of sepsis, with a markedly increased erythrocyte sedimentation rate and leukocytosis. Ocular involvement, ranging from diplopia to complete blindness, occurs in about half the subjects. The disease occurs exclusively in older persons, and is often associated with polymyalgia rheumatica.

Huchard's d., continued arterial hypertension, thought to be a cause of arteriosclerosis.

Hunger d., hungry d., excessive hunger accompanied by weakness and nervousness caused by the hypoglycemia of hyperinsulinism.

Hunt's d., 1. Dyssnergia cerebellaris myoclonica—dyssynergia cerebellaris progressive associated with myoclonus epilepsy. 2. see Ramsay Hunt syndrome, def. 1.

Huntington's d., chorea—a relatively common autosomal dominant disease characterized by chronic progressive chorea and mental deterioration terminating in dementia; the age of onset is variable but usually occurs in the fourth decade of life. Death usually follows within 15 years.

Hurler's d., see under syndrome.

Hutchinson's d., 1. Prurigo estivalis—a papular dermatosis regarded as a form of polymorphous light eruption, usually occurring in childhood during the summer months and sometimes improving or resolving after puberty. 2. Angioma serpiginosum—generalized essential telangiectasia characterized by a group of tiny copper colored to bright red angiomatous puncta that enlarge by forming new puncta at the periphery with central clearing, which produces annular or serpiginous patterns. The eruption usually occurs on the lower extremities 3. Tay's choroiditis—degeneration of the choroid marked by irregular yellow spots around the macula lutea, and believed to be due to an atheromatous state of the arteries.

Hutchinson-Gilford d., progeria—a syndrome of uncertain genetic inheritance, characterized by precocious senility of striking degree, with dead from coronary artery disease frequently occurring before 10 years of age.

Hutinel's d., tuberculous pericarditis with cirrhosis of the liver in children.

Hyaline membrane d., a disorder affecting newborn infants (usually premature) characterized pathologically by the development of a hyaline-like membrane lining the terminal respiratory passages. Extensive atelectasis is attributed to lack of surfactant. See respiratory distress syndrome of newborn under syndrome.

Hydatid d., an infection, usually of the liver, caused by larval forms (hydatid cysts) of tapeworms of the genus *Echinococcus*, and characterized by the development of expanding cysts. See hydatid d., alveolar and hydatid d., unilocular. Also called hydatidosis, *Echinococcus* d. and echinococcosis.

Hydatid d., alveolar, infection with larval forms (hydatid cysts) of *Echinococcus multilocularis*, characterized by invasion and destruction of the host's tissues as the cysts undergo endogenous budding to form an aggregate of innumerable small cysts which honey-comb the affected organ (the liver in over 90 percent of cases) and may metastasize.

Hydatid d., unilocular, infection with the larval forms (hydatid cysts) of *Echinococcus granulosis*, characterized by the formation of single or multiple expanding cysts which are unilocular in nature; as the cysts expand, they may give rise to symptoms of related space-occupying lesions in the tissues or organs affected.

Hydrocephaloid d., a condition similar to hydrocephalus, but marked by depression of the fontanels, due to diarrhea or some other wasting disease with dehydration.

Hyperendemic d., a disease equally endemic in all age groups of a population. Cf: holoendemic d.

Hypopigmentation-immunodeficiency d., see Griscelli syndrome.

Iceland d., Icelandic d., epidemic neuromyasthenia—a disease somewhat resembling poliomyelitis, usually occurring in epidemics, characterized by headache, muscle pain, cervical lymphadenopathy, fever, and sometimes paralysis but without atrophy and with hyper-reflexia rather than hyporeflexia.

I-cell d., mucolipidosis II—a rapidly progressive disease of young children, characterized histologically by abnormal fibroblast containing a large number of dark inclusions which fill the central part of the cytoplasm except for the juxtanuclear zone (I-cells), and clinically by severe growth impairment, minimal hepatomegaly, extreme mental and motor retardation, and clear corneas; inherited as an autosomal recessive trait, it is due to deficiency of multiple acid hydrolases.

Idiopathic d., one not consequent upon any other disease, and of which the cause is unknown.

Immune-complex d., diseases caused by the formation of immune complexes in tissues or by the deposition of circulating immune complexes in tissues resulting in acute or chronic inflammation. Deposition of circulating immune complexes is generally associated with glomerulonephritis, vasculitis synovitis endocarditis, neuritis, and dermatitis. Locally formed complexes are involved in the pathogenesis of some autoimmune diseases. Circulating complexes may result from administration of heterologous antigens (as in serum sickness) or from the immune response to microbial antigens or tumor antigens.

Immunodeficiency d., any of a group of disorders resulting from the functional impairment of components of the immune system, which may include deficiency or malfunction of a cell population (e.g. phagocytic cells; subpopulations of T lymphocytes), lack of an antibody response, or complement abnormality. Also called immunodeficiency disorder or syndrome.

Immunoproliferative small intestine d., a condition characterized by diarrhea, malabsorption, abdominal pain, clubbing, plasma cell infiltration of the lamina propria of the small bowel, and presence of an abnormal alpha heavy chain fragment in the serum, occurring predominantly in young adults living around the Mediterranean sea; it frequently evolves into primary malignant lymphoma. Also called alpha-chain d.

Inborn lysosomal d' s., see lysosomal storage d.

Inclusion d., any disease in which cell inclusions are found.

Infantile celiac d., the infantile form of celiac disease, or nontropical sprue—see Gee-Hertet d.

Infectious d., a disease caused by a pathogenic microorganism; the etiologic agent may be a bacterium, virus, fungus, or animal parasite, and may be transmitted from another host or arise from the host's own indigenous microflora. See communicable d. and contagious d.

Infectious bursal d., a highly contagious acute disease of chickens, caused by virus provisionally classified as an orbivirus, characterized by a propensity of infected birds to pick at their own vents (cloacal apertures), edema and swelling of the cloacal bursa, soiled wet feathers whitish watery diarrhea, listlessness, trembling, extreme kidney damage, damage of the bursa of Fabricius and death. Also called Gumboro disease and avian nephrosis.

Inflammatory bowel d., a general term for those inflammatory diseases of the bowel of unknown etiology, including Crohn's disease and ulcerative colitis.

Inherited d., one transmitted genetically, from parents to offspring.

Intercurrent d., a disease occurring during the course of another disease with which it has no connection.

Interstitial d., one in which the stroma of an organ is mainly affected.

Interstitial lung d., a heterogeneous group of noninfectious, nonmalignant disorders of the lower respiratory tract, affecting primarily the alveolar wall structures but also often involving the small airways and blood vessels of the lung parenchyma; slowly progressive loss of alveolar-capillary units may lead to respiratory insufficiency and death.

Iron storage d., hemochromatosis—a disorder due to deposition of hemosiderin in the parenchymal cells, causing tissue damage and dysfunction of the liver, pancreas, heart, and pituitary. Other clinical signs include bronze pigmentation of skin, arthropathy, diabetes, cirrhosis, hepatosplenomegaly, hypogonadism, and loss of body hair. Full developement of the disease among women is restricted by menstruation, pregnancy, and lower dietary intake of iron. Acquired hemochromatosis may be the result of blood transfusions, excessive dietary iron, or secondary to other disease, e.g., thalassemia or sideroblastic anemia. Idiopathic or genetic hemochromatosis is an autosomal recessive disorder of metabolism associated with gene tightly linked to the A locus of the HLA complex on the chromosome 6.

Isambert's d., acute miliary tuberculosis of the larynx and pharynx.

Island d., scrub typhus—an acute typhus-like infectious disease caused by *Rickettsia tsutsugamushi*, transmitted by the bite of infected larval trombiculit mites (chiggers), occurring chiefly in Asia and the southern and western Pacific, and characterized chiefly by the formation of a pathognomonic primary cutaneous lesion or eschar at the site of inoculation (tache noire) accompanied by regional lymphadenopathy, fever, and a maculopapular rash.

Isle of Wight d., paralysis of the muscles of flight in honeybees caused by the presence of the mite *Acarapis woodi* in the tracheas of the bees.

Itch d., a dermatomycosis of horses probably caused by the mold *Microsporum canis*.

Jaffe-Lichtenstein d., cystic osteofibromatosis—a form of polyostotic fibrous dysplasia characterized by an enlarged medullary cavity with a thin cortex, which is filled with fibrous tissue (fibroma).

Jakob's d., Jakob-Creutzfeldt d., see Creutzfeldt-Jakob disease.

Jaksch's d., anemia pseudoleukemica infantum—a condition originally as a specific entity in children under age three, with anisocytosis, poikilocytosis, peripheral red blood cell immaturity, leukocytosis, lymphadenopathy, and hepatosplenomegaly; now considered to be a syndrome produced by many factors such as malnutrition, chronic infection, malabsorption, and hemoglobinopathies.

Janet's d., psychasthenia—a term used by Janet to cover all psychoneuroses not classified as hysteria; it mainly included what would now be called phobias and anxiety neuroses.

Jansen's d., metaphyseal dysostosis—a skeletal abnormality in which the epiphyses are normal, or nearly so, and the metaphyseal tissues are replaced by masses of cartilage, producing interference with enchondral bone formation, and expansion and thinning of the metaphyseal cortices.

Jansky-Bielschowsky d., amaurotic idiocy—a term for several lipidoses differing biochemically in clinical manifestation; the congenital form may be lethal within less than one month from birth; a disialonganglioside, G(D3), is present in tissue, and there is three-fold concentration of cholesterol in the brain. The infantile type is Tay-Sachs disease. The late infantile type begins between three and four years of age, shows no racial or ethnic preference, no fundus changes, cherry-red spot, or optic atrophy

Jensen's d., retinochoroiditis juxtapapillaris—a condition seen in young healthy subjects marked by a small inflammatory area on the fundus close to the papilla.

Johne's d., a usually fatal form of chronic enteritis due to *Mycobacterium paratuberculosis* chiefly affecting cattle but also sheep, goats, and deer. It remotely resembles a tuberculous infection, and is marked by intermitted or persistent diarrhea, progressive emaciation, anemia, and extreme weakness. Also called chronic dysentery of cattle, bovine leprosy, and paratuberculosis.

Johnson-Stevens d., see Stevens-Johnson syndrome.

Joseph d., see Azorean d.

Jumping d., see Gilles de la Tourette's syndrome.

Juvenile Paget d., hyperostosis corticalis deformans juvenilis—an autosomal recessive disorder beginning in childhood and marked by multiple fractures and bowing of all extremities, by thickening of the frontal parietal, and occipital bones, by osteoporosis and by elevated concentrations of serum alkaline phosphatase and of urinary hydroxyproline.

Kahler's d., multiple myeloma—a disseminated malignant neoplasm of plasma cells characterized by multiple bone marrow tumor foci and secretion of an M component (a monoclonal immunoglobulin or immunoglobulin fragment), associated with widespread osteolytic lesions appearing radiographically as punched out defects, resulting in bone pain, pathological fractures, hypercalcemia and normochromic mormocytic anemia; spread to extraosseous sites occurs frequently in advanced disease. Depression of immunoglobulin levels results in increased susceptibility to infection. Bence Jones proteinuria is present in many cases and results in systemic amyloidosis. Renal failure, resulting from calcium nephropathy or extensive case formation, occurs in about 20 percent of cases.

Kaiserstuhl d., a form of chronic arsenic poisoning that occurred in the Kaiserstuhl wine district of Germany.

Kaschin-Beck d., see Kashin-Bek d.

Kashin-Bek d., a slowly progressive, chronic, disabling, degenerative disease of the peripheral joints and spine, which principally occurs in children and is endemic in eastern Siberia, northern China, and Korea. It is believed to be caused by the ingestion or cereal grains infected with *Fusarium sporotrichiella*. Also called osteoarthritis deformans endemica.

Katayama's d., acute systemic schistosomiasis causing a distinct serum sickness-like syndrome, usually associated with heavy infection by *Schistosoma japonicum*, characterized by fever, chills, nausea and vomiting, cough, headache, urticaria, hepatosplenomegaly, lymphadenopathy, marked eosinophilia, and usually increased level of IgE and IgG. It was first reported from the Katayama river valley in Japan.

Kawasaki d., see mucocutaneous lymph node syndrome.

Keshan d., a fatal, congestive cardiomyopathy of selenium in the diet and occurs in areas with low selenium content in the soil, especially China, New Zealand, and Finland.

Kienböck's d., 1. Slowly progressive osteochondrosis of the semilunar (carpal lunate) bone; it may affect other bones of the wrist. Also called lunatomalacia. 2. Traumatic cavity formation in the spinal cord; also called traumatic syringomyelia.

Kimberley horse d., a disease of horses in the Kimberley district of northeastern Western Australia occurring during the wet season (January to April), due to grazing on *Crotolaria* spp. It is marked by cirrhosis of the liver, dullness, wasting, irritability, biting of other horses, gnawing fence posts, constant yawning, and muscular spasms leading to uncontrollable galloping, which gradually merges into aimless walking with a slow staggering gait and low stiff carriage of the head. Also called walk-about d.

Kimura's d., angiolymphoid hyperplasia—one or more erythematous dermal or subcutaneous nodules occurring primarily on the head and neck of young adults, sometimes associated with lymphadenopathy and peripheral eosinophilia. The more superficial, usually larger, lesions have been called pseudopyogenic granuloma.

Kinky hair d., see Menkes' syndrome.

Kinnier Wilson d., hepatolenticular degeneration. See Wilson's disease.

Kirkland's d., an acute infection of the throat with regional lymphadenitis.

Kissing d., see Filatov's d.

Klebs' d., glomerulonephritis.

Klemperer's d., see Banti's d.

Klippel's d., arthritic general pseudoparalysis—a condition resembling general paralysis, dependent on intracranial atheroma in arthritic persons.

Knight's d., infection of the perianal region following a minute abrasion of skin, so called historically because of the frequency of its occurrence in horsemen.

Köhler's bone d., 1. Osteochondrosis of the tarsal navicular bone in children; also called tarsal scaphoiditis, epiphysitis juvenilis, osteoarthrosis juvenilis, and os naviculare pedis retardatum. **2.** A disease of the second metatarsal bone with thickening of its shaft and changes about its articular head, characterized by pain in the second metatarsophalangeal joint on walking or standing. Also called Kohler's second d., and juvenile deforming metatarsophalangeal osteochondritis.

Köhler's second d., see Kohler's bone d., def. 2.

Köhler-Pellegrini-Stieda d., see Pellegrini's d.

Koshevnikoff's (Koschewnikow's, Kozhevnikov's) d., epilepsia partialis continua—continous clonic movements of the limited part of the body, due to an abnormal neuronal discharge.

Krabbe's d., a lysosomal storage disease due to deficient galactosylceramidase. It begins in infancy with irritability, fretfulness and rigidity, followed by tonic seizures, convulsions, quadriplegia, blindness, deafness, dysphagia and progressive mental deterioration. Pathologically, there is rapidly progressive cerebral demyelination and large globoid bodies in the white substance. Also called galactosylceramide lipidosis, galactosylceramide β-galactosidase deficiency, globoid, globoid cell, and Krabbe's leukodystrophy.

Krishaber's d., a neurosis characterized by tachycardia, insomnia, lightheadedness or vertigo, and hyperesthesia; Also called cerebrocardiac syndrome.

Kufs' d., see Jansky-Bielschowsky d.

Kugelberg-Welander d., a hereditary juvenile form of muscular atrophy, usually transmitted as an autosomal recessive trait, due to lesions of the anterior horns of the spinal cord. It is marked by onset in the first or second decade principally between two and seventeen years, and atrophy and weakness of the proximal muscles of the lower extremities and pelvic girdle, followed by involvement of the distal muscle and muscular twitchings. Cf: Werdnig-Hoffman paralysis.

Kuhnt-Junius d., disciform macular degeneration—a form of macular degeneration occurring in persons above 40 years of age, in which sclerosis involving the macula and retina is produced by hemorrhages between Bruch's membrane and the pigment epithelium.

Kümmell's d., compression fracture of vertebra; a complex of symptoms coming on in a few weeks after spinal injury, and consisting of pain in the spine, intercostal neuralgia, motor disturbances of the legs, and a gibbus of the spine which is painful on pressure and easily reduced by extension; post-traumatic spondylitis. Also called Kümmell-Verneuil d.

Kümmell-Verneuil d., se Kümmell's d.

Kuru d., It's a chronic, progressive, uniformly fatal nervous system disorder characterized by a long incubation period and transmissible to subhuman primates. It is found only among the fore and neighbouring peoples of New-guinea and is thought to be associated with cannibalism. The chief symptoms are truncal and limb atoxia, a shivering like tremors, and dysarthria, but strabismus and extrapyramidal symptoms may also be found. Pathologically the brain shows the changes of the spongiform encephalopathies, neuronal loss, gliosis and status spongiosus, amyloid plaques are also present in 2/3rd of the cases.

Kussmaul's d., Kussmaul-Maier d., periarteritis nodosa—classically, a form of systemic necrotizing vasculitis involving the small-and medium-sized arteries with signs and symptoms resulting from infarction and scarring of the affected organ system.

Kyasanur Forest d., a severe hemorrhagic fever marked by fever, hemorrhagic manifestation, and rash, occurring in the Mysore, Karnataka of India, first found in an epidemic among forest workers and monkeys in the Kyasanur Forest, caused by a flavivirus and transmitted to humans from monkey and vole reservoirs by ticks of the genus *Haemophysalis*, especially *H. spinigera*.

Kyrle's d., a rare chronic disorder of keratinization characterized by a papular eruption and the development of hyperkeratotic cone-shaped plugs in the hair follicles and eccrine ducts, which project through the epidermis into the dermis, producing a foreign body giant cell reaction and pain. The usually discrete lesions leave a crateriform depression on removal; they may coalesce to form circinate patches, and coalescing plaques are often seen. Also called hyperkeratosis follicularis et parafollicularis in cutem penetrans, hyperkeratosis follicularis in cutem penetrans, and hyperkeratosis penetrans.

Laennec's d., 1. Cirrhosis—cirrhosis of the liver closely associated with chronic excessive alcohol ingestion. In the early stages, liver enlargement may reflect fatty infiltration of liver cells (fatty c.), with necrosis and inflammation due to acute alcohol injury; progressive fibrosis extending from portal areas separates uniform small regeneration nodules. 2. Dissecting aneurysm—one resulting from hemorrhage that causes longitudinal splitting of the arterial wall, producing a tear in the intima and establishing communication with the lumen. It usually affects the thoracic aorta.

Lafora's d., myoclonus epilepsy—a slowly progressive autosomal recessive form of epilepsy beginning in childhood and characterized by attacks of intermittent or continuous clonus of muscle groups resulting in voluntary movements; there is mental deterioration, sometimes progressing to complete dementia, and the presence of Lafora's bodies in various cells, including those of the nervous system, retina, heart, muscle, and liver.

Lancereaux-Mathieu d., see Weil's syndrome.

Landouzy's d., see Weil's syndrome.

Landry's d., acute, febrile polyneuritis—rapidly progressive ascending motor neuron paralysis of unknown etiology, frequently following an enteric or respiratory infection. An autoimmune mechanism following viral infection has been postulated. It begins with paresthesias of the feet, followed by flaccid paralysis and weakness of the legs, ascending to the arms, trunk, and face, and is attended by slight fever, bulbar palsy, absent or lessened tendon reflexes, and an increase in the protein of the cerebrospinal fluid without corresponding increase in cells.

Lane's d., chronic intestinal stasis; small bowel obstruction in chronic constipation.

Larsen's d., Larsen-Johansson d., a disease of patella in which the X-ray shows an accessory center of ossification in the lower pole of the patella.

Lauber's d., fundus albipunctatus—a disorder in which gray or white mottling of the fundus of the eye is associated with night blindness.

Laughing d., see kuru d.

Leaf-curl d., a viral disease of plants characterized by curling or crinkling of the leaves.

Leber's d., 1. Leber's optic atrophy—a hereditary disorder of males, characterized by bilateral progressive atrophy, with onset usually at about the age of twenty. It is thought to be an X-linked trait. 2. Leber's congenital amaurosis—a characteristic and a rare type of blindness transmitted as an autosomal recessive trait, occurring at or shortly after birth and associated with an atypical form of diffuse pigmentation and commonly with optic atrophy and attenuation of the retinal vessels.

Legal's d., a disease affecting the pharyngotympanic region, and marked by headache and local inflammatory changes; Also called pharyngotympanic cephalalgia.

Legg's d., Legg-Calvé d., Legg-Calvé-Perthes d., Legg-Calvé-Waldenström d., osteochondrosis of the capitular epiphysis of the femur—a disease of the growth or ossification centers in children which begins as a degeneration or necrosis followed by regeneration or recalcification; also called epiphyseal ischemic necrosis. When it affects the capitular epiphysis (head) of the femur, it is called Legg-Calvé-Perthes disease.

Legionnaires' d., a highly fatal disease caused by a gram-negative bacillus (*Legionella pneumophila*), which is not spread by person-to-person contact and is characterized by high fever, gastrointestinal pain, headache, and penumonia; there may also be involvement of the kidneys, liver, and nervous system. The etiologic agent was identified after an outbreak occurred in the summer of 1976 at an American Legion convention in Philadelphia, Pennsylvania.

Leigh's d., subacute necrotizing encephalomyelopathy—an encephalopathy of unclear clinical and pathological criteria, causing neuropathologic and brainstem damage like that from the Wernicke-Korsakoff syndrome. It occurs in two forms: In the infantile, which may be same as pyruvate carboxylase deficiency, the chief pathological finding is degeneration of the gray matter with foci of necrosis and capillary proliferation in the brainstem, and chief biological findings are high lactate and pyruvate in the blood and low glucose in blood and CSF. There is a wide variety of manifestation, including anorexia and vomiting, slow or arrested development, hypotonia, seizures, abnormal movements, ocular and respiratory disorders, and dementia, with death usually occurring before age 3. In the adult form, the fist manifestation is bilateral optic atrophy with central scotoma and color blindness, which is followed by quiescent period of up to 30 years, after which ataxia, spastic paresis, clonic jerks, grandmal seizures, psychic lability, and mild dementia, appear.

Leiner's d., a disorder of infancy characterized principally by generalized seborrheic-like dermatitis and erythroderma, intractable, severe diarrhea, recurrent infections, and failure to thrive. The cause is unclear, but familial cases associated with a dysfunction of the C5 component of complement, which results in decreased phagocytosis of the patient's serum (opsonic activity), have been reported. Also called erythroderma de squamativum.

Lenegre's d., acquired complete heart block due to primary degeneration of the conduction system.

Leriche's d., post-traumatic osteoporosis—loss of bone substance following an injury in which there is damage to a nerve, sometimes due to an increased blood supply caused by the neurogenic insult, or to disuse secondary to pain.

Letterer-Siwe d., a nonlipid, autosomal recessive reticuloendotheliosis of early childhood, characterized by hemorrhagic tendency, eczematoid skin eruption, hepatosplenomegaly with lymph node enlargement, and progressive anemia. Also called L-S d. and acute disseminated histiocytosis X.

Lev's d., acquired complete heart block due to sclerosis of the cardiac skeleton.

Lewandowsky-Lutz d., epidermodysplasia verruciformis—the widespread and persistent, sometimes for decades, dissemination of verruca plana associated with a tendency to malignant degeneration. It typically begins in early childhood with the development of flat-topped papules, varying in color from pink and flesh to grey or brown, which increases in number and coalesces to form large plaques, especially on the knees, elbows, and trunk. Familial occurrence, parental consanguinity, and mental retardation are often associated with the disorder.

Leyden's d., a form of periodic vomiting.

Libman-Sacks d., atypical verrucous endocarditis—nonbacterial endocarditis found in association with systemic lupus erythematosus, in which the vegetations consist of necrotic debris, fibrinoid material, and trapped, disintegrating, fibroblastic and inflammatory cells.

Lichtheim's d., subacute combined degeneration of the spinal cord—degeneration of both the posterior and lateral columns of the spinal cord caused by vitamin B_{12} deficiency; a progressive disease, most often affecting persons over forty years of age, it is usually associated with pernicious anemia. The symptoms include paresthesias, ataxia, unsteadiness of gait, and sometimes emotional disorders.

Lignac's d., Lignac-Fanconi d., see Fanconi syndrome, def. 2.

Lindau's d., Lindau-von Hippel d., see von Hippel-Lindau d.

Lipid storage d., lipidosis—a term for several of the lysosomal storage diseases in which there is an abnormal accumulation of lipids in the reticuloendothelial cells.

Lipschütz's d., ulcus vulvae acutum—a nonvenereal, rapidly growing lesion of the vulva. The etiology is uncertain, but *Bacillus crassus*, a normally nonpathogenic species sometimes found in vaginal cultures, has been implicated.

Little's d., congenital spastic stiffness of the limbs, a form of cerebral spastic paralysis dating from birth and due to lack of development of the pyramidal tracts; it may be associated with various disorders, including birth trauma, fetal anoxia, or illness of the mother during pregnancy. Clinically, it is characterized by muscular weakness, walking difficulties, and, usually, by convulsions, bilateral athetosis, and mental deficiency. Also called spastic diplegia.

Lobo's d., keloidal blastomycosis—an infection caused by *Loboa loboi*, characterized by the appearance of red, smooth, hard cutaneous nodules which histologically, have the appearance of a keloid.

Lobstein's d., osterogenesis imperfecta, type I—see Durante's disease.

Local d., a condition which originates in and remains confined to one part.

Loco d., locoism—a disease of horses, cattle, and sheep caused by poisoning by loco and marked by locomotor disturbances, trembling, depression and, in pregnant animals, absorption.

Lorain's d., hypophysia infantilism—a type of dwarfism, with retention of infantile characteristics, due to undersecretion of the growth hormone and the gonadotrophic hormones of the anterior pituitary gland (adenohypophysis).

Lowe's d., see oculocerebrorenal syndrome.

L-S d., see Letterer-Siwe d.

Luft's d., a hypermetabolic disorder of striated muscle caused by an abnormal quantity and type of mitochondria producing excessive cellular respiration; it is characterized by profuse perspiration, asthenia, progressive weakness, and an abnormally increased basal metabolic rate.

Lumpy skin d., a highly infectious poxvirus disease indigenous to African cattle, which may result in permanent sterility or death, marked by the formation of nodules in the skin and sometimes in the mucous membranes. It resembles dermopathic herpesvirus disease (qv).

Lung fluke d., parasitic hemoptysis—a disease caused by infection of the lungs with *Paragonimus westermani* and other lung flukes of the genus *Paragonimus*. It is marked by cough and spitting of blood and by gradual deterioration of health.

Lunger d., pulmonary adenomatosis—a chronic progressive pneumonia of sheep, probably of viral region, with adenomatous proliferation in the alveoli and small bronchioles.

Lutembacher's d., see Lutembacher's syndrome.

Lutz-Splendore-Almeida d., paracoccidoidomycosis—an often fatal infection caused by *Paracoccidiodes brasiliensis*. The primary infection begins in the lungs and spreads to the mucocutaneous areas, particularly the buccal mucosa, and may extend to the adjacent skin, tonsils, gastrointestinal lymphatics, liver, and spleen.

Lyell's d., toxic epidermal necrolysis—an exfoliative skin disease seen primarily in adults, occurring as a severe cutaneous reaction to various etiologic factors, including primarily drugs but also infections (viral, bacterial, and fungal), neoplastic disease, graft-versus-host reaction, and chemical exposures. It is characterized histopathologically by full-thickness epidermal necrosis, resulting in subepidermal separation and bulla formation along with dermal inflammatory changes, and clinically by widespread loss of the skin leaving raw, denuded areas that make the skin surface look scalded.

Lyme d., a recurrent multisystemic disorder first reported in Old Lyme, Connecticut, beginning with the lesions of erythema chronicum migrans and followed by arthritis of the large joints, myalgia, malaise, and neurologic and cardiac manifestations. It is caused by the spirochete *Borrelia burgdorferi* with the vector being the tick *Ixodes dammini*. Also called Lyme arthritis.

Lymphocystic d. of fish, a disease of fish marked by the formation on the skin of spherical nodules caused by a virus.

Lymphoproliferative d's., lymphoproliferative—pertaining to or characterized by proliferation of the cells of the lymphoreticular system. The lymphoproliferative disorders compromise a group of malignant neoplasms arising from cells related to the common multipotential, primitive lymphoreticular cell that includes among others the lymphocytic, histiocytic, and monocytic leukemias, multiple myeloma, plasmacytoma, Hodgkin's disease, all lymphocytic lymphomas, and immunosecretory disorder associated with monoclonal gammopathy. An interrelationship with the myeloproliferative (qv) disorders is thought to exist.

Lymphoreticular d's., lymphoreticular—pertaining to the cells of the lymphoreticular system. The lymphoreticular disorders are characterized by the proliferation of lymphocytes or lymphoid tissues and may be either benign (e.g., lymphocytosis or lymphoid hyperplasia) or malignant (e.g., lymphocytic leukemias, multiple myeloma, and nonHodgkin's lymphoma).

Lysosomal storage d., any inborn error of metabolism having four characteristics: (i) a defect in a specific lysosomal hydrolase; (ii) intracellular accumulation of the unmetabolized substrate, (iii) clinical progression affecting multiple tissues and organs; (iv) considerable phenotypic variation within a disease. All but two of the lysosomal storage disorders are of autosomal recessive inheritance. The term comprises the mucolipidoses, mucopolysaccharidoses, glycoprotein storage diseases, and lipase deficies, ceramidase deficiency (Farber's lipogranulomatosis), α-galactosidase A deficiency (Fabry's disease), lipidoses and gangliosidoses. Also called lysosomal enzymopathy and inborn lysosomal d.

Machado-Joseph d., see Azorean d.

Mackenzie's d., see X disease.

MacLean-Maxwell d., a chronic condition of the calcaneus marked by enlargement of its posterior third and attended by pain on pressure.

Madelung's d., 1. Radial deviation of the hand secondary to overgrowth of distal ulna or shortening of the radius; also called carpus curvus. 2. Diffuse symmetrical lipomas of the neck.

Maher's d., paracolpitis—inflammation of the tissue around the vagina.

Majocchi's d., purpura anularis telangiectodes—a rare purpuric eruption, commonly beginning on the lower extremities and becoming generalized, the original punctate erythematous lesions coalescing to form an annular or serpiginous pattern; involution is gradual, sometimes followed by atrophy and loss of hair in the area.

Malassez's d., cyst of the testis.

Malibu d., surfers' nodules—hyperplastic, fibrosing, rarely ulcerated granulomas 1 to 3 cm in diameter, occurring over bony prominences of the feet and legs of surfers, occurring as a result of repeated trauma from kneeling on surfboards.

Manson's d., a species found in Egypt and elsewhere in Africa as well as in South America and West Indies, including Puerto Rico, which causes schistosomiasis mansoni by penetrating the skin of persons coming in contact with infested waters; the transmitting hosts are planorbid snails, especially of the genus *Biomphalaria*.

Maple bark d., a granulomatous interstitial pneumonitis caused by inhalation of spores from *Coniosporium corticale*, a mold found beneath the bark of maple logs.

Maple syrup urine d. (MSUD), a genetic aminoacidopathy due to an enzyme deficiency in the second step in branched-chain amino acid (BCAA) catabolism; the BCAAs and their analogues accumulate in the blood and urine, causing severe ketoacidosis soon after birth, death in about half the newborns, seizures, coma, physical and mental retardation, and a characteristic smell of maple syrup or curry in the urine and on the body. There are five clinical phenotypes of MSUD: classic, intermittent, intermediate, thiamine-responsive and dihydrolipoyl dehydrogenase (E_3) deficiency. Also called ketoacid decarboxylase deficiency and branched-chain ketoaciduria or ketoaminoacidemia.

Marburg d., Marburg virus d., a severe, acute, often fatal, viral hemorrhagic fever, characterized by fever, prostration, hemorrhagic manifestations, pancreatitis, and hepatitis, the first reported primary cases of which were in Marburg and Frankfurt, Germany, and Belgrade, Yugoslavia, in laboratory workers handling infected African green monkeys or their organs; secondary infection is acquired through direct physical contact with infected patients. It has been reported as occurring in Kenya, Zimbabwe, and South Africa.

March's d., see Graves'd.

Marchiafava-Bignami d., progressive degeneration of the corpus callosum, characterized by progressive intellectual deterioration, emotional disturbances, confusion, hallucinations, tremor, rigidity, and convulsions. It is a very rare disorder affecting chiefly middle-aged male alcoholics, especially those who consume excessive amounts of crude red wine.

Marchiafava-Micheli d., paroxysmal nocturnal hemoglobinuria—a chronic aquired blood cell dysplasia in which there is proliferation of clone of stem cells producing erthrocytes, platelets, and granulocytes that are abnormally susceptible to lysis by complement; it is marked by episodes of intravascular hemolysis, particularly following infections; and by venous thromboses, particularly of the hepatic veins; diagnosis is based on acidified serum test (Ham's test) or the sucrose lysis test.

Marek's d., lymphoproliferative disease of chickens caused by a herpesvirus. Lymphoid cell infiltrations are most common in the peripheral nerves and gonads, but widespread infiltrations may also be found in any of the visceral organs, skin, muscle, and the iris of the eye. Perivascular cuffing of blood vessels in the brain and spinal cord frequently occurs. The location of the lesions dictates the clinical signs, such as paralysis, general depression, and blindness. It was once included in the avian leukosis complex. Also called, according to the symptoms manifested, acute leukosis, fowl paralysis, ocular lymphomatosis, neural lymphomatosis, neurolymphomatosis gallinarum, range paralysis, and skin leukosis.

Margarine d., erythema multiforme (a symptom complex representing reaction pattern of the skin and mucous membranes secondary to various known, suspected, and unknown factors, including infections, ingestants, physical agents, malignancy, and pregnancy. The conditions in the complex are characterized by sudden onset of an erythematous macular, bullous, papular, nodose, or vesiuclar eruption, the characteristic lesion being the iris, bull's eye, or target lesion, which consist of central papule with two or more concentric rings. The complex comprise a mild self-limited mucocutaneous form, i.e., multiforme minor; see Hebra's d; and a severe sometimes fatal, multisystem form, i.e. multiforme minor; see Stevens-Johnson syndrome) due to an emulsifier in oleomargarine; it occurred as an explosive epidemic outbreak in Germany and Holland, thought at the time to be infectious in origin.

Marie's d., 1. Acromegaly—a chronic disease of adult caused by hypersecretion of pituitary growth hormone and characterized by enlargement of many parts of the skeleton, especially the distal portion—the nose, ears, jaws, fingers, and toes. 2. Hypertrophic pulmonary osteoarthropathy—symmetrical enlargement of the four limbs chiefly localized to the phalanges and terminal epiphyses of the long bones of the forearms and leg, sometimes extending to the proximal ends of the limbs and the flat bones, and accompanied by dorsal kyphosis and some affection of the lungs and heart.

Marie-Bamberger d., hypertrophic pulmonary osteoarthropathy—see Marie's d. (2).

Marie-Strümpell d., rheumatoid spondylitis—see Bekhterev's d.,

Marie-Tooth d., progressive neuropathic (peroneal) muscular atrophy—a hereditary form of muscular atrophy, beginning in the muscles supplied by the peroneal nerves, progressing slowly to involve the muscles of the hands and arms.

Marion's d., congenital obstruction of the posterior urethra due to muscular hypertrophy of the bladder neck or absence of the plexiform dilator fibers in the urinary tract.

Marsh's d., see Graves'd.

Martin's d., periosteoarthritis of the foot from excessive walking.

McArdle's d., see glycogen storage d. (type v).

Medin's d., poliomyelitis—an acute viral disease, occurring sporadically and in epidemics, and characterized clinically by fever, sore throat, headache, and vomiting, often with stiffness of back and neck. In the minor illness these may be the only symptoms. The major illness, which may or may not be preceded by the minor illness, is characterized by involvement of the central nervous system, stiff neck, pleocytosis in the spinal fluid, and perhaps paralysis. There may be subsequent atrophy or groups of muscles, ending in contraction and permanent deformity.

Mediterranean d., β-thalassemia caused by diminished synthesis of beta chains of hemoglobin. The homozygous form, in which hemoglobin A is completely absent and which appears in the newborn period, is a severe form marked by hemolytic, hypochromic-microcytic anemia, pronounced hepatosplenomegaly, skeletal deformation, mongloid facies, and cardiac enlargement.

Medullary cystic d., familial juvenile nephronophthisis—a progressive hereditary disease of the kidneys characterized clinically anemia, polyuria, and renal loss of sodium, progressing to chronic renal failure; pathologically, there is tubular atrophy, interstitial fibrosis, glomerular sclerosis, and medullary cysts.

Meige's d., see Milroy's d.

Ménétrier's d., giant hypertrophic gastritis—excessive proliferation of the gastric mucosa, producing diffuse thickening of the stomach wall; inflammatory changes may be associated.

Méniére's d., hearing loss, tinnitus, and vertigo resulting from nonsuppurative disease of the labyrinth with the histapathologic feature of endolymphatic hydrops (distention of the membranous labyrinth).

Menkes' d., see under syndrome.

Mental d., see under disorder.

Merzbacher-Pelizaeus d., see Pelizaeus-Merzbacher d.

Metabolic d., general term for diseases caused by disruption of a normal metabolic pathway because of a genetically determined enzyme defect.

Metazoan d., a disease caused by metazoan parasites, such as nematodes, cestodes, trematodes, and arthropods.

Meyer's d., adenoid vegetations of the pharynx.

Meyer-Betz d., a rare, familial disease of unknown etiology, marked by attacks of myoglobinuria, which may be precipitated by strenuous exertion or possibly by an infection, and which results in tenderness, swelling, and weakness of muscles of varying intensity. It may occur with or without diffuse chronic myopathy or dystrophy. Also called idiopathic, spontaneous or familial myoglobinuria.

Microdrepanocytic d., see sickle cell-thalassemia d.

Mikulicz's d., originally, a chronic, benign, and usually painless inflammatory swelling of the lacrimal and salivary glands; some authorities have broadened the entity to include lacrimal and salivary gland enlargement associated with other diseases, such as Sjögren's syndrome, sarcoidosis, lupus erythematosus, leukemia, lymphoma, and tuberculosis, which they designate Mikulicz's syndrome (see under syndrome).

Milky d., milky-white d., a fatal infection of beetle larvae due to *Bacillus papilliae* or *B. lentimorbus* in which the "blood" of the larvae appears milky white as a result of the profuse multiplication and sporulation of the bacilli. The infection may be produced deliberately in Japanese beetle to control their population.

Miller's d., osteomalacia—a condition marked by softening of the bones (due to impaired mineralization, with excess accumulation of osteoid), with pain, tenderness, muscular weakness, anorexia, and loss of weight, resulting from deficiency of vitamin D and calcium.

Mills' d., ascending hemiplegia that eventually develops into quadriplegia; its etiology is unknown.

Milroy's d., congenital hereditary lymphedema of the legs, caused by chronic lymphatic obstruction; other areas, including the arms, trunk, and face may be involved. Also called Meige's d., Milroy's edema, Nonne-Milroy-Meige syndrome, and congenital lymphedema.

Milton's d., angioneurotic edema—a vascular reaction involving the deep dermis or subcutaneous or submucosal tissues, representing localized edema caused by dilatation and increased permeability of the capillaries. and characterized by development of giant wheals. Hereditary angioedema, transmitted as an autosomal dominant trait, tends to involve more visceral lesions than the sporadic form and is caused by deficiency or functional impairment of complement component C1 estrase inhibitor (CIINH) resulting in increased levels of several vasoactive mediators of anaphylaxis. Urticaria (qv) is the same physiologic reaction occurring in the superficial portions of the dermis.

Minamata d., a severe, neurologic disorder caused by alkyl mercury poisoning, usually characterized by peripheral and circumoral paresthesia, ataxia, dysarthria, and loss of peripheral vision, and leading to severe permanent neurologic and mental disabilities or death. It was prevalent between 1953 and 1958 among those who ate sea food from Minamata Bay, Japan, which contained an excess of alkyl mercury compounds.

Minor's d., hematomyelia (hemorrhage into the spinal cord, usually confined to the gray substance most often due to trauma, and marked by the sudden onset of flaccid paralysis with sensory disturbances) involving the central parts of the spinal cord.

Mitchell's d., see Gerhardt's disease.

Mixed connective tissue d., a disorder combining features or scleroderma, myositis, systemic lupus erythematosus, and rheumatoid arthritis, and marked serologically by the presence of antibody against extractable nuclear antigen.

Möbius' d., periodic migraine with paralysis of the oculomotor muscles.

Moeller-Barlow d., subperiosteal hematoma in rickets.

Molecular d., any disease in which the pathogenesis can be traced to a single molecule, usually a protein, which is either abnormal in structure or present in reduced amounts; the classical example is abnormal hemoglobin in sickle cell anemia.

Molten's d., see Pictou's d.

Mondor's d., phlebitis affecting the large subcutaneous veins normally crossing the lateral chest region and breast from the epigastric or hypochondriac region to the axilla, occurring in both males and females.

Monge's d., see Andes disease.

Morgagni's d., hyperostosis frontalis intern—thickening of the inner table of the frontal bone, which may be associated with hypertrichosis and obesity; it most commonly affects women near menopause.

Morquio's d., see Morquio's syndrome.

Morquio-Ullrich d., see Morquio's syndrome.

Morton's d., a form of metatarsalgia due to compression of a branch of the plantar nerve by the metatarsal heads; chronic compression may lead to formation of a neuroma.

Morvan's d., 1. Syringomyelia—a slowly progressive syndrome in which cavitation occurs in the central segments of the spinal cord, generally involving the cervical region, but the lesions may extend up into medulla oblongata (syringobulbia) or down into the thoracic region; it may be of developmental origin, arise secondary to tumor, trauma, infarction, or hemorrhage, or be without known cause. It results in neurological deficits that generally consists of segmental muscular weakness and atrophy accompanied by a dissociated sensory loss (loss of pain touch) and thoracic scoliosis is often present. Sometimes, the use of the term syringomyelia is restricted to the condition, with the terms segmental sensory dissociation with brachial muscular atrophy, and syndrome of sensory dissociation with brachial amyotrophy being used to denote a similar clinical condition that may be associated with other pathological lesions or states. 2. see under syndrome, def. 2.

Mosaic d., infectious diseases of plants caused by viruses and characterized by mottling of the foliage.

Moschcowitz's d., thrombotic thrombocytopenic purpura—a disease of undefined cause, characterized by thrombocytopenia, hemolytic anemia, bizarre neurological manifestations, azotemia, fever and thromboses in terminal arterioles and capillaries.

Motor neuron d., any disease of a motor neuron, including spinal muscular atrophy, progressive bulbar paralysis, amyotrophic lateral sclerosis and lateral sclerosis.

Mountain d., see, Acosta's disease and Andes disease and Monge's disease.

Moyamoya d., (Jap moyamoya puff of smoke, from the angiographic appearance) cerebral ischemia due to occlusion and small hemorrhages from rupture of an abnormal network of vessels at the base of the brain, causing progressive neurologic disability; it occurs predominantly in the Japanese.

Mozer's d., 1. Sclerosis of the spinal cord. 2. A condition characterized by obliteration of the normal marrow cavity by the formation of small spicules of bone, the pathogenesis possibly being similar to that of myelofibrosis.

Muchain d., the rarest heavy chain disease, found in patients with chronic lymphocytic leukemia, with symptoms of hepatomegaly and splenomegaly.

Mucha's d., Mucha-Habermann d, see Haberman's disease.

Mucosal d., a disease of cattle, due to the virus of bovine virus diarrhea; ulcerations in the mouth may be the only sign, but often there is fever, diarrhea, loss of appetite, and a drop in milk yield.

Mule spinner's d., warts or ulcers of the skin, especially of the scrotum, which tend to become malignant; so called because they were found chiefly among the operators of spinning mules in cotton mills.

Münchmeyer's d., a diffuse progressive ossifying polymyositis.

Murray Valley d., a viral encephalitis that occurred epidemically in 1950 and 1951 in the Murray Valley, Victoria, Australia, believed to be a recrudescence of Australian X-disease; a few cases occurred in 1956 and it has been reported in the New Guinea.

Mushroom picker's d., Mushroom worker's d., an allergic respiratory disease closely resembling farmer's lung, developing in persons working with moldy compost prepared for growing mushrooms in closed areas, especially in those handling the dried material after harvesting.

Mushy chick d., omphalitis of birds—infection of the yolk sac with the bacteria normally found in the alimentary and on the skin of the hen, leading to the death of the embryos and chicks, occurring up to 10 days after hatching.

Nairobi d., an infectious disease of sheep and goats in Africa, especially in the region around Nairobi, marked by acute hemorrhagic gastroenteritis, green, watery diarrhea, mucopurulent nasal discharge, and breathing difficulty; it is caused by a virus transmitted by the ticks *Rhipicephalus appendiculatus* and *Amblyomma variegatum*.

Nanukayami d., nanukayami—a leptospirosis marked by fever and jaundice, first reported in Japan and caused by *Leptospira interrogans* serogroups hebdomidis; the animal host is the field vole, *Microtus montebelli*.

Navicular d., necrotic inflammation of the navicular bone in horses, causing intermittent lameness; also called grog.

Newcastle d., an influenza-like viral disease of birds, including domestic fowl, characterized by respiratory and gastrointestinal or pneumonic and encephalitis symptoms. First seen near Newcastle, England, the infection is also transmissible to man by contact with infected birds. Also called avain influenza.

New duck d., infectious avian serositis in ducklings.

Nicolas-Favre d., see Durand-Nicolas-Favre d.

Niemann's d., Niemann-Pick d., sphingolipidosis due to sphingomyelinase deficiency with sphingomyelin accumulation in the reticuloendothelial system. There are five types distinguished by age of onset and by the amount of CNS involvement and of sphingomyelinase activity. Type A (acute neuronopathic) in the classic type, accounting for 85 percent of the patients; onset is in early infancy; CNS damage is severe; death occurs by 4 years. Type B (chronic non-neuronopathic) has onset in early infancy but does not affect the CNS or intelligence; normal lifespan is possible. Type C (chronic neuronopathic) has variable CNS involvement. Type D (the Nova Scotia variant) resembles type C; type E (the adult, non-neuronopathic form may be a late-onset variant of type C. Also called sphingolipidosis, sphingomyelin lipidosis, and sphingomyelinase deficiency.

Nodule d., nodular worm d., a disease of sheep and cattle, caused by a minute worm, *Oesophagostomum columbianum*, which infests the intestines, becoming embedded in the mucous membrane, where it causes the formation of nodules of varying size.

Norrie's d., a congenital, X-linked disorder consisting of bilateral blindness from retinal malformation with possible mental retardation and deafness developing later; also called atrophic bulborum hereditaria.

Norum-Gjone d., familial lecithin-cholesterol acyltransferase deficiency.

Nosema d., a disease of bees caused by *Nosema apis* characterized by dysentery and paralysis.

Notifiable d., one required to be reported to federal, state, or local health officials when diagnosed, because of infectiousnes, severity, or frequency of occurrence; also called reportable d.

Novy's rat d., a viral disease discovered by Novy in his stock of experimental rats.

Oasthouse urine d., see methionine malabsorption syndrome.

Occupational d., one due to factors involved in one's employment, e.g., various forms of pneumocioniosis or dermatitis.

Oguchi's d., a form of congenital night blindness occurring in Japan.

Ohara's d., see Francis d.

Oid-Oid d., (from discoid and lichenoid), exudative discoid and lichenoid dermatitis—a form of neurodermatitis occurring predominantly in middle aged or older men of the Jewish origin, characterized by intense pruritus with exudative, weeping discoid and oval patches scattered irregularly over most of the body, many of which are of the eczematous type and undergo lichenification, or they may resemble lesion seen in various other cutaneous disorders such as mycosis fungoides or lichen planus.

Ollier's d., enchondromatosis—a condition characterized by hamartomatous proliferation of cartilage cells within the metaphysis of several bones, causing thinning of the overlying cortex and distortion of the growth in length. In combination with multiple cutaneous or visceral hemangiomas, the disorder is known as Maffucci's syndrome.

Ondiri d., bovine infectious petechial fever—a disease of cattle in Kenya, characterized by hemorrhages of the visible mucous membranes, fever, and diarrhea; there may be severe conjunctivitis and protrusion of the eyeball, and death within one to three days is not uncommon. The cause is believed to be a rickettsial-like organism, *Cytoectes ondiri* spread by biting insect.

Opitz's d., thrombophlebitic splenomegaly—enlargement of the spleen due to thrombosis of the splenic vein.

Oppenheim's d., amyotonia congenital—any of several rare congenital diseases of children marked by general hypotonia of the muscles.

Organic d., one associated with demonstrable change in a bodily organ or tissue.

Oriental lung fluke d., parasitic hemoptysis—a disease caused by infection of the lungs with *Paragonimus westermani* and other lung flukes of the genus *Paragonimus*. It is marked by cough and spitting of blood and by gradual deterioration of health.

Ormond's d., retroperitoneal fibrosis—deposition of fibrous tissue in the retroperitoneal space, producing vague abdominal discomfort, and often causing blockage of the ureters, with resultant hydronephrosis and impaired renal function, which may result in renal failure.

Osgood-Schlatter d., osteochondrosis of the tuberosity of the tibia; also called apophysitis tibialis adolescentium, Schlatter's d. and Schlatter-Osgood d.

Osler's d., 1. Polycythemia vera—a myeloproliferative disorder of unknown etiology, characterized by abnormal proliferation of all hematopoietic bone marrow elements and an absolute increase in red cell mass and total blood volume, associate frequently with splenomegaly, leukocytosis and thrombocythemia. Hematopoiesis is also reactive in extramedullary sites (liver and spleen). In time, myelofibrosis occurs. 2. Hereditary hemorrhagic telangiectasia—an autosomal dominant vascular anomaly characterized by the presence of multiple small telangiectases of the skin, mucous membranes, gastrointestinal tract, and other organs, associated with recurrent episodes of bleeding from affected sites and gross or occult melena.

Osler-Vaquez d., see Osler's d.,

Osler-Weber-Rendu d., see Osler's d. and Goldstein's d.

Otto's d., osteoarthritic protrusion of the acetabulum; arthrokatadysis—a sinkin in or subsidence of the floor of the acetabulum with protrusion of the femoral head through it (intrapelvic protrusion) resulting in limitation of movement of the hip joint.

Overeating d., see pulpy kidney d.

Owren's d., Factor V deficiency—an autosomal recessive trait, leads to a rare hemorrhagic tendency, known as parahemophilia, which varies greatly in severity.

Ox-warble d., see larva migrans*.

Paas' d., a familial disorder marked by skeletal deformities such as coxa valga, shortening of phalanges, scoliosis, spondylitis, etc.

Paget's d., 1. Intraductal carcinoma of the breast extending to involve the nipple and areola, characterized clinically by eczema-like inflammatory skin changes, and histologically by infiltration of the epidermis by malignant cells (Paget's cells). 2. A neoplasm of the vulva and sometimes the perianal region histologically and clinically quite similar to Paget's disease of the breast, but having less of a tendency to be associated with underlying invasive carcinoma. 3. Osteitis deformans—a disease of the bone marked by repeated

---

*See Appendix

episodes of increased bone resorption followed by excessive attempts at repair, resulting in weakened deformed bones of increased mass. There may be bowing of the long bones and deformation of flat bones; pain and pathological features are associated. When if affects the bones of the skull, deafness may result.

Paget's d. extramammary, see Paget's d., def 2.

Panner's d., osteochondrosis of the capitellum of the humerus.

Parenchymatous d., one which attacks the parenchyma of an organ.

Parkinson's d., paralysis agitans—a form of parkinsonism of unknown etiology usually occurring in late life, although a juvenile form has been described. It is a slowly progressive disease characterized by mask-like facies, a characteristic tremor of resting muscles, a slowing of voluntary movements, a festinating gait, peculiar posture, and weakness of the muscles. There may be excessive sweating and feelings of the heat. Pathologically, there is degeneration within the nuclear masses of the extrapyramidal system and a characteristic loss of melanin-containing cells from the substantia nigra and a corresponding reduction in dopamine levels in the corpus striatum.

Parrot's d., psittacosis—primarily an acute or chronic respiratory and systemic disease of various wild and domestic birds, originally thought to be seen only in psittacine birds, which is caused by *Chlamydia psittaci* and is transmissible to humans and the other animals. Human infection, generally acquired by inhalation of dried bird excreta containing the pathogen or rarely by handling feathers or tissue of infected birds or through an open lesion or the bite of an infected bird, may be asymptomatic, or it may be manifested by mild influenza-like symptoms or sometimes by a severe and highly fatal pneumonia.

Parrot's d., pseudoparalysis of one or more of the extremities in infants caused by syphilitic osteochondritis of an epiphysis.

Parry's d., toxic nodular goiter, see Graves' disease.

Patella's d., pyloric stenosis in tuberculosis patients, following fibrous stenosis.

Pavy's d., cyclic proteinuria—a term once used to denote the appearance at stated times each day of a small amount of protein in the urine; it is observed principally in young persons.

Payr's d., constipation with left upper quadrant pain attributed to kinking of a andhesion between the transverse and descending colon with obstruction; probably a manifestation of the irritable colon syndrome rather than an organic lesion. Also called splenic flexure syndrome.

Pearl d., tuberculosis of the peritoneum and mesentery of cattle.

Pearl-worker's d., recurrent inflammation of bone with hypertrophy seen in persons who work in pearl dust.

Pel-Ebstien d., see Hodgkin's d.

Pelizaeus-Merzbacher d., a familial form of leukoencephalopathy (qv) occurring in early life and running a slowly progressive course into adolescence or adulthood. It is marked by nystagmus, ataxia, tremor, choreoathetotic movements, parkinsonian facies, dysarthria, and mental deterioration. Pathologically, there is diffuse demyelination in the white substance of the brain, which may involve the brainstem, cerebellum, and spinal cord.

Pellegrini's d., Pellegrini-Stieda d., a condition characterized by a semilunar bony formation in the upper portion of the medial lateral ligament of the knee, due to traumatism; also called Kohler-Pellegrini-Stieda d. and Stieda's d.

Pelvic inflammatory d., any ascending pelvic infection involving the upper female genital tract beyond the cervix.

Periodic d., a condition characterized by regularly recurring and intermittent episodes of fever, edema, arthralgia, or gastric pain and vomiting, continuing for years without further development in otherwise healthy individuals.

Periodontal d., any of a group of pathological conditions that affect the surrounding and supporting tissues of the teeth, generally classified as inflammatory (gingivitis and periodontitis), dystrophic (periodontal trauma and periodontosis), and anomalies.

Perrin-Ferraton d., snapping hip—a condition marked by slipping around of the hip joint, sometimes with an audible snap, due to slipping tendinous band over the greater trochanter.

Perthes' d., osteochondrosis of the capital femoral epiphysis; see Legg-Calve'-Perthes d.

Peyronie's d., induration of the corpora cavernosa of the penis, producing a fibrous chordee; also called fibrous cavernitis, penis plastica, and penile induration.

Pfeiffer's d., infectious mononucleosis, see Filatov's d.

Phocas' d., chronic glandular mastitis with the formation of numerous small nodules.

Phytanic acid storage d., see Refsum's d.

Pick's d., 1. (Arnold Pick) a rare, progressive degenerative disease of the brain very similar in clinical manifestations and course of Alzeimer's disease but having distinctive histopathology; cortical atrophy is confined to the frontal and temporal lobes; degenerating neurons contain globular intracytoplasmic filamentous inclusions (Pick's bodies). Also called circumscribed cerebral aytophy. 2. (Friedel Pick) (obs). pericardial pseudocirrhosis of the liver; congestive cirrhosis resulting from constrictive pericarditis. 3. (Ludwig Pick) see Niemann-Pick d.

Pictou's d., cirrhosis of the liver in horses and cattle in Nova Scotia due to ingestion of *Senecio jacobeus*, the ragwort; also called Molten's d. and Winton's d.

Pink d., acrodynia, see Feer's d.,

Plaster of Paris d., atrophy of a limb which has been enclosed in a plaster of Paris splint.

Plummer's d., toxic multinodular goiter, see Graves' d.

Pneumatic hammer d., vasospastic disease in the hands resulting from use of a pneumatic hammer.

Policeman's d., tarsalgia—pain in the ankle or foot.

Polycystic d. of kidneys, a heritable disorder marked by cysts scattered throughout both kidneys. It occurs in two unrelated forms: The infantile form, transmitted as an autosomal recessive trait, may be congenital or appear at any time during childhood. There is a high perinatal mortality rate, and almost all cases lead to hypertension. In older children cystic and fibrotic disease of the liver may be associated. The adult form, transmitted as an autosomal dominant trait, is marked by progressive deterioration of renal function. Also called polycystic kidneys and polycystic renal d.

Polycystic ovary d., see Stein-Leventhal syndrome.

Polycystic renal d., see polycystic kidney d.

Polyendocrine autoimmune d., the combination of endocrine and nonendocrine autoimmune diseases. In type I, which occurs in infants and children, candidiasis, hypoparathyroidism, and adrenal insufficiency are associated, and pernicious anemia, vitiligo, gonadal failure, alopecia, insulin-dependent diabetes, and thyroid autoimmune disease may also occur; also called autoimmune polyendocrine-candidiasis syndrome. Type II is known as Schmidt's syndrome.

Polyhedral d., infectious diseases of insects, especially caterpillars, caused by viruses.

Pompe's d., glycogen storage d. (type II).

Poncet's d., tuberculous rheumatism—a bacterial arthritis occurring secondary to tuberculosis; it usually affects a single joint and is characterized by chronic inflammation with effusion and destruction of contiguous bone.

Portuguese-Azorean d., see Azorean d.

Posada-Wernicke d., coccidioidomycosis, see California d.

Pott's d., tuberculosis of the spine—osteitis or caries of the vertebrae usually occurring as a complication of tuberculosis of the lungs; it is marked by stiffness of the vertebral column, pain on motion, tenderness on pressure, prominence of certain of the vertebral spines, and occasionally abdominal pain, abscess formation and paralysis.

Pregnancy d., pregnancy toxemia in ewes—an acute disorder leading to impaired nervous function, coma, and death, occurring during the last few pregnancies in ewes that are typically twins, triplets, or a particularly large single lamb; the principal predisposing cause is undernutrition association with stress.

Preiser's d., osteoporosis and atrophy of the carpal scaphoid due to trauma or fracture which has not been kept immobilized.

Pringle's d., adenoma sebaceum—nevoid hyperplasia of sebaceous glands, forming multiple yellow papules or nodules of the face (Balzer type); a cutaneous malformation or hamartoma of the face involving blood vessels and connective tissue associated with the tuberous sclerosis complex (Pringle type). In the pringle type, the term adenoma sebaceum is a misnomer since the sebaceous glands are rarely involved.

Profichet's d., see under syndrome

Pullet d., pyelonephritis of young hens of unknown etiology, characterized by loss of appetite, diarrhea with watery or whitish evacuations, and sometimes darkening of the comb; affected birds appear drowsy.

Pullorum d., an infectious disease of young chickens marked by loss of appetite, dullness, and diarrhea, the discharge of which leaves white clumps around the cloaca; it is caused by *Salmonella pullorum*.

Pulpy kidney d., a fatal enterotoxemia usually seen in young animal, chiefly lambs, but which may affect sheep, goats, and cattle of any age; it is caused by *Clostridium perfringens* type D. Pathologically, the kidneys are mottled and soft in consistency and the cortex is jelly-like or almost semifluid; the liver is severely congested with small hemorrhages diffusely scattered over its surface.

Pulseless d., progressive obliteration of the brachiocephalic trunk and the left subclavian and left common carotid arteries above their origin in the aortic arch, leading to loss of pulse in both arms and carotids and to symptoms associated with ischemia of the brain (syncope, transient hemiplegia, etc), eyes (transient blindness, retinal atrophy, etc.), face (muscular atrophy, etc.), and arms (claudication, etc.). Also called arteritis brachiocephalica or brachiocephalic arteritis. Martorell's syndrome, reversed coarctation, and Takayasu's disease or syndrome.

Purtscher's d., traumatic angiopathy of the retina with edema, hemorrhage, and exudation, usually following crush injuries of the chest; Also called Purtscher's angiopathic retinopathy.

Pyle's d., metaphyseal dysplasia. see Jansen's d.

Pyramidal d., buttress foot—a condition of periostitis or ostitis in the region of the pyramidal process of the os pedis of the horse, with fracture of the process, deformity of the hoof, and alteration of the normal angle of the joint.

Quervain's d., see de Quervain's d.

Quincke's d., angioedema, see Milton's d., or Bannister's d.

Ragpicker's d., ragsorter's d., inhalational anthrax—a highly fatal form of anthrax due to inhalation of dust contaning anthrax spores, which are transported by the alveolar pneumocytes to the regional lymph nodes where they germinate, multiply, and produce toxin, and characterized by hemorrhagic edematous mediastinitis, pleural effusions, dyspnea, cyanosis, stridor, and shock. It is usually an occupational disease, most often affecting those who handle and sort contaminated wools and fleeces.

Railroad d., transit tetany—a condition usually affecting well-fed cows and ewes in advanced pregnancy and in lactating mares that have been shipped long distances, which may result in paralysis, unconsciousness, and death unless treatment is begun early in the course of disease. The etiology is unknown, but may be due to acute hypocalcium associated with improper feeding and care.

Ramsay Hunt d., see under syndrome, def 1.

Rat bite d., either of two clinically similar but etiologically distinct, acute infectious disease, usually transmitted through bite of rat, and occurring in a bacillary form caused by *Streptobacillus monilliformis*, and in a spirally form caused by *Spirillum minus*. In the bacillary form, there is a latent period of a week to ten days, during which time the original wound heals promptly without inflammation, but then the bite site becomes inflammed, painful, and indurated, followed by adenitis, chills, vomiting, headache, high fever, morbilliform eruption, especially on the hands and feet, and polyarthritis that is often severe. This form may also be associated with ingestion of contaminated raw milk or its products (Haverhill fever), in which case there is no initial wound, the first symptoms being systemic. In the spirally form, the latent period is most commonly greater than ten days, inflammation recurs at the primary wound site, the rash is less evident than in the bacillary form, arthritis is rare, and the fever is commonly of the relapsing type.

Raynaud's d., 1. A primary or idiopathic vascular disorder characterized by bilateral attacks of Raynauds's phenomenon. The disease affects females more frequently than males. Also called Raynaud's gangrene. See Raynauds' phenomenon, under phenomenon. 2. Paralysis of the throat muscle following parotiditis; also called local asphyxia.

Recklinghausen's d., neurofibromatosis—a familial condition characterized by developmental changes in the nervous system, muscles, bones and skin and marked superficially by the formation of multiple pedunculated soft tumors (neurofibromas) distributed over the entire body associated with areas of pigmentation.

Recklinghausen's d. of bone, osteitis fibrosa cystica—rarefying osteitis with fibrous degeneration and formation of cysts, and with the presence of fibrous nodules on the affected bones; it is due to marked osteoclastic activity secondary to hyperfunction of the parathyroid gland.

Recklinghausen-Applebaum d., hemochromatosis—a disorder due to deposition of hemosiderin in the parenchymal cells, causing tissued damage and dysfunction of the liver, pancreas, heart, and pituitary. Other clinical signs include bronze pigmentation of skin, arthropathy, diabetes, cirrhosis, hepatosplenomegaly, hypogonadism, and loss of body hair. Full development of the disease among women is restricted by menstruation, pregnancy, and lower dietary intake of iron. Acquired hemochromatosis may be the result of blood transfusions, excessive dietary iron, or secondary to other disease, e.g., thalassemia or sideroblastic anemia. Idiopathic or genetic hemochromatosis is an autosomal recessive disorder of metabolism associated with a gene tightly linked to the A locus of the HLA complex on chromosome 6.

Reclus' d., 1. A painless, cystic enlargement of the mammary glands, marked by multiple dilatations of the acini and ducts. 2. Cellulitis with induration.

Redwater d., bacillary hemoglobinuria—an infectious disease caused by *Clostridium haemolyticum*—affecting primarily cattle, occasionally sheep, and rarely dogs. In cattle, it is marked by inappetance, by cessation of rumination, lactation, and defecation, by fever, bloody diarrhea, and dark-red urine, and by anemia and hemoglobinuria.

Reed-Hodgkin d., see Hodgkin's d.

Refsum's d., an inborn error of metabolism caused by accumulation of phytanic acid, and manifested chiefly by chronic polyneuritis, retinitis pigmentosa, cerebellar ataxia, and persistent elevation of protein in cerebrospinal fluid; there may also be ichthyosis, nerve deafness, and electrocardiographic abnormalities. Also called phytanic acid storage d, heredopathia atactica polyneuritiformis, and Refsum's syndrome.

Reichmann's d. (of cs.), gastrosuccorrhea—excessive and continuous secretion of gastric juice.

Reiter's d., see under syndrome.

Rendu-Osler-Weber d., hereditary hemorrhagic telangiectasia, see Osler-Rendu-Weber d.

Renikhet d. (obs.), see Newcastle d. in chickens.

Reportable d., see notifiable d.

Rheumatic heart d., the most important manifestation of and sequel to rheumatic fever (qv), consisting chiefly of valvular deformities.

Rheumatoid d., a systemic condition best known by its articular involvement (rheumatoid arthritis) but emphasizing nonarticular changes, e.g., pulmonary interstitial fibrosis, pleural effusion, and lung nodules.

Ribas-Torres d., variola minor—a mild form of smallpox, confined to certain world such as South America and West Africa, asociated with a much lower (about 1 to 2%) rate than classic small pox (v.major).

Rice d., beriberi—a disease caused by a deficiency of thiamine (vitamin B_1) characterized by polyneuritis, cardiac pathology, and edema. The epidemic form is found primarily in areas in which white (polished) rice is the staple food, as in Japan, China, the Philippines, India, and other countries of Southeast Asia.

Riedel's d., thyroiditis—a rare, chronic proliferating, fibrosing, inflammatory process of unknown etiology involving usually one but sometimes both lobes of the thyroid as well as the trachea and other structures adjacent to the gland.

Riga-Fede d., a small sublingual ulceration in infants with natal or neonatal teeth d. rubbing the lower central incisors; most often observed in whooping cough.

Riggs' d., marginal periodontitis, see Fauchard's d.

Ritter's d., staphylococcal scalded skin syndrome.

Robles' d., name for onchocerciasis in Central America.

Roger's d., a ventricular septal defect; the term is usually restricted to small asymptomatic defects.

Rokitansky's d. (obs), massive hepatic necrosis—massive necrosis of the liver, a rare complication of viral hepatitis (fulminant hepatitis) that may also result from exposure to hepatotoxins or from drug hypersensitivity. A lobe or the entire liver shrinks, becoming a soft, flabby, yellow-brown to green mass with a wrinkled capsule; there is confluent necrosis of hepatocytes, often with fatty change. Mortality is 60 to 90%.

Rolling d., a disease of laboratory mice characterized by lateral rolling movements, by neurolysis and by a polymorphonuclear leukocytic reaction in the brain; it is caused by a potent neurolytic exotoxin produced by *Mycoplasma neurolyticum*.

Romberg's d., facial hemiatrophy—atrophy of one-half of the face which is sometimes progressive, and is of unknown cause.

Rose d., the urticarial form of swine erysipelas.

Rossbach's d., hyperchlorhydria—excessive secretion of hydrochloric acid by the stomach cells.

Rot's d., Rot-Bernhardt d., meralgia paresthetica, see Bernhardt's d.

Roth's d., meralgia paresthetica, see Bernhardt's d.

Roth-Bernhardt d., meralgia paresthetica, see Bernhardt's d.,

Rougnon-Heberden d., angina pectoris—a paroxysmal thoracic pain, with a feeling of suffocation and impending death, due, most often to anoxia of the myocardium and precipitated by effort or excitement.

Round heart d., a disease of unknown etiology which causes sudden death in apparently healthy poultry; a greatly enlarged heart is seen postmortem.

Roussy-Lévy d, see under syndrome.

Rubarth's d., hepatitis contagiosa canis—an infectious hepatitis of the dog caused by adenovirus.

Runt d., graft-versus-host disease produced by injection of allogenic lymphocytes into immunologically immature experimental animals.

Rust's d., tuberculous spondylitis of the cervical vertebrae.

Ruysch's d., see Hirschsprung's d.

Saccharine d., a term proposed for any disease resulting from the overconsumption of refined carbohydrate foods in combination with the removal of dietary fiber and protein including diabetes, cardiovascular disease, constipation, obesity, peptic ulcer, etc.

Sachs' d., see Tay-Sachs d.

Sacroiliac d., chronic tuberculous inflammation of the sacroiliac joint.

Salivary gland d., see cytomegalic inclusion d.

Sanders' d., epidemic keratoconjunctivitis—a highly infectious disease characterized by relatively little ocular excludate, development of round subepithelial corneal opacities in association with the keratitis, and often swelling of regional lymph nodes; systematic symptoms, especially headache, may also be present. Adenovirus type 8 has been repeatedly isolated from patients with the disease.

Sandhoff's d., a type of GM_2 gangliosidosis with clinical features similar to Tay-Sachs disease although it has been observed only among non-Jews. The underlying defect is deficiency of both hexosaminidase A and hexosaminidase B.

Sandworm d., larva migrans—skin disease marked by thin, pruritic, erythematous, serpiginous, papular, or vesicular lines of eruption corresponding to the movements of parasitic larvae beneath the skin. It is most often due to the presence of larvae of the cat and dog hookworm, *Ancylostoma braziliense*, which burrow beneath the skin but cannot complete their migration to the gut (also called creeping eruption). The terms larva migrans and creeping eruption are also applied to similar lesions caused by other parasites such as those seen in gnathostomiasis and cutaneous migratory myiasis (dermamyiasis, dermatomyiasis).

San Joaquin Valley d., coccidioidomycosis, see California d.

Saunders' d., a dangerous condition seen in infants having digestive disturbances to whom is given a large percentage of carbohydrates: it is marked by vomiting, cerebral symptoms, and depression of circulation.

Schamberg's d., a chronic, asymptomatic dermatosis occurring in adolescent and young adult males, localized to the shin, ankles, and dorsa of the feet and toes, and characterized by an eruption of orange- to fawn-colored macules with red puncta (cayenne pepper spots) within or on their border. Also called progressive pigmentary dermatosis, Schamberg's dermatosis, and Schamberg's progressive pigmented purpuric dermatosis.

Schanz's d., traumatic inflammation of the tendo-Achillis.

Schaumann's d., sarcoidosis, see Boeck's d.

Scheuermann's d., a disease of the growth or ossification centers in children which begins a degeneration or necrosis followed by regeneration or recalcification. Also called epiphyseal ischemic necrosis. Osteochondrosis of vertebral epiphyses in juveniles is called Scheuermann's d.

Schilder's d., a subacute or chronic form of leukoencephalopathy of children and adolescents. Clinical symptoms include blindness, deafness, bilateral spasticity, and progressive mental deterioration. There is massive destruction of the white substance of the cerebral hemispheres, cavity formation, and glial scarring. The disease usually occurs sporadically, but a familial form has been reported. Also called encephalitis periaxialis diffusa, Flatau-Schilder disease, and Schilder's encephalitis.

Schimmelbusch's d., see cystic d. of breast.

Schlatter's d., Schlatter-Osgood d., see Osgood-Schlatter d.

Schmorl's d., 1. Herniation of the nucleus pulposus into an adjacent ventral body. 2. Necrobacillosis of wild and domestic rabbits, rats, and other wild animals, due to infection with *Fusobactem necrophrum* (Schmorl's bacillus); it is characterized by abscesses on various parts of the body, or by areas of necrosis around the mouth, nose, eyelids, throat, and chest.

Scholz's d., metachromatic leukodystrophy (juvenile form), see Greenfield's disease.

Schönlein's d., Schönlein-Henoch purpura with articular symptoms and without gastrointestinal symptoms.

Schönlein-Henoch d., a form of nonthrombocytopenic purpura probably due to a vasculitis of unknown cause, most commonly observed in children and associated with a variety of clinical symptoms including urticaria and erythema, arthropathy and arthritis, gastrointestinal symptoms and renal involvement.

Schottmüller's d., paratyphoid fever.

Schroeder's d., a condition characterized by hypertrophic endometrium and excessive uterine bleeding, probably due to deficiency of the gonadotropic hormone.

Schüller's d., 1. see Hand-Schüller-Christian disease. 2. osteoporosis circumscripta cranii—demineralization of the bones of the skull, characteristic of the destructive or osteolytic phase of Paget's d.

Schüller-Christian d., see Hand-Schüller-Christian d.

Schultz's d., agranulocytosis—a symptom complex characterized by marked decrease in the number of granulocytes and by lesions of the throat and other mucous membranes, of the gastrointestinal tract, and of the skin.

Schwediauer's d., see Swediaur's d.

Secondary d., 1. A morbid condition occurring subsequent to or as a consequence of another disease. 2. One due to introduction of incompatible immunologically competent cells into a host rendered incapable of rejecting them by heavy exposure to ionizing radiation.

Seitelberger's d., infantile neuroaxonal dystrophy—a progressive hereditary degenerative encephalopathy transmitted as an autosomal recessive trait beginning in infancy with muscular hypotonia and arrest of development in late infancy, followed by dementia, blindness, spasticity and ataxia. Pathologically, it is characterized by widespread focal swellings and degeneration of the axons with scattered spheroids in the brain.

Self-limited d., one which by its very nature runs a limited and definite course.

Senecio d., cirrhosis of the liver occurring as the result of poisoning by the plant Senecio.

Septic d., one which arises from the development of pyogenic or putrefactive organisms.

Serum d., a hypersensitivity reaction to the administration of foreign serum or serum proteins characterized by fever, urticaria, arthralgia, edema, and lymphadenopathy. It is caused by the formation of circulating antigen-antibody complexes that are deposited in tissues and trigger tissue injury mediated by complement and polymorphonuclear leukocytes. Serum sickness is classed with the Arthur's reaction and immune complex disease as type III in the Gell and Coombs' classification of immune reaction. Although most animal derived antisera with human immune globulins, an identical illness (serum sickness-like reaction or syndrome) can be produced by hypersensitivity reactions to penicillin and other drugs.

Setter's d., acrodynia, see Pink d.

Sever's d., epiphysitis (inflammation of an epiphysis or of the cartilage that separates it from the main bone) of the calcaneus.

Severe combined immunodeficiency d. (SCID), a group of rare congenital disorder is characterized by gross impairment of both humoral and cell-mediated immunity manifested by lack of antibody formation response to antigenic challenge, absence of delayed hypersensitivity and inability to reject transplants of foreign tissue. In most cases, all classes of immunoglobulins are nearly or completely absent, and there is marked lymphocytopenia. Blood transfusions can result in graft-versus-host (GVH) disease and routine vaccinations in fatal infection. Unless immune function is restored by a histocompatible bone marrow or fetal tissue transplant or the patient is kept in gnotobiotic isolation; death from opportunistic infection usually occurs before the first birth-day. Four major forms are distinguished. Swiss type agamma-globulinemia, the first form to be described in 1958 is marked by nearly complete absence of lymphocytes and immunoglobulin and by autosomal recessive inheritance. One form is associated with a specific metabolic defect, adenosine deaminase (ADA) deficiency. In another form, B cells are presented normal levels but antibody response is absent owing to lack of T cells; and the pattern of inheritance may be either autosomal recessive or X-linked. The last form, that results in absence of granulocytes and macrophages as well as lymphocytes.

Sexually transmitted d., any of a diverse group of infections caused by biologically dissimilar pathogens and transmitted by sexual contact, which includes both heterosexual and homosexual behavior; sexual transmission is the only important mode of spread of some of the diseases in the group (e.g., the classic venereal diseases), while others (e.g., hepatitis viruses, shigellosis, amebiasis, giardiasis) can also be acquired by nonsexual means. See also venereal d.

Shaver's d., bauxite pneumoconiosis—a rapidly progressive pneumoconiosis leading to extreme pulmonary emphysema, frequently accompanied by pneumothorax, caused by inhalation of bauxite fumes containing fine particles of alumina and silica.

Shimamushi d., scrub typhus—an acute typhus-like infectious disease caused by *Rickettsia tsutsugamushi* transmitted by the bite of infected larval trombiculid mites (chiggers), occurring chiefly in Asia and the southern and western Pacific, and characterized chiefly with the formation of a pathognomic primary cutaneous lesion or eschar at the site of sinnoculation (tache noir) accompanied by regional lymphadenopathy, fever, and a maculopapular rash.

Shuttlemaker's d., a condition in shuttlemakers, marked by faintness, shortness of breath, headache, nausea, etc. attributed to inhaling the dust of poisonous wood from which the shuttles (devices used in weaving) are made.

Sickle cell d., any of the diseases associated with the presence of hemoglobin S, including sickle cell anemia, sickle cell-hemoglobin C or D disease, and sickle cell-thalassemia disease.

Sickle cell-hemoglobin C d., a genetically determined anemia in which the red cells contain both hemoglobin S and hemoglobin C.

Sickle cell-hemoglobin D d., a genetically determined anemia characterized by the presence of both hemoglobin S and hemoglobin D in red blood cells.

Sickle cell-thalassemia d., a hereditary anemia involving simultaneous heterozygosity for hemoglobin S and thalassemia. Also called microdrepanocytosis, microdrepanocytic d., hemoglobin S-thalassemia, sickle cell-thalassemia, and thalassemia-sickle cell disease.

Silo-filler's d., pulmonary inflammation, often with acute pulmonary edema, caused by inhalation of the irritant gases (especially oxides of nitrogen) which collect in recently filled silos.

Simmonds' d., panhypopituitarisrr—generalized hypopituitarism due to absence of or damage to the pituitary gland, which, in its complete form, leads to absence of gonadal function and insufficiency of thyroid and adrenal cortical function. Dwarfism, regression of secondary sex characters and loss of libido weight loss, fatigability, bradycardia, hypotension, pallor, depression, and many other manifestations may occur. When cachexia is a prominent feature, it is called hypophysial or pituitary cachexia and Simmond's disease.

Simons' d, see Barraquer's d.

Sixth d., exanthema subitum—an acute, short lived probably viral, disease of infants and young children in which after a high fever of 3 to 4 days duration the temperature suddenly drops to normal and a macular or maculopapular rash appears on the trunk and spreads to other areas shortly before, simultaneously with or shortly after the subsidence of the fever.

Sixth venereal d., lymphogranuloma venereum, see fifth venereal d.

Sjögren's d., see under syndrome.

Skevas-Zerfus d., see sponge-diver's d.

Sleeping d., narcolepsy.

Sleepy foal d., a form of equlosis affecting foals within the first three days of life, due to infection with *Actinobacillus equuli*, characterized by sudden onset, extreme prostration, and death usually within 12 hours.

Smith-Strang d., see methionine malabsorption syndrome.

Sneddon-Wilkinson d., subcorneal pustular dermatosis—a chronic, superficial, pustular disorder with a chronic relapsing course, resembling dermatitis herpetiformis, and chiefly affecting women in middle life, with sterile pustular blebs beneath the horny layer of the epidermis on the trunk and in the skin folds.

Sod d., vesicular dermatitis—a sometimes fatal disease, believed to be eczematous in nature, affecting young poultry that range over unbroken prairie sod, marked by the formation of blisters and scabs on the feet and legs.

Specific d., any disease, such as syphilis, due to a characteristic morbific agency.

Spencer's d., a form (probably viral) of epidemic gastroenteritis.

Spielmeyer-Vogt d., see Kufs' disease.

Sponge-diver's d., a condition encountered by divers in the Mediterranean who come in contact with the stinging tentacles of sea anemones of the genera *Sagartia* and *Actinia*, which are frequently attached to the base of sponges; it is marked by burning, itching, erythema, necrosis, and ulceration. Also called Skevas-Zerfus d.

Stargardt's d., hereditary degeneration of the macula lutea occurring between the ages of six and twenty, marked by rapid loss of visual acuity and by abnormal appearance and pigmentation of the macular area.

Steinert's d., myotonic dystrophy—rare, slowly progressive, hereditary disease transmitted as an autosomal dominant trait, characterized by myotonia followed by atrophy of the muscles (especially those of the face and neck), cataracts, hypogonadism, frontal balding and cardiac abnormalities.

Sterility d., a deficiency disease observed in experimental animals and due to lack of vitamin E in the diet.

Steinberg's d., see Hodgkin's d.

Sticker's d., erythema infectiosum, see fifth d.

Stieda's d., see Pellegrini's d.

Stiff lamb d., polyarthritis of lambs called by a chlamydial organism, with stiffness of the legs, reluctance to move, and recumbency.

Still's d., a variety of chronic polyarthritis affecting children and marked by enlargement of lymph nodes, generally of the spleen, and irregular fever; also called juvenile rheumatoid arthritis.

Stokes-Adams d., see Adams-Stokes d.

Storage d., a metabolic disorder in which some substances accumulate or are stored in certain cells in unusually large amounts; the stored substances may be lipids, proteins, carbohydrates, or other substances. See, for example, glycogen storage d., mucopolysaccharidosis and proteinosis. Formerly called thesaurismosis.

Storage pool d., a blood coagulation disorder due to failure of the platelets to release ADP in response to aggregating agents (collagen, epinephrine, exogenous ADP, thrombin, etc.). It is characterized by mild bleeding episodes, prolonged bleeding time, and reduced aggregation response to collagen or thrombin.

Structural d., any disease in which there are microscopic changes.

Strümpell's d., 1. A hereditary form of lateral sclerosis in which the spasticity is principally limited to the legs; also called Strümpel's type. 2. Polioencephalomyelitis—inflammation of the gray matter of the brain and spinal cord and of the meninges covering it.

Strümpell-Leichtenstern d., hemorrhagic encephalitis—herpes encephalitis in which there is inflammation of the brain with hemorrhagic foci and perivascular exudate.

Strümpell-Marie d., rheumatoid spondylitis—the form of rheumatoid arthritis that affects the spine. It is a systemic illness of unknown etiology, affecting young males predominantly, and producing pain and stiffness as a result of inflammation of the sacroiliac, intervertebral and costovertebral joints; paraspinal calcification with ossification and ankylosis of the spinal joints, may cause complete rigidity of the spine and thorax.

Sturge's d., see Sturge-Weber syndrome.

Stuttgart d., a nonjaundiced type of canine leptospirosis caused by *Leptospira interrogans* serogroup *canicola*, also called canine typhus.

Sudeck's d., post-traumatic osteoporosis.

Sutton's d., 1. (R. L. Button, Sr.) (a) halo nevus—a pigmented lesion (usually a compound or intradermal nevocytic nevus but sometimes a neuronevus, blue nevus, or malignant melanomal) surrounded by annular depigmented area (b) periadenitisi mucosa necrotica recurrens—a recurrent disease of the mucous membranes of unknown etiology, generally considered to be a severe form of recurrent aphthous stomatitis, which is marked by development of deep crateriform ulcers with inflamed borders that leave scars after healing. The mucosa of the lips, cheeks, tongue, palate, and anterior tonsillar pillars are most commonly involved, but the pharynx, larynx, and genitalia may also be affected. 2. (R L Sutton, Jr) granuloma fissuratum—a circumscribed, firm, reddish fissured, fibrotic granuloma of the gum and buccal mucosa, occurring on an edentulous alveolar ridge and in the fold between the ridge and cheek; it is caused by an ill-fitting denture.

Sutton-Gull d. (oos.), arteriocapillary fibrosis.

Swediaur's (Schwediauer's) d., inflammation of the calcaneal bursa.

Sweet clover d., a hemorrhagic disease of animals, especially cattle, caused by ingestion of spoiled sweet clover which contains the anticoagulant dicumarol.

Swift's d., see Pink d.

Swift-Feer d., see Pink d.

Swineherd's d., leptospirosis, manifested as a benign meningitis, caused by *Leptospira interrogans* serogroups *hyos* or *pomona*, and affecting those who work with swine or pork or come in contact with the urine of carriers.

Sylvest's d., see Bornholm's d., and Daae's d.,

Symmers' d., see Brill-Symmer d.,

Systemic d., one affecting a number of organs and tissues.

Takahara's d., a rare, autosomal recessive disease caused by congenital absence of the catalase and observed mainly in Japan and Switzerland. It is usually characterized by gingivitis and infections of associated oral structures.

Takayasu's d., see pulseless d.

Taltan d., infectious porcine encephalomyelitis.

Talma's d., myotonia acquisita—tonic muscular spasm developed after injury or in inconsequence of disease.

Tangier d., it is caused by a decreased synthesis and increased catabolism of the apolipoprotein components A-I and A-ll (apoA-l and apoA-ll) of HDL; HDL is absent from plasma, and the other lipoproteins are abnormal; cholesteryl esters accumulate in the reticuloendothelial cells. Clinical signs include enlarged orange tonsils and pharyngeal and rectal mucosa, recurrent peripheral neuropathy, splenomegaly, and corneal infiltration.

Tartanc d., gout and calculus (Paracelsus).

Tarui's d., see glycogen storage d. (type VII).

Tay's d., degeneration of the choroid marked by irregular yellow spots around the macula lutea, and believed to be due to an atheromatous state of the arteries; seen in advanced life.

Tay-Sachs d. (TSD), the most common ganglioside storage disease, occurring almost exclusively among northeast European Jews. TSD is a GM_2 gangliosidosis specifically characterized by infantile onset (3-6 months), doll-like facies, cherry-red macular spot (90 percent of the infants), early blindness, hyperacusis. macrocephaly, seizures, and hypotonia; the children die between 2 and 5 years of age. See also gangliosidosis: Sandhof's disease., and amaurotic familial idiocy*.

Teart d. in cattle, a diarrhea that affects cattle that graze on certain pastures in England, due to the presence of molybdenum in the herbage.

Teschen's d., infectious porcine encephalomyelitis.

Thalassemia sickle cell d., see sickle cell-thalassemia d.

Thaysen's d., see Gee's d.

Theiler's d., spontaneous encephalomyelitis of mice, caused by invasion of the nervous system by a common viral infection of the intestinal tract; also called Theiler's mouse encephalomyelitis and marine encephalomyelitis.

Thiemann's d., familial avascular necrosis of the phalangeal epiphysis, beginning in childhood or adolescence and resulting in deformity of the interphalangeal joints; also called familial osteoarthropathy of the fingers. Similar lesions may occur in the great toes and first tarsometatarsal joints, in which case it is known as osteochondritis ossis metacarpi et metatarsi.

Thomsen's d., myotonia congenita—congenital genetic disease characterized by tonic spasm and rigidity of certain muscles when an attempt is made to move them after a period of rest or when mechanically stimulated. The stiffness disappears as the muscles are used. They are in autosomal dominant and autosomal recessive forms.

Thomson's d., an autosomal recessive skin disorder similar to Rothmund-Thomson syndrome except that saddle nose and cataract are not manifestations.

Thyrocardiac d., see Thyrotoxic heart d.

Thyrotoxic heart d., heart disease associated with hyperthyroidism, marked by atrial fibrillation, cardiac enlargement, and congestive heart failure; also called thyrocardiac d.

Tietze's d., see under syndrome.

Tillaux's d., mastitis with the formation of multiple tumors in the breast.

Tommaselli's d., pyrexia and hematuria due to excessive use of quinine.

Tooth's d., progressive neuropathic (peroneal) muscular atrophy, see Charcot-Marie-Tooth d.

Tornwaldt's (Thornwaldt's) d., chronic inflammation of the pharyngeal bursa, attended with formation of a pus-containing cyst, and naso-pharyngeal stenosis.

Tourette's d., see Gilles de la Tourette's syndrome.

Traum's d., infectious abortion (brucellosis) in swine.

Trevor's d., dysplasia epiphysealis hemimelica—a rare condition characterized by swellings of the extremities, usually on the inner and outer aspects of the ankles and knees, made up of bone covered with epiphyseal cartilage, and leading to limitation of movements of joints.

Trophoblastic d., a group of disorder that has its origin in the placenta, including hydatidiform mole, chorioadenoma destruens, and gestational choriocarcinoma.

Tsutsugamushi d., scrub typhus—see Shimamushi d.

Tunnel d., 1. See Hookworm d. 2. Decompression sickness, see Caisson's d.

Twin-lamb d., see Pregnancy d.

Twist d., see whirling d.

Tyzzer's d., a disease caused by *Bacillus piliformis* and characterized by necrotic lesions of the liver and intestine; originally described in Japanese waltzing mice, it also affects rats, rabbits, gerbils, dogs, and man.

Tzaneen d., a tickborne protozoal disease, reported in Tzaneen, South Africa, due to *Theileria mutans*, and occurring in cattle and water buffalo, which may manifest as a mild febrile disease or may be severe and fatal.

Underwood's d., scleroma—a hardened patch or induration, especially of the nasal or laryngeal tissues.

Unna-Thost d., diffuse palmoplantar keratoderma—an autosomal dominant disorder characterized by the presence of well-demarcated, usually bilateral and symmetrical confluent areas of scalling on the palms and soles, sometimes involving adjacent skin of the hands and feet, which is usually present early but may appear later in life. Striate and punctate variants have also been reported; the latter may be associated with focal gingival hyperkeratosis.

Unverricht's d., see Lafora's d.

Urbach-Wiethe d., lipoid proteinosis—an autosomal recessive disorder of lipid metabolism characterized by the deposition of hyaline material in the skin and mucosa of the mouth, pharynx, hypopharynx, and larynx, resulting in prolonged hoarseness, often from birth, due to infiltration of the vocal cords. Skins lessions are first manifested as recurrent pustules or bullae on the face and distal exposed surface of the arms and legs, which heal and leave white varioliform scars, and later by waxy yellow ivory papules, nodules, or verrucoid plaques primarily located on the face, eyelids, nape, hands, fingers, elbows, and knees.

Vagabonds' d., vagrants' d., discoloration of the skin in persons subjected to louse (*Pediculus humanus corporis*) bites over long periods; also called parasitic melanoderma.

van Buren's d., see Peyronie's d.

Vaquez' d., Vaquez-Osler d., polycythemia vera, see Osler's d.

Veld d., veldt d., see heartwater d.

Venereal d., classically, five infectious diseases (**gonorrhea, syphilis, chancroid lymphogranuloma venereum, granuloma inguinale**) that were known to be transmitted by sexual contact, principally sexual intercourse. Infections caused by *Chlamydia trachomatis* are now also included. See sexually transmitted d.

Veno-occlusive d. of the liver, symptomatic occlusion of the small hepatic venules, first seen in children in Jamaica where it resulted from ingestion of Senecio tea, also caused by other hepatotoxins and by radiation. Many patients recover after withdrawal of the offending toxin; some progress to portal hypertension and liver failure, as in Budd-Chiari syndrome.

Vent d., rabbit syphilis.

Verneuil's d., syphilitic disease of the bursae.

Verse's d., calcinosis intervertebralis—deposit of calcium in one or more intervertebral disks.

Vibration d., blanching and diminished flexion of the fingers with loss of perception of cold, heat, and pain and osteoarthritic changes in joints of the arm, due to continuous use of vibrating tools.

Vogt's d., see under syndrome.

Vogt-Spielmeyer d., see amaurotic idiocy*, see Jansky-Bielschowsky d.; Batten d.; Kuf's d.

Volkamann's d., a congenital deformity of the foot due to a tibiotarsal dislocation; also called Volkmann's deformity.

Voltolini's d., an acute, purulent inflammation of the internal ear with violent pain, followed by involvement of the meninges with subsequent fever, delirium, and unconsciousness.

von Economo's d., lethargic encephalitis, see Economo's d.

von Gierke's d., glycogen storage d. (type I).

von Hippel's d., hemangiomatosis confined principally to the retina; when associated with hemangioblastoma of the cerebellum, it is known as von Hippel-Lindau d.

von Hippel-Lindau d., hereditary phakomatosis, characterized by congenital angiomatosis of the retina and cerebellum; there may also be similar lesions of the spinal cord and cysts of the pancreas, kidneys, and other viscera. Neurologic symptoms, including seizures and mental retardation, may be present. Also called cerebroretinal or retinocerebral angiomatosis, and Lindau-von Hippel d.

von Jaksch's d., anemia pseudoleukemica infantum—a condition originally described as a specific entity in children under age three, with anisocytosis, poikilocytosis, peripheral red blood cell immaturity, leukocytosis, lymphadenopathy, and hepatosplenomegaly; now considered to be a syndrome produced by many factors such as malnutrition, chronic infection, malabsorption, and hemoglobinopathies.

von Recklinghausen's d., see Recklinghausen's d.

von Willebrand's d., a congenital hemorrhagic diathesis, inherited as an autosomal dominant trait, characterized by prolonged bleeding time, deficiency of coagulation Factor VIII, and often impairment of adhesion of platelets on glass beads, associated with epistaxis and increased bleeding after trauma or surgery, menorrhagia, and postpartum bleeding. Also called angiohemophilia, Minot-von Willebrand syndrome, pseudohemophilia, vascular hemophilia, and Willebrand's syndrome.

Vrolik's d., osteogenesis imperfecta congenita, see Durante's d.

Waldenström's d., osteochondrosis of the capital femoral epiphysis; see Legg-Calvé-Perthes d.

Walkabout d., see Kimberley horse d.

Wartenberg's d., 1. Cheiralgia paresthetica—isolated neuralgia of the superficial ramus of the radial nerve. 2. Brachialgia statica paresthetica—painful paresthesias in the arm and hand during sleep due to compression of the blood vessels. 3. Partial thenar atrophy.

Wasting d., any disease marked especially by progressive emaciation and weakness.

Weber's d., see Sturge-Weber syndrome.

Weber-Christian d., relapsing, febrile, nodular, nonsuppurative panniculitis, see Christian-Weber d.

Wegner's d., osteochondrotic separation of the epiphyses in hereditary syphilis.

Weil's d., see under syndrome.

Weir Mitchell's d., erythromelalgia, see Gerhardt's d.

Wenckebach's d., cardioptosis—downward displacement of the heart.

Werdnig-Hoffmann d., Werdnig-Hoffmann spinal muscular atrophy—a progressive, infantile, autosomal recessive form of muscular dystrophy, usually occurring in siblings rather than in successive generations, and resulting from degeneration of the anterior horn cells of the spinal cord. It is marked by early onset (usually at about six months of age, but sometimes in fetal life), hypotonia and wasting of the muscles, complete flaccid paralysis, and death, usually in early life.

Werlhof's d., idiopathic thrombocytopenic purpura—thrombocytopenic purpura unassociated with any definable systemic disease but often accompanied by presence of a serum antiplatelet factor, now characterized as an IGg immunoglobulin.

Werner-His d., see His' d.

Werner-Schultz d, see Schultz's d.

Wernicke's d., encephalopathy.

Wesselsbron's d., a mosquito-borne viral disease causing death of lambs and abortion and death in ewes in Africa; it is communicable to man, in whom it causes a mild febrile, illness.

Westphal-Strümpell d., see Wilson's d.

Whipple's d., a malabsorption syndrome characterized by diarrhea, steatorrhea, skin pigmentation, arthralgia and arthritis, lymphadenopathy, and central nervous system lesions. The intestinal mucosa is infiltrated with macrophages containing PAS-positive material (the remnants of bacillary microorganisms which invade the lamina propria).

Whirling d., a highly fatal protozoal disease of young salmonid fish caused by *Myxosoma cerebralis*, characterized chiefly by cartilaginous damage in the axial skeleton and granuloma formation involving the auditory-equilibrium apparatus of the fish, causing it to swim rapidly in a circular pattern. Also called twist d.

White heifer d., a condition reputed to most commonly occur in white heifers usually of the shorthorn breed, in which there is a rubber-like sheet of fibrous tissue and membrane stretching across the posterior part of the vagina; the coverage may be partial or complete. Also called persistent hymen.

White muscle d., skeletal muscle degeneration in animals, produced by calcification of muscle fibers, the result of deficiency of selenium in the diet.

White-spot d., 1. Lichen sclerosus et atrophicus see Csillag's d., 2. Guttate morphea—a form characterized by multiple small, rounded, atrophic macules, sometimes surrounded by a violaceous zone, and arranged in clusters or lines; it is difficult to distinguish from and believed by some authorities to be the same as lichen sclerosus et atrophicus. 3. A pustular eruption involving the skin, gills, and eyes of marine and fresh water fishes both in the wild and in aquaria, caused by the protozoan *Ichthyophthirius multifiliis*, and often leading to death, and sometimes to great econornic loss. Also called ich, ichthyophthiriasis, and ick.

Whitmore's d., melioidosis—a rare infection of humans and animals, clinically resembling glanders, caused by *Pseudomonas pseudomallei*, which occurs worldwide although most cases of disease are seen in

Southeast Asia. Human diseases, which are usually acquired through contact of a break in the skin with contaminated soil or water, may range from an inapparenet dormant infection to localized abscess formation to a relatively benign pneumonia or overwhelming and highly fatal septicemia; late activation of inapparent disease or recrudescene of previous symptoms may occur many years after the initial infection.

Whytt's d., tuberculous meningitis causing acute hydrocephalus.

Wilson's d., a rare, progressive disease, inherited as an autosomal recessive trait and due to a defect in the metabolism of copper, with accumulation of copper in the liver, brain, kidney, cornea, and other tissues. The disease is characterized by cirrhosis of the liver and degenerative changes in the brain, particularly the basal ganglia. Liver disease is the most likely presenting manifestation in children: neurologic disease is most common in young adults. The characteristic ophthalmic feature is a pigmented ring (Kayser-Fleischer ring) at the outer margin of the cornea. Also called hepatolenticular degeneration or disease, familial hepatitis, and Westphal-Strümpell disease or pseudosclerosis.

Winckel's d., a fatal disease of newborn infants characterized by jaundice, hemoglobinuria, hemorrhage, bloody urine, cyanosis, polyuria, collapse, and convulsions.

Winiwarter-Buerger d., thromboangiitis obliterans, see Buerger's d.

Winkler's d., chondrodermatitis nodularis chronica helices—a condition seen principally in middle-aged men marked by the presence of a small painful skin-colored, grayish or waxy and translucent, firm, scaly, nodular region on the helix of the ear, most often the right one; multiple lesion may occur along the rim of the ear.

Winton's d., see Pictou's d.

Wolman's d., a lysosomal storage disease due to acid lipase deficiency, with onset in early infancy and death before one year of age. Clinical features include hepatosplenomegaly, steatorrhea, abdominal distension, anemia, inanition, and adrenal calcification. Also called primary familial and Wolman's xanthomatosis.

Woolsorters' d., inhalational anthrax, see Ragpicker's or Ragsorter's d.

Woringer-Kolopp d., pagetoid reticulosis—a solitary skin lesion of long duration and slow growth characterized histologically by large numbers of abnormal mononuclear cells infiltrating the epidermis with an underlying reactive mixed dermal infiltrate, which is considered by some authorities to represent an indolent, epidermotropic form of cutaneous T cell lymphoma, although some studies suggest that the characteristic cells are not T cells but are of the monocyte-macrophage series or Merkel's cells.

X d., 1. Hyperkeratosis—a skin disease of cattle marked by inflammation and thickening of the horny layer, and caused by the ingestion of grease containing high levels of chlorinated hydrocarbons. 2. Aflatoxicosis—a form of mycotoxicosis affecting turkeys and other farm animals fed on groundnut meal contaminated with the molds *Aspergillus flavus*, and realated species, which produce aflatoxins; widespread epidemics with high mortality rates have been reported from all parts of the world.

X-linked lymphoproliferatative d., see under syndrome.

Zahorsky's d., exanthema subitum—an acute short-lived, probably viral, disease of infant and young children in which after a high fever of 3 to 4 day duration temperature suddenly drops to normal and a macular or maculopapular rash appears on the trunk and spreads to other areas shortly before, simultaneously with, or shortly after the subsidence of fever.

Ziehen-Oppenheim d., dystonia musculorum deformans—a rare, chronic, genetic disease marked by involuntary, irregular, clonic contortions of the muscles of the trunk and extremities. The symptoms appear chiefly on walking, at which time the contortions twist the body forward and sideways in a grotesque fashion (tortipelvis). An autosomal recessive form occurs before puberty, principally among Jews; the autosomal dominant form has a later onset and is not as consistent in severity.

3
Disorders

Disorder: A derangement or abnormality of function; a morbid physical or mental state.

Adjustment d., (DMR III-R), a maladaptive reaction to identifiable stressful life events, such as divorce, loss of job, physical illness, or natural disaster; this diagnosis assumes that the condition will remit when the stress ceases or when the patient adapts to the situation.

Affective d's., see Mood d's.

Amnestic d., (DSM III-R), either of two DSM III-R diagnostic categories: alcohol amnestic disorder (amnestic syndrome due to prolonged alcohol use, Korsakoff's syndrome) and sedative, hypnotic, or anxiolytic amnestic disorder (a transient amnestic syndrome due to prolonged use of a sedative, hypnotic, or anxiolytic).

Anxiety d's., (DSM III-R), a group of mental disorders in which anxiety and avoidance behavior predominate. Included are panic disorder with and without agoraphobia, agoraphobia without history of panic disorders, social phobia, simple phobia, obsessive compulsive disorder, post-traumatic stress disorder, and generalized anxiety disorder.

Anxiety d's of childhood or adolescence., (DSM III-R), a group of mental disorders of children and adolescents in which the predominant clinical feature is anxiety, either focused on specific situations (separation anxiety disorder, avoidant disorder of childhood or adolescence) or generalized (overanxious disorder).

Attention deficit hyperactivity d., (DSM III-R), a controversial childhood mental disorder with onset before age seven characterized by fidgeting and squirming, difficulty in remaining seated, easy distractibility, difficulty awaiting one's turn and refraining from blurting out answers to questions before they have been completed, and inability to follow instruction excessive talking and other disruptive behavior. Called also minimal brain dysfunction (based on the unproven assumption that brain damage causes the syndrome and the neurological abnormalities) and hyperkinetic reaction or syndrome and hyperactive child syndrome.

Autistic d., (DSM III-R), a severe mental disorder with onset in infancy characterized by qualitative impairment in reciprocal social interaction (e.g. lack of awareness of the existence of feelings of other, failure to seek comfort at time of distress, lack of imitation) and in verbal and nonverbal communication and restricted repertoire of activities and interest. If differs from childhood schizophrenia in its early onset and in the lack of delusions, hallucinations, incoherence, or loosening of associations and from mental retardation in the presence of intelligent, responsive facies and in that the full syndrome of infantile autism is not produced by mental retardation.

Avoidant d., of childhood or adolescence (DSM III-R), persistent and excessive shrinking from contact with strangers.

Behavior d., 1. see Conduct d. 2. (obs) mental disorder characterized by socially unacceptable behavior.

Bipolar d., 1. (DSM III-R), a mood disorder characterized by the occurrence of one or more manic episodes (qv) will eventually occur. Bipolar disorder is further classified as mixed if; manic and depressive episodes alternate every few days and otherwise as manic or ; depressed according to the type of the most recent episodes. Also called manic depressive disorder, illness, or psychosis. 2. Cylothymia - (DSM III-R), a mood disorder characterized by numerous hypomanic and depressive periods with symptoms like those of manic and major depressive episodes but of lesser severity.

Body dysmorphic d., (DSM III-R), a mental disorder characterized by preoccupation with some imagined defect in appearance of an normal appearing person.

Character d., see Personality disorder.

Collagen d., any inborn error of metabolism in involving abnormal structure or metabolism collagen; the term includes the Ehlers-Danlos syndrome, the Marfan's syndrome, cutis laxa; osteogenesis imperfecta, and epidermolysis bullosa.

Conduct d., (DSM III-R), a mental disorder of childhood and adolescence characterized b persistent pattern of conduct in which rights of others and age-appropriate societal norms rules are violated.

Conversion d., (DSM III-R), a mental disorder characterized by conversion symptoms (loss or alteration of physical function suggesting physical illness, usually of the sensorimotor system, such as seizures, paralysis, dyskinesia, anesthesia, blindness, or aphonia) having no demonstrable physiological basis and whose psychological basis is suggested by (i) exacerbation of symptoms at times of psychological stress (ii) relief from tension or inner conflicts (primary gain) provided by the symptoms, or (iii) secondary gain (support, attention avoidance of unpleasant responsibilities) provided by the symptoms. Many patients exhibit "la bell indifference," a lack of concern about the impairment caused by the symptoms; histerionic (hysterical) personality traits are also common. This diagnosis excludes patients whose symptoms are under voluntary control (as in factitious disorder with physical symptoms or malingering), patients with the full syndrome of somatization disorder (qv) and patients whose predominant complaint is pain (as in psychogenic pain disroder).

Cyclothymic d., see Bipolar disorder.

Delusional (paranoid) d., (DSM III-R]), a psychotic disorder marked by persistent delusions of persecution or delusional jealousy and behavior like that of the paranoid personality such as suspiciousness, mistrust, and combativeness. It differs from paranoid schizophrenia, in which hallucinations or formal thought disorders are present, in that the delusions are logically consistent and that there are no other psychotic features. The designations in DSM III-R is delusional (paranoid) disorders with five types: persecutory, jealous, erotomanic somatic and grandiose.

Depersonalization d., (DSM III-R), a dissociate disorder characterized by one or more episodes of depersonalization (feelings of unreality and strangeness in one's perception of the self or one's body image) not due to another mental disorder, such as schizophrenia. Episodes of depersonalization are usually accompanied by dizziness, anxiety, fears of going insane, and derealization called also depersonalization neuroses or syndrome.

Dissociative d's (DSM III-R), hysterical neuroses, dissociate type; mental disorder characterized by sudden, temporary alterations in identity, memory, or consciousness, segregating normally integrated memories or parts of the personality from the dominant identity of the individual. This category includes multiple personality disorder, psychogenic fugue, psychogenic amnesia, and depersonalization disorder.

Dysthymic d., (DSM III-R), a mood disorder characterized by depressed feeling (sad, blue low down in the dumps) and loss of interest or pleasure in one's usual activities and in which the associated symptoms have persisted for more than two years but are not severe enough to meet the criteria for major depression.

Emotional d., (DSM III-R), a colloqualism roughly equivalent to mental disorder but not usually applied to organic mental disorders or mental retardation.

Factitious d., (DSM III-R), a mental disorder characterized by repeated knowing simulation of physical and psychological symptoms for no apparent purpose other than obtain treatment. It differs from malingering in that there is no recognizable motive feigning illness. DSM III distinguishes two main types; chronic factitious disorder with physical symptoms (called also Munchausen syndrome) and factitious disorder with psychological sympto (called also Ganser syndrome.).

Functional d., a disorder of function having no known organic basis. In psychiatry, the term is roughly equivalent to "psychogenic disorder" in other branches medicine to "idiopat disorder"

Generalized anxiety d., (DSM III-R), a neurotic mental disorder characterized by the presence of unrealistic or excessive anxiety and worry about two or more life circumstances for six months or longer.

Genetic d., see under disease.

Identity d., (DSM III-R), severe subjective distress, lasting 3 months or longer, about inability to reconcile aspects of the self into a relatively coherent whole and acceptable sense of self with uncertainty about career choice, sexual orientation, and behavior, moral value, and the like, occurring most commonly in late adolescence.

Immunodeficiency d., see under disease.

Induced psychotic d., (DSM III-R), a delusional system that develops in a second person; a result of a close relationship with another person who already has a psychotic disorder with prominent delusions. Also called folie a deux.

Intermittent explosive d., (DSM III-R), a functional mental disorder characterized by multiple discrete episode of loss of control of aggressive impulses resulting in serious assualt .destruction of property that are out of keeping with the individual's normal personality.

Isolated explosive d., (DSM III-R), a functional mental disorder characterized by a single violent catastrophic act performed for no apparent reason and not attributable to a underlying psychotic or mental disorder.

LDL-receptor d., familial hyperlipoproteinemia, type lla.

Major mood d., [DSM III-R], bipolar d.

Mendelian d., a genetic disease, showing a mendelian pattern of inheritance, and caused by a single mutation in the structure of DNA, which causes a single basic defect that some pathological consequences or consequences. Called also monogenic or single-gene d.

Mental d., any clinically significant behavioral or psychological syndrome characterized by the presence of distressing symptoms or significant impairment of functioning. Mental disorderes are assumed to result from some psychological or organic dysfunction of the individual: the concept does not include disturbance that the essentially conflicts between the individual and society (social deviance).

Monogenic d., see Mendelian disease.

Mood d's (DSM III-R), mental disorder whose essential features is a disturbance of mood manifested as a full or partial manic or depressive syndrome. Functional mood disorders are subclassified as bipolar disorders, including bipolar disorder and cyclothymia, and depressive disorders, including major depression and dysthymia.

Multifactorial d., a disorder caused by interaction of genetic factors and perhaps also non-genetic, environmental factors, e.g. some forms of birth defects and diabetes mellitus. See also genetic disease.

Multiple personality d., a functional mental disorder characterized by the existence in an individual or two or more distinct personalities, each having unique memories, characteristic behavior, and social relationship that determines the individual's actions when that personality is dominant. Transitions from one personality to another are abrupt. The original personality usually is totally unaware of the other personalities (subpersonalities) experiencing only gaps of time when the others are in control. Subpersonalities may or may not have awareness of the others.

Organic mental d., a particular organic brain syndrome in which the etiology is known or presumed, such as delirium tremens or Alzheimer's disease.

Overanxious d., (DSM III-R), an anxiety disorder of childhood or adolescence characterized by excessive worrying and fearful behavior not related to specific situation or due recent.

Panic d., (DSM III-R), a neurotic mental disorder characterized by recurrent panic (anxiety) attacks, episodes of intense apprehension, fear, or terror associated with somatic symptoms such as dyspnea, palpitations, dizziness, vertigo, faintness, shakiness and with psychological symptoms such as feelings of unreality (depersonalization or derealization) or fears of dying, going crazy, or loosing control; there is usually chronic nervousness and tension between attacks. It may be associated with agoraphobia. This disorder does not include panic attacks that may occurs in phobias when the patient is exposed to the phobic stimulus.

Paranoid d's. see Delusional (paranoid) disorder.

Pervasive development d., (DSM III-R), a subclass of disorder in which there is impairment in development of reciprocal social interaction and of verbal and nonverbal communication skills and in imaginative activity: included is autistic disorder.

Post-traumatic stress d., (DSM III-R), a mental disorder caused by a traumatic event outside the range of normal human experience, such as rape or assault, military combat or bombing of civilians, natural disasters or terrible accidents, torture, or death camps, and characterized by re-experiencing the traumatic event in recurrent intrusive recollections, nightmares, or flashbacks, by "psychic numbness" or "emotional aesthesia," by hyperalertness and difficulty in sleeping, remembering, or concentrating, and guilt about surviving and other have not or about things that had to be done in order to survive: classified as acute, chronic or delayed depending on the duration of symptoms and on whether there is a latent period, which may be months or years, between the trauma and the onset of symptoms.

Psychoactive substance-induced organic mental d's (DSM III-R), organic brain syndromes associated with use of psychoactive substance; DSM III-R includes ten specific syndromes, intoxication, withdrawal, delirium, dementia, amnestic disorder, delusional disorder, hallucinosis, mood disorder, perception disorder, and personality disorder, when the causative substance is known, it is specified, e.g. "alcohol intoxication."

Psychoactive substance used's (DSM III-R), mental disorders involving maladaptive behavior associated with regular use of mood, or behavior-altering substance, psychoactive substance abuse, and psychoactive substance dependence.

Psychogenic pain d., see somatoform pain d.

Psychophysiologic d., psychosomatic d.

Psychosomatic d., a disorder in which the physical symptoms are caused or exacerbated by psychological factors, such as migraine headache, lower back pain, gastric ulcer or irritable bowel syndrome. The term psychophysiologic disorders used in previous officials nomenclatures and defined as "physical disorder of presumably psychogenic origin" has been replaced in DSM III-R by the more neutral phrase psychological factors affecting physical condition, which may be applied to "any physical condition to which psychological factors are judged to be contributory," and reflects the exiting lack of certainty about the actual etiological role of psychological factors in these conditions.

Schizoaffective d. (DSM III-R), a diagnostic category for mental disorder that have features of both schizophrenia and mood disorder (mania or depression).

Schizophreniform d. (DSM III-R), a mental disorder with the signs and symptoms of schizophrenia but duration of less than 6 months. Formerly called acute schizophrenia.

Seasonal mood d., depression with increased need for sleep and increased carbohydrate intake occurring during winter months.

Separation anxiety d. (DSM III-R), distress and apprehension in a child on being removed from parents, home, or familiar surroundings.

Shared paranoid d., induced psychotic d.

Single-gene d., mendelian d.

Sleep terror d. (DSM III-R), repeated episode of awakening shortly after sleep onset with intense anxiety, autonomic symptoms, and unresponsiveness to comforting efforts. Called also pavor nocturnus.

Sleepwalking d., (DSM III-R), repeated episodes of somnambulism.

Somatization d., (DSM III-R), classic hysteria (Briquet's syndrome); a mental disorder characterized by multiple somatic complaints that are not caused by a real physical illness; the complaints may involve a general complaint of being sickly or specific conversion (pseudoneurological) symptoms, gastrointestinal symptoms, female reproductive symptoms, psychosexual symptoms, cardiopulmonary symptoms, or pain. Complaints are often presented in a dramatic, vague, or exaggerated way; many physicians become involved in the medical care; and numerous diagnostic evaluations and unnecessary medical treatment or surgery may be performed. Most patients have symptoms of anxiety and depression and a wide range of interpersonal difficulties; many have histerionic (hysterical) personality traits.

Somatoform d's (DSM III-R), mental disorders characterized by symptoms suggesting a physical disorder that are of psychogenic origin but not under voluntary control; this category includes body dysmorphic disorder, conversion disorder (the pain is inconsistent with neuroanatomy and known pathophysiological mechanism or far exceeds what would be expected from what organic pathologic change is present, and there are signs indicating the psychological origin of the symptoms).

Substance use d., see psychoactive substance use d's.

Tourette's d., Gilles de La Tourette's syndrome.

Unipolar d's., major depression and dysthymic disorder (depressive neurosis), Cf: bipolar d's.

4
Signs

Sign: An indication of the existence of something; any objective evidence of a disease, i.e., such evidence as is perceptible to the examining physician, as opposed to the subjectives sensations (symptoms) of the patient.

Aaron's s., a sensations of pain or distress in the epigastric or precor-dial region on pressure over McBurney's point in appendicitis.

Abadie's s., 1. Spasm of the levator palpebrae superioris muscle; a sign of Graves' disease. 2. Insensibility of the Achilles tendon to pressure; seen in tabes dorsalis.

Abrahams's s., 1. A sound between dull and flat obtained on percussion over the acromion process in early tuberculosis of the apex of the lung. 2. Acute pain produced in vesical lithiasis when pressure is applied midway between the umbilicus and the ninth right costal cartilage.

Accessory s., any nonpathognomonic sign of disease.

Air-cushion s., see Klemm's.

Allis's s., relaxation of the fascia between the crest of the ilium and the greater trochanter a sign of fracture of the neck of the femur.

Amoss's., in painful flexure of the neck of the spine, the patient, when rising to a sitting posture from lying in bed, does so by supporting himself with his hands placed far behind him in the bed.

Andral's s., decubitus on the sound side, a position assumed in early stages of pregnancy.

Andre-Thomas s., if during the finger to nose test, the patient is directed to raise his arm over his head and is then suddenly ordered to let it fall to his head, the arm will rebound; seen in disease of the cerebellum.

Anghelescu's s., inability to bend the spine while lying on the back so as to rest on the head and heels alone, seen in tuberculosis of the vertebrae.

Antecedent s., any precursory indication of an attack of disease.

Anterior tibial s., involuntary contraction of the tibialis anterior muscle when the thigh is forcibly flexed on the abdomen; seen in spastic paraplegia.

Anticus s., see Piotrowski's s.

Argyll Robertson pupil s., one which is miotic and which responds to accommodation effort, but not to light.

Arroyo's s., asthenocoria—a condition in which the pupillary light reflex is sluggish seen in hypoadrenalism.

Aschner's s., oculocardiac reflex—a slowing of the rhythm of the heart following compression of the eyes or pressure on the carotid sinus. A slowing of from 5 to 13 beats per minute is normal; one of from 13 to 50 or more is exaggerated; one of from 1 to 5 is diminished. If ocular compression produces acceleration of the heart.

Assident s., see Accessory s.

Auenbrugger's s., a bulging of the epigastrium, due to extensive pericardial effusion.

Aufrecht's s., noisy breathing heard just above the suprasternal notch, indicative of tracheal stenosis.

Babinski's s., 1. Loss or lessening of the Achilles tendon reflex in sciatica—this distinguishes it from hysteric sciatica. 2. Babinski's reflex—dorsiflexion of the big toe on stimulating the sole of the foot; it occurs in lesions of the pyramidal tract, and indicates organic, as distinguished from hysteric hemiplegia. 3. In hemiplegia, the contraction of the platysma muscle in the healthy side is more vigorous than on the affected side, as seen in opening the mouth, whistling, blowing, etc. 4. The patient lies supine on the floor, with arms crossed upon his chest, and then makes an effort to rise to the sitting posture.

On the paralyzed side, the thigh is flexed upon the pelvis and the heel is lifted from the ground, while on the healthy side the limb does not move. This phenomenon is repeated when the patient resumes the lying posture. It is seen in organic hemiplegia, but not in hysterical hemiplegia. 5. When the paralyzed forearm is placed in supination, it turns over to pronation: seen in organic paralysis. Called also pronation sign.

Babinski's toe s., see Babinski's s., (2).

Baccelli's s., whisper heard over the chest in pleural effusion.

Bail-larger's s., inequality of the pupils in paralytic dementia.

Ballance's s., resonance of right flank when the patient lies on the left side; said to be present in splenic rupture.

Ballet's s., external ophthalmoplegia, with loss of all voluntary eye movements, the pupillary movements and reflex eye movements persisting; seen in Graves' disease and hysteria.

Bamberger' s., 1. Allochiria—a condition in which, if one extremity is stimulated, the sensation is referred to the opposite side. 2. Presence of signs of consolidation at the angle of the scapula, which disappear when the patient leans forward; a sign of pericardial effusion.

Barany's s., see caloric test.

Bard's s., in organic nystagmus the oscillations of the eye increase as the patient's attention follows the finger moved alternately from one side to the other: but in congenital nystagmus the oscillations disappear in like condition.

Barre's s., contraction of the iris is retarded in mental deterioration.

Barre's pyramidal s., the patient lies face down and the legs are flexed at the knee; he is unable to hold the legs in this vertical position if there is disease of the pyramidal tracts.

Baruch's s., resistance of the temperature in the rectum to a bath of 75° F for fifteen minutes; a sign of typhoid fever.

Bastian-Bruns' s., if there is complete transverse lesion in the spinal cord cephalad to the lumbar enlargement, the tendon reflexes of the lower extremities are abolished.

Battle's s., discoloration in the line of the posterior auricular artery, the ecchymosis first appearing near the tip of the mastoid process; seen in fracture of the base of the skull.

Becker's s., see under phenomenon.

Beclard's s., a sign of the maturity of the fetus consisting of a center of ossification in the lower epiphysis of the femur.

Beevor's s., 1. A sign of functional paralysis consisting in inability of the patient to inhibit the antagonistic muscles. 2. Upward deviation of the umbilicus on attempting to lift the head, a sign of weakness of the lower abdominal muscles.

Behier-Hardy s., aphonia in the early stages of pulmonary gangrene.

Bekhterev's s., 1. In tabes dorsalis, anesthesia of the popliteal space. 2. Bekhterev's reflex—(i) deep: passive flexion of the toes and foot in plantar direction is followed by flexion in dorsal direction and by flexive movements of hip and knee, (ii) hypogastric: contraction of muscles of the lower abdomen on stroking skin of the inner surface of the thigh, (iii) pupil: dilatation of the pupil on exposure to light; sometimes seen in tabes and general paralysis, (iv) tickling of the nasal mucosa of the nasal cavity with a feather or piece of paper produces contraction of the facial muscles on the same side of the face.

Bell's s., see under phenomenon.

Berger's s., an irregularly shaped or elliptical pupil in the early stages of tabes dorsalis, paralytic dementia, and certain paralyses.

Bergman's s., in urologic radiography, (a) the ureter is dilated immediately below a neoplasm, rather than collapsed as below an obstructing stone and (b) the ureteral catheter tends to coil in this dilated portion of the ureter.

Bethea's s., when the examiner, standing in back of the patient, places his fingers so that the tips rest on the upper surfaces of corresponding ribs high up in the patient's axillae, unilateral impairment of chest expansion is indicated by the lessened degree of respiratory movement of the ribs on the side affected.

Bezold's s., an inflammatory swellig below the apex of the mastoid process; evidence of mastoiditis.

Biederman's s., a dark red color (instead of the normal pink) of the anterior pillars of the throat, seen in some patients with syphilis.

Biermer's s., the metallic resonance over hydropneumothorax varies in pitch with change of position of the patient; seen in pneumothorax. Called also change of sound and Gerhardt's sign.

Biernacki's s., analgesia of the ulnar nerve in paralytic dementia and tabes dorsalis.

Binda's s., a sudden movement of the shoulder when the head is passively and sharply turned toward the other side, an early sign of tuberculous meningitis.

Biot's s., breathing characterized by irregular periods of apnea alternating with periods in which four or five breaths of identical breath are taken seen in patients with increased intracranial pressure.

Bird's s., a definite zone of dullness with absence of the respiratory sounds in hydatid disease of the lung.

Bjerrum's s., a further development of the Siedel's scotoma [a further development of arcuate scotoma (a scotoma arising at or near the blind spot and arching inferiorly or superiorly towards the nasal field, following the paths of retinal nerve fibers), which extends at either or both ends, the concavity of the prolongation always being directed towards the fixation point] the sickle shaped defect contiguous to the blind spot extending above and below the fixation point and encircling it more or less completely.

Blatin's s., hydatid thrill—a tremulous impulse sometimes felt on palpation of the body surface over a hydatid cyst.

Blumberg's s., pain on abrupt release of steady pressure (rebound tenderness) over the site of a suspected abdominal lesion; seen in peritonitis.

Bonnet's s., pain on thigh adduction in sciatica.

Bordier-Frankel d., an outward and upward rolling of the eye in peripheral facial paralysis.

Borsieri's s., when the fingernail is drawn along the skin in early stages of scarlet fever, a white line is left which quickly turns red; called also Borsieri's line.

Boston's s., in Graves' disease, when the eyeball is turned downward there is arrest of descent of the lid, spasm, and continued descent.

Bouchard's s., a few drops of Fehling's solution are added to the urine and the mixture is shaken; if pus from the kidney is present, fine bubbles will form, which push to the surface the coagulum formed by heating.

Bouillaud's s., permanent retraction of the chest in the precordial region; a sign of adherent pericardium.

Boyce's s., a gurgling sound heard on pressure by the hand on the side of the neck, in diverticulum of the esophagus.

Bozzolo's s., a visible pulsation of the arteries within the nostrils; said to indicate aneurysm of the thoracic aorta.

Bragard's s., with the knee stiff, the lower extremity is flexed at the hip until the patient experiences pain; the foot is then dorsiflexed. Increase of pain points to disease of the nerve root.

Branham's s., bradycardia produced by digital closure of an artery proximal to an arteriovenous fistula.

Braunwald s., occurrence of a weak pulse instead of a strong one immediately after a premature ventricular contraction.

Braxton Hicks's., light, usually painless irregular in intensity and frquency and becoming more rhythmic during the third trimester.

Brickner's s., diminished oculoauricular associated movements seen in impairment of function of the facial nerve.

Broadbent's s., a retraction seen on the left side of the back, near the eleventh and twelfth ribs, related to pericardial adhesion.

Broadbent's inverted s., pulsations synchronizing with ventricular systole on the posterior lateral wall of the chest in gross dilatation of the left atrium.

Brockenbrough's s., occurrence of a weak pulse instead of a strong one immediately after a premature ventricular contraction.

Brodie's s., 1. A black spot on the glans penis—a sign of urinary extravasation into the spongiosum. 2. Brodie's pain—pain induced by folding a skin near joint affected with neuralgia.

Brown-Sequard's s., see under syndrome.

Brudzinski's s., 1. In meningitis, flexion of the neck usually results in flexion of the hip and knee. 2. In meningitis, when passive flexion of the lower limb on one side is made, a similar movement will be seen in the opposite limb; called also contralateral sign.

Brunati's s., the appearance of opacities in the cornea during the course of pneumonia or typhoid fever.

Bruns' s., see under syndrome.

Bryant's s., lowering of the axillary folds in dislocation of the shoulder.

Burger's s., see Heryng's s.

Burghart's s., fine rales over the anterior inferior edge of the lung; an early sign of pulmonary tuberculosis.

Burton's s., leadline—a gray or bluish black line at the gingival margin in lead poisoning, seen especially in patients with bad oral hygiene.

Cantelli's s., dissociation between the movements of the head and eyes; as the head is raised the eyes are lowered, and vice versa. Called also doll's eye s.

Capps' s.,

Carabelli's s., an accessory cusp on the lingual aspect of the mesiolingual cusp of an upper molar, which may be unilateral or bilateral and may vary considerably in size, present in some form of Caucasians, but virtually never present in those of mongoloid race.

Cardarelli's s., transverse pulsation of the laryngotracheal tube in aneurysm and in dilatation of the arch of the aorta.

Cardinals's., (of inflammation), dolor, calor, rubor, tumor, and functio laesa.

Cardiorespiratory s., a change in the normal pulse-respiration ratio from 4:1 to 2:1; seen in infantile scurvy.

Carman's s., see meniscus s.

Carnett's s., the test for demonstrating parietal tenderness consists of palpation during a period in which the patient holds his anterior abdominal muscles as tense as possible. The tense abdominal muscles prevent the examiner's fingers from coming in contact with the underlying viscera and any tenderness that is elicited over them will be parietal in location. Tenderness elicited over relaxed muscles may be either parietal or intra-abdominal in origin. Tenderness present with relaxed muscles and absent with tense muscles is due to a subparietal lesion and its cause should be sought inside of the abdomen. Tenderness found both when the muscles are relaxed and when voluntarily tensed is due to an anterior parietal lesion and its cause should be sought outside the abdominal cavity.

Carvallo s., in tricuspid regurgitation, augmentation of the pansystolic murmur by inspiration.

Castellino's s., see Cardarelli's s.

Cegka's s., invariability of the cardiac dullness during the different phases of respiration; a sign of adherent pericardium.

Chaddock's s., stimulation below the external malleolus produce extension of the great toe; it occurs in lesion of the pyramidal tract.

Charcots s., 1. The raising of the eyebrow in peripheral facial paralysis, and the lowering of the same part in facial contraction. 2. Intermittent limping in arteriosclerosis of the legs and feet.

Cheyne-Stokes s., breathing characterized by rhythmic waxing and waning of the depth of respiration, with regularly recurring periods of apnea; seen especially in coma resulting from affection of the nervous centers.

Chilaiditi s., hepatoptosis—positioning of the colon between liver and diaphragm on the X-ray.

Chin-retraction s., a sign of the third stage of anesthesia: the chin and larynx move downward during inspiration.

Chvostek's s, Chvostek-Weiss s., spasm of the facial muscles elicited by tapping the facial nerve in the region of the parotid gland; seen in tetany.

Claude's hyperkinesis s., reflex movements of paretic muscles elicited by painful stimuli

Clavicular s., a tumefaction at the inner third of the right clavicle; seen in congenital syphilis. Called also Higoumenakis's s.

Cleeman's s., creasing of the skin just above the patella, indicative of fracture of the femur with overriding of fragments.

Cloquet's needle s., a clean needle is plunged into the biceps muscle; if life is not extinct, the needle oxidizes in 20 to 60 minutes.

Codman's s., in rupture of the supraspinatus tendon, the arm can be passively abducted without pain, but when support of the arm is removed and the deltoid contracts suddenly, pain occurs again.

Cogwheel s., see under phenomenon.

Coin s., see under test.

Coles' s., deformity of the duodenal contour as seen in the roentgenogram, a sign of the presence of duodenal ulcer.

Commemorative s., any sign of a previous disease.

Comolli's s., a sign of scapular fracture consisting in the appearance in the scapular region, shortly after the accident, of a triangular swelling reproducing the shape of the body of the scapula.

Complementary opposition s., see Grasset-Gaussel-Hoover s.

Contralateral s., see Brudzinski's s., def. 2.

Coopernail s., ecchymosis on the perineum and scrotum or labia— a sign of fracture of the pelvis.

Cope's s., see psoas s.

Corrigan's s., 1. A purple line at the junction of the teeth and gum in chronic copper poisoning. 2. A peculiar expanding pulsation indicative of aneurysm of the abdominal aorta; 3. A shallow and frequent blowing respiration in a low fever.

Coughing s., see Huntington's s.

Courvoisier's s., when the common bile duct is obstructed by a stone dilatation of the gallbladder is rare; when the duct is obstructed in some other way, dilatation is common.

Cowen's s., jerky constriction of the contralateral pupil when light is shown into the pupil, a sign of Graves' disease.

Crichton-Browne's s., tremor of the outer angles of the eyes and of the labial commissures in the earlier stages of paralytic dementia.

Cruveilhier's s., a swelling in the groin is palpated when the patient coughs: in saphenous varix there is felt a tremor as of a jet of water entering and filling the pouch.

Cullen's s., a bluish discoloration of the skin around the umbilicus sometimes associated with intraperitoneal hemorrhage, especially following rupture of the uterine tube in ectopic pregnancy. A similar discoloration is seen in acute hemorrhagic pancreatitis.

Dalrymple's s., abnormal wideness of the palpebral opening in Graves' disease.

D'Amato's s., in pleural effusion, the location of dullness is altered from the vertebral area in the sitting position to the heart region when the patient assumes a lateral position on the side opposite the effusion.

Damoiseau's s., Ellis' line—an S-shaped line on the chest, showing the upper border of pleural effussions.

Darier's s., urtication and itching occurring on rubbing the lesions of urticaria pigmentosa.

Davidsohn's s., decrease of illumination of the pupil on transillumination with an electric light placed in the mouth; indicates tumor or fluid in the maxillary antrum.

Davis's., an empty state and a yellowish or pale tint of the pulseless arteries; a sign of death.

Dawbarn's s., in acute subacromial bursitis, when the arm hangs by the side palpation over the bursa causes pain, but when the arm is abducted this pain disappears.

Dejerine's s., aggravation of symptoms of radiculitis produced by coughing, sneezing, and straining at stool.

De la Camp's s., relative dullness over and at each side of the fifth and sixth vertebrae in tuberculosis of the bronchial lymph nodes.

Delbet's s., in aneurysm of the main artery of a limb, if the nutrition of the part distal to the aneurysm is maintained, although the pulse may have disappeared, the collateral circulation is sufficient.

Delmege's s., deltoid flattening; said to be an early sign of tuberculosis.

Demarquay's s., fixation or lowering of the larynx during phonation and deglutition; a sign of syphilis of the trachea.

Demianoff's s., a sign that permits the differentiation of pain originating in the sacrolumbalis muscles from lumbar pain of any other origin. The sign is obtained by placing the patient in dorsal decubitus and lifting his extended leg. In the presence of lumbago this produces a pain in the lumbar region which prevents raising the leg high enough to form an angle of 10 degrees, or even less, with the table or bed on which the patient reposes. The pain is due to the stretching of the sacrolumbalis.

De Mussets s., see Musset's s.

De Mussy's s., a point, exceedingly painful on pressure on the line of the left border of the sternum, at the level of the end of the tenth rib; it is a symptom of diaphragmatic pleurisy.

Dennie's s., Morgan's line—a secondary crease in the lower eyelids in atopic dermatitis.

Desault's s., a sign of intracapsular fracture of the femur, consisting of alteration of the arc described by rotation of the great trochanter, which normally describes the segment of a circle, but in this fracture rotates only as the apex of the femur as it rotates about its own axis.

D'Espine's s., in the normal person, on auscultation over the spinous processes, pectoriloquy ceases at the bifurcation of the trachea, and in infants opposite the seventh cervical vertebra. If pectoriloquy is heard lower than this, it indicates enlargement of the bronchial lymph nodes.

Dew's s., in diaphragmatic hydatid abscess beneath the right cupola, the area of resonance moves caudally with the patient on hands and knees.

Dixon Mann's s., see Mann's s.

Doll's eye s., see Cantelli's s.

Dorendorf's s., fullness of the supraclavicular groove one side in aneurysm of the aortic arch.

Drummond's s., a whiff heard at the open mouth during respiration is cases of aortic aneurysm.

DTP s., (distal tingling on percussion), see Tinel's s.

Du Bois's., shortness of the little finger in congenital syphilis.

Duchenne's s., the sinking in of the epigastrium on inspiration in paralysis of the diaphragm or in certain cases of hydropericardium.

Duckworth's s., see under phenomenon.

Dugas' s., see under tests.

Duncan-Bird s., see Bird's s.

Dupuytren's s., 1. A crackling sensation on pressure over a sarcomatous bone. 2. In congenital dislocation of the head of the femur, there is a free up-and-down movement of the head of the bone.

Duroziez's s., a double murmur over the femoral or other large peripheral artery, due to aortic insufficiency.

Echo s., 1. A percussion sound resembling an echo which is heard over a hydatid cyst. 2. The repetition of the last word or clause of a sentence, seen in certain brain diseases; echolalia.

Elliot's s., 1. Induration of the edge of a syphilitic skin lesion. 2. A scotoma extending from the blind spot and made up of numerous points or spots.

Ellis' s., the peculiar curved line of dullness discoverable during resorption of a pleuritic exudate.

Ely's s., see under tests.

Enroth's s., abnormal fullness of the eyelids in Graves' disease.

Erb's s., 1. Increased electric irritability of motor nerves in cases of tetany. 2. Dullness in percussion over the manubrium of the sternum in acromegaly.

Erben's s., slowing down of the pulse upon bending the head and trunk. Strongly forward; said to indicate vagal excitability.

Erichsen's s., when the iliac bones are sharply pressed toward each other pain is felt in sacroiliac disease but not in hip disease.

Emi's s., the cavernous tympany developed over an apical cavity that has previously been filled with fluid. Sometimes gently rapping over such a filled cavity with a hard instrument will excite coughing, which will expel the secretion, and thus the cavernous signs are developed.

Escherich's s., in tetany, percussion of the inner surface of the lips or tongue produces contraction of the lips, tongue, and masseter muscles.

Ether s., a sign of death—1 or 2 ml of ether is injected subcutaneously. If the ether spurts back when the needle is withdrawn, death has occurred. Its absorption indicates that life still persists.

Eustace Smith's., see Smith's s.

Ewart's s., 1. Undue prominence of the sternal end of the first rib in certain cases of pericardial effusion. 2. Bronchial breathing and dullness on percussion at the lower angle of the left scapula in pericardial effusion.

Ewing's., tenderness at the upper inner angle of the orbit: a sign of obstruction of the outlet of the frontal sinus.

External malleolar s., Chaddock's reflex—stimulation below the external malleolus produces extension of the great toe; it occurs in lesions of the pyramidal tract.

Fabere s., see Patrick's test, under tests.

Facial s., see Chvostek's s.

Fajersztajn's crossed sciatic s., in sciatica, when the leg is flexed, the hip can also be flexed, but not when the leg is held straight; flexing the sound thigh with the leg held straight causes pain on the affected side.

Fan s., spreading apart of the toes following the stroking of the sole of the foot; it forms part of the Babinski's reflex.

Federici's s., on auscultation of the abdomen, the cardiac sounds can be heard in cases of intestinal perforation with gas in the peritoneal cavity.

Filipovitch's s., the yellow discoloration of prominent parts of the palms and soles in typhoid fever; called also palmoplantar s.

Fischer's s., 1. On auscultation over the manubrium with the patient's head bent backward, there is sometimes heard, in tuberculosis of the bronchial glands, a murmur due to pressure of the glands on the innominate veins. 2. A presystolic murmur in certain cases of adherent pericardium.

Flag s., dyspigmentation of the hair occurring as a band of light hair, seen in children who have recovered from kwashiorkor.

Flush-tank s., the passage of a large amount of urine and the coincident temporary disappearance of a lumbar swelling; a sign of hydronephrosis.

Forearm s., see Leri's s.

Formication s., see Tinel's s.

Frankel's s., excessive range of passive movement of the hip joint, indicating diminished tone of the surrounding musculature in tabes dorsalis.

Friedreich's s., 1. Diastolic collapse of the cervical veins due to adherent pericardium. 2. Lowering of the pitch of the percussion note over an area of cavitation during forced inspiration; called also Friedreich's change of note.

Froment's paper s., flexion of the distal phalanx of the thumb when a sheet of paper is held between the thumb and index finger; seen in affections of the ulnar nerve.

Furbringer's s., in cases of subphrenic abscess, the respiratory movements will be transmitted to a needle inserted into the abscess, which is thus distinguished from abscess above the diaphragm.

Gaenslen's s., with the patient on his back on the operating table, the knee and hip of one leg are held in flexed position by the patient, while the other leg, hanging over the edge of the table, is pressed down by the examiner to produce hyperextension of the hip: pain occurs on the affected side in lumbosacral disease.

Galeazzi s., in congenital dislocation of the hip, apparent shortening of the femur, as shown by the difference of knee levels with the knees and hips flexed at right angles with the patient lying on a flat table.

Garel's s., see Heryng's s.

Gerhardt's s., see Biermer's s.

Gianelli's s., see Toumay's s.

Gifford's s., inability to evert the upper lid; seen in Graves' disease.

Gilbert's s., opsiuria indicative of hepatic cirrhosis.

Glasgow's s., a systolic sound in the brachial artery in latent aneurysm of the aorta.

Goggia's s., in health, the fibrillary contraction produced by striking and then pinching the brachial biceps extends throughout the whole muscle: in debilitating disease, such as typhoid fever, the contraction is local.

Goldstein's s., wide space of distance between the great toe and the adjoining toe seen in cretinism and Down's syndrome.

Goldthwait's s., the patient lying supine, his leg is raised by the examiner with one hand, the other hand being placed under the patient's lower back; leverage is then applied to the side of the pelvis. If pain is felt by the patient before the lumbar spine is moved, the lesion is a sprain of the sacroiliac joint. If pain does not appear until after the lumbar spine moves, the lesion is in the sacroiliac or lumbosacral articulation.

Golonbov's s., tenderness on percussion over the tibia in chlorosis (a disorder, especially common during the nineteenth century and disappearing abruptly soon thereafter, generally affecting adolescent females, believed to be associated with iron deficiency anemia, and characterized by greenish yellow discoloration of the skin and by hypochromic erythrocytes).

Goodell's s., if the woman's cervix uteri is soft she is pregnant; if it is hard she is not.

Gordon's s., finger phenomenon, see phenomenon.

Gottron's s., 1. A cutaneous sign pathognomonic of dermatomyositis, consisting of symmetrical macular violaceous erythema, with or without edema, overlying the dorsal aspect of the interphalangeal joints of the hands, olecranon processes, patellas, and medial malleoli. 2. A cutaneous manifestation pathognomonic of dermatomyositis, consisting of flat-topped violaceous papules on the dorsal aspect of the interphalangeal joints of the hand, which develop central atrophy with hypopigmen-tation and telangiectasia.

Gower's s., 1. Abrupt intermittent oscillation of the iris under the influence of light; seen in certain stages of tabes dorsalis. 2. A sign of pseudohypertrophic muscular dystrophy; to stand from the supine position, the patient rolls to the prone position, kneels, and raises himself to a standing position by pushing with his hands against shins, knees, and thighs. Called also Gower's maneuver and Gower's phenomenon.

Graefe's s., failure of the upper lid to move downward promptly and evenly with the eyeball in looking downward, instead it moves tardily and jerkingly; seen in Graves' disease.

Grancher's s., equality of pitch between expiratory and inspiratory murmurs; a sign of obstruction to expiration.

Granger's s., it in the radiograph of an infant two years old or less, the anterior wall of the lateral sinus is visible, extensive destruction of the mastoid is indicated.

Grasset's s., Grasset-Bychowski s., see Grasset's phenomenon.

Grasset-Gaussel-Hoover s., when the patient in a recumbent position attempts to lift the paretic limb, there is greater downward pressure on the examiner's hand with the sound limb than is observed in the test with a normal person.

Greene's s., outward displacement of the free cardiac border by the expiratory movement in pleuritic effusion; it is detected by percussion.

Grey Turner's s., see Turner's s.

Griesinger's s., edematous swelling behind the mastoid process; seen in thrombosis of the transverse sinus.

Griffith's s., lower lid lag on upward gaze, a sign of Graves' disease.

Grisolle's s., the papule of smallpox can be felt beneath the skin when the skin over the lesion is stretched; to the contrary, if the papule becomes impalpable, it is a lesion of measles.

Grocco's s., 1. A sign of pleural effusion consisting of the presence of a triangular area of dullness (Grocco's, Koranyi-Grocco, paravertebral or Rauchfuss' triangle) on the back, on the side opposite to that on which the effusion is present. Called also Grocco's triangular dullness. 2. Extension of the liver dullness to the left of the midspinal line indicating enlargement of the organ.

Grossman's s., dilatation of the heart as a sign of pulmonary tuberculosis.

Gubler's s., a tumor on the back of the wrist, with paralysis of the extensors of the hand, in case of lead poisoning.

Guilland's s., brisk flexion at the hip and knee joint when the contralateral quadriceps muscle is pinched; a sign of meningeal irritation.

Gunn's s., a raising of a ptosed eyelid on opening the mouth and moving the jaw toward the opposite side in the Gunn syndrome.

Gunn's crossing s., a crossing of an artery over a vein in the fundus of the eye, indicative of essential hypertension.

Gunn's pupillary s., see Swinging flashlight s.

Guyon's s., the ballottement and palpation of a floating kidney.

Hahn's s., persistent rotation of head from side to side in cerebellar disease of childhood.

Hall's s., a tracheal diastolic shock felt in aneurysm of the aorta.

Halo s., a halo effect produced in the roentgenogram of the fetal head between the subcutaneous fat and the cranium; said to be indicative of intrauterine death of the fetus.

Hamman's s., a precordial crunching, clicking, or knocking sound, synchronous with each heartbeat, heard on ausculation in such conditions as acute mediastinitis, pneumomediastinum, and pneumothorax.

Harlequin s., reddening of the lower half of the laterally recumbent body and blanching of the upper half, due to temporary vasomotor disturbance in newborn infants.

Hatchcock's s., tenderness on running the finger toward the angle of the jaw in mumps.

Haudek's s., a projecting shadow in radiographs of penetrating gastric ulcer, due to settlement of bismuth in pathologic niches of the stomach wall: called also Haudek's niche.

Heberden's s., small hard nodules, formed usually at the distal interphalangeal articulations of the fingers, produced by calcific spurs of the articular cartilage and associated with interphalangeal osteoarthritis. Heredity is an important etiologic factor.

Hefke-Turner s., a widening and change in contour of the normal obturator X-ray shadow, indicative of pathologic condition of the hip joint; called also obturator s.

Hegar's s., softening of the lower segment of the uterus, an indication of pregnancy.

Heilbronner's s., broadening and flattening of the thigh; seen in cases of organic paralysis when a patient lies on his back on a hard mattress; it does not appear in hysterical paralysis.

Heim-Kreysig s., a depression of the intercostal spaces occurring along with the cardiac systole in adherent pericarditis.

Helbing's s., medialward curving of the Achilles tendon as viewed from behind; seen in flatfoot.

Hellat's s., (obs), in mastoid suppuration, a tuning fork placed on the diseased area is heard for a shorter time than when placed on any other part.

Hellendall's s., see Cullen's s.

Hennebert's s., in the labyrinthitis of congenital syphilis, compression of the air in the external auditory canal produced a rotatory nystagmus to the diseased side; rarefaction of the air in the canal produces a nystagmus to the opposite side. Called also pneumatic s. or test.

Henning's s., an angular deformiy of the angulus of the stomach, in which it assumes a Gothic arch shape: a sign of chronic gastric ulcer. Called also Gothic arch formation.

Heryng's s., an infraorbital shadow produced by fluid or by a hypertrophied, hyperplastic, or neoplastic membrane in the maxillary antrum and observable by electric illumination of the buccal cavity; seen in diseases of the antrum of Highmore (maxillary sinus).

Hicks' s., light, usually painless, irregular uterine contraction during pregnancy, gradually increasing in frequency and intensity and becoming more rhythmic during third trimester.

Higoumenakis's., see clavicular s.

Hill's s., disproportionate femoral systolic hypertension.

Hirschberg's s., adduction, inversion, and slight plantar flexion of the foot on stroking the inner aspect (not the sole) of the foot from the great toe to the heel; called also adductor reflex of foot.

Hochsinger's s., 1. Indicanuria in the tuberculosis of childhood. 2. see under phenomenon.

Hoehne's., absence of uterine contractions during delivery despite repeated injections of oxytocics, regarded as a sign of rupture of the uterus.

Hoffmann's s., 1. Increased mechanical irritability of the sensory nerves in tetany; the ulnar nerve is usually tested. 2. A sudden nipping of the nail of the index, middle, or ring finger produced flexion of the terminal phalanx of the thumb and of the second and third phalanx of some other finger; called also digital reflex. Hoffmann's reflex, and Trammer's s.

Holmes's s., see rebound phenomenon.

Homans' s., pain on passive dorsi flexion of the foot; a sign of thrombosis of deep calf veins.

Hoover's s., 1. In the normal state or in genuine paralysis, if the patient, lying on a couch, is directed to press the leg against the couch, there will be a lifting movement seen in the other leg, this phenomenon is absent in hysteria and malingering. 2. Movement of the costal margins toward the midline in inspiration, occurring bilaterally in pulmonary emphysema and unilaterally in conditions causing flattening of the diaphragm, such as pleural effusion and pneumothorax.

Hope's s., double heart beat in aortic aneurysm.

Horn's s., pain produced by traction on the right spermatic cord in the acute appendicitis.

Homer's s., see Spalding's s.

Horsley's s., if there is a difference in the temperature in the two axillae, the higher temperature will be on the paralyzed side.

Howship-Romberg s., pain passing down in the inner side of the thigh to th knee due to pressure on the obturator nerve by an obturator hernia.

Hoyne's s., a sign elicited in paralytic or nonparalytic poliomyelitis: with the patient in the supine position, his head falls back when his shoulders are elevated.

Huchard's s., paradoxic percussion resonance in pulmonary edema.

Hueter's s., the absence of the transmission of osseous vibration in cases of fracture with fibrous material interposed between the fragments.

Human's s., see chin-retraction s.

Huntington's s., the patient is recumbent, with his legs hanging over the edge of a table, and is told to cough. If the coughing produces flexion of the thigh and extension of the leg in the paralyzed limb, it indicates that the paralysis is due to an upper motor neuron lesion.

Hutchinson's s., 1. Interstitial keratitis and a dull-red discoloration of the cornea in inherited syphilis. 2. A tooth abnormality seen in congenital syphilis, in which the incisors have a screw-driver like shape, sometimes associated with notching of the incisal edges or depressions in the labial surfaces above the cutting edge. 3. Diffuse interstitial keratitis, labrynthine disease, and hutchison teeth seen in inhertited syphilis.

Hyperkinesis s., see Claude's hyperkinesis s.

Interossei s., see Souques's phenomenon.

Itard-Cholewa s., anaesthesia of the tympanic membrane in otosclerosis.

Jaccoud's s., prominence of the aorta in the suprasternal notch.

Jackson's s., 1. (Chevalier Jackson) A sound similar to the wheezing heard when the ear is placed close to the mouth of an asthmatic; heard in cases of foreign body in the trachea or bronchus, 2. (James

Jackson, Jr.) Prolongation of the expiratory sound over the affected area in pulmonary tuberculosis.

Jellinek's s; the pigmentation, usually brownish, occurring on the lid margins in many cases of hyperparathyroidism. Called also Rosin's s.

Jendrassik's s., paralysis of the extraocular muscles in Graves' disease.

Joffroy's s., absence of forehead wrinkling in Graves' disease when the patient suddenly turns his eye upward.

Jugular s., see Queckenstedt's s.

Jurgensen's s., delicate crepitation sometimes heard in auscultation in acute pulmonary tuberculosis.

Kanavel's s., a point of maximum tenderness in the palm 1 inch proximal to the base of the little finger in infection of tendon sheath.

Kantor's s., a thin stringlike shadow in the roentgenogram of the colon through the filling defect; seen in colitis and regional ileitis.

Karplus s., a modification of the vocal resonance, in which, on auscultation over a pleural effusion, the vowel u spoken by the patient is heard as a.

Kashida's s., spasm of muscles and hyperesthesia produced by applying heat or cold; seen in tetany.

Keen's s., increased diameter of the leg at the malleoli in Pott's fracture of the fibula.

Kehr's s., severe pain in the left shoulder in some cases of rupture of the spleen.

Kellock's s., increase of the vibration of the ribs on sharp percussion with the right hand, the left hand being placed firmly on the thorax under the nipple; a sign of pleural effusion.

Kelly's s., if the ureter is teased with an artery forceps, it will contract like a snake or worm.

Kerandel's s., deep hyperesthesia accompanied by pain, often retarded, after some slight blow upon a bony projection of the body; seen in African trypanosomiasis. Called also Kerandel's symptom.

Kergaradec's s, uterine souffle—a sound made by the blood within the arteries of the gravid uterus.

Kernig's s., in dorsal decubitus, the patient can easily and completely extend the leg; in the sitting posture or when lying with the thigh flexed upon the abdomen, the leg cannot be completely extended; it is a sign of meningitis.

Kerr's s., alteration of the texture of the skin below the somatic level in lesions of the spinal cord.

Kestenbaum's s., a decrease in number of arterioles traversing the optic disk margin as a criterion for optic atrophy.

Kleist's s., the fingers of the patient when gently elevated by the fingers of the examiner will hook into the examiner's fingers; indicative of frontal and thalamic lesions.

Klemm's s., in the roentgenogram in chronic appendicitis, there is often an indication of tympanites in the right lower quadrant.

Klippel-Feil s., flexion and adduction of the thumb when the patient's flexed fingers are quickly extended by the examiner; indicative of pyramidal tract disease.

Knie's s., unequal dilatation of the pupils in Graves' disease.

Kocher's s., a sign of Graves' disease: the examiner places his hand on a level with the patient's eyes and then lifts it higher; the patient's upper lid springs up more quickly than does his eyeball.

Koplik's s., small irregular, bright red spots on the buccal and lingual mucosa, with a minute bluish white speck in the center of each; seen in the prodromal stage of measles.

Koranyi's s., increase of resonance over the dorsal segment on percussion of the spinal processes of the thoracic vertebrae; a sign of pleural effusion.

Kreysig's s., see Heim-Kreysig s.

Krisovski's (Krisowski's) s., cicatricial lines which radiate from the mouth in congenital syphilis.

Kussmaul's s., 1. Distention of the jugular veins on inspiration, seen in constrictive pericarditis and mediastinal tumor. 2. Convulsions and coma in gastric disease as a result of toxin absorption. 3. Paradoxical pulse—a pulse that markedly decreases in size during inspiration, as that which often occurs in constrictive pericarditis.

Kustner's s., a cystic tumor on the median line anterior to the uterus in cases of ovarian dermoids.

Laborde's s., see Cloquet's needle s.

Ladin's s., a sign of pregnancy, consisting of a circular elastic area, which offers a sensation of fluctuation to the examining finger, situated in the median line of the anterior surface of the body of the uterus just above the junction of the body and the cervix. This area increases in size as pregnancy advances.

Laennec's s., the occurrence of rounded, gelatinous masses (Laennec's pearls) in the sputum of bronchial asthma.

Lafora's s., picking of the nose regarded as an early sign of cerebrospinal meningitis.

Langoria's s., relaxation of the extensor muscles of the thigh, a symptom of intracapsular fracture of the femur.

Larcher's s., grayish, cloudy discoloration of the conjunctivae that are speedily blackened; a sign of death.

Lasegue's s., in sciatica, flexion of the hip is painful when the knee is extended, but painless when the knee is flexed. This distinguishes the disorder from disease of the hip joint.

Laugier s s., a condition in which the styloid processes of the radius and of the ulna are on the same level; seen in fracture of the lower part of the radius.

Leg s., 1.see Schlesinger's s. 2.see Neri's s.

Leichtenstern's s., in cerebrospinal meningitis, tapping lightly any bone of the extremities causes the patient to wince suddenly.

Lennhoffs s., a furrow appearing on deep inspiration below the lowest rib and above an echinococcus cyst of the liver.

Leri's s., passive flexion of the hand and wrist of the affected side in hemiplegia shows no normal flexion at the elbow.

Leser-Trelat s., the sudden appearance and rapid increase in size and number of seborrheic keratoses may be a sign of internal malignancy, especially of the gastrointestinal tract.

Leudet's s., a cracking sound in the ear, audible also to an observer, produced by involuntary contraction of an internal muscle, coinciding with a tic of some of the fibers of the mandibular division of the trigeminal (fifth cranial) nerve.

Levasseur's s., the failure of the scarificator and cupping-glass to draw blood; a sign of death.

Lhermitte's s., the development of sudden, transient, electric-like shocks spreading down the body when the patient flexes the head forward; seen mainly in multiple sclerosis but also in compression and other disorders of the cervical cord.

Libman's s., extreme tenderness, but without pain on pressure of the tips of the mastoid bones.

Lichtheim's s., in subcortical aphasia, although the patient cannot speak, he is able to indicate with his fingers the number of syllables in the word he is thinking of.

Ligature s., in hematuria, the development of ecchymoses in the distal part of a limb to which a ligature has been applied.

Linder's s., with the patient recumbent or sitting with outstretched legs, passive flexi of the head will cause pain in the leg or the lumbar region in sciatica.

Litten's s., see under phenomenon.

Liverato's s., vasoconstriction when the abdominal sympathetic nerve is irritated by striking the anterior abdomen along the xiphoumbilical line.

Lloyd's s., a symptom of renal calculus, consisting of pain in the loin on deep percussion over the kidney, even when pressure causes no pain.

Lombardi's s., the appearance of venous varicosities in the region of the spinous processes of the seventh cervical and first three thoracic vertebrae; seen in early pulmonary tuberculosis.

Lucas's., distention of the abdomen in the early stages of rickets.

Ludloff's s., swelling and ecchymosis at the base of Scarpa's triangle together with inability to raise the thigh when in a sitting posture, a sign of traumatic separation of the epiphysis of the greater trochanter.

Lust's s., see under phenomenon.

McBurney's s., tenderness at a point two-thirds the distance from the umbilicus to the anterior superior spine of the ilium; indicative of appendicitis.

Macewen's s., on percussion of the skull behind the junction of the frontal, temporal, and parietal bones, there is a more resonant note than normal in internal hydrocephalus and cerebral abscess.

McGinn-White s., a Q wave and late inversion of the T wave in lead III, low S-T intervals and T waves in lead II, and inverted T waves in chest leads V_2 and V_3 the electrocardiographic evidence of right ventricular dilatation due to massive pulmonary embolism, plus the clinical signs of acute cor pulmonale.

McMurray s., occurrence of a cartilage click during manipulation of the knee; indicative of meniscal injury.

Magendie's s., Magendie-Hertwig s., skew deviation—downward and inward rotation of the eye on the side of the cerebellar lesion and upward and outward deviation on the opposite side.

Magnan's s., a sensation as of a round body beneath the skin, sometimes experienced in chronic cocainism.

Mangus' s., after death, light ligation of a finger causes no visible change in its distal portion.

Mahler's s., a steady increase of pulse rate without corresponding elevation of temperature; seen in thrombosis.

Maisonneuve's s., marked hyperextensibility of the hand; a symptom of Colles' fracture.

Mann's s., 1. In Graves' disease the two eyes appear not to be on the same level. 2. Lessened resistance of the scalp to a constant electric current; seen in certain traumatic neuroses. Called also Dixon Mann's s.

Mannkopf' s s., increase in the frequency of the pulse on pressure over a painful spot; not present in simulated pain.

Marcus Gunn's pupillary s., see swinging flashlight s.

Marfan's s., a red triangle at the tip of a coated tongue indicates typhoid fever; a rarely observed phenomenon.

Marie's s., tremor of the body or extremities in Graves' disease.

Marie-Foix s., withdrawal of lower leg on transverse pressure of tarsus or forced flexion of toes, even when the leg is incapable of voluntary movement.

Mayo's s., relaxation of the muscles controlling the lower jaw, indicative of profound anesthesia.

Means's., lag of the eyeball on upward gaze in Graves' disease.

Meltzer's s., loss of the normal second sound, heard on auscultation of the heart after swallowing; symptomatic of occlusion or contraction of the lower part of the esophagus.

Mendel-Bekhterev s., percussion of the dorsum of the foot normally causes dorsal flexion of the second to fifth toes; in certain organic nervous condition it causes plantar flexion of the toes.

Meniscus s., the radioscopic appearance of a crescentic shadow made by the crater of a gastric ulcer: when the convexity of the crescent points outward the ulcer is on the lesser curvature; when the convexity points downward the ulcer is distal to the angular incisure.

Mennell's s., an examining thumb is placed over the posterosuperior spine of the sacrum and then made to slide, first outward and then inward. If on pressure over the former point tenderness is detected, it is due to a sensitive deposit in the structures of the gluteal aspect of the posterosuperior spine. If the tenderness is over the inner point, it is probable that the superior ligaments of the sacroiliac joint are strained and sensitive. If the tenderness is increased by pressure backward on the anterosuperior aspect of the ilium and decreased by pulling forward the crest from behind, this is positive proof that it is caused by the sensitive ligaments.

Minor's s., the method of rising from a sitting position characteristic of the patient with sciatica: he supports himself on the healthy side, placing one hand on the back, bending the affected leg and balancing on the healthy leg.

Mirchamp's s., when a sapid substance, such as vinegar, is applied to the mucous membrane of the tongue, a painful reflex secretion of saliva in the gland about to be affected is indicative of sialadenitis, e.g., mumps.

Mobius's., inability to keep the eyeballs converged in Graves' disease; due to insufficiency of the internal recti muscles.

Moebius's., see Mobius, s.

Monteverde's s., failure of any response to the subcutaneous injection of ammonia; a sign of death.

Morquio's s., the patient lying supine resists all attempts to raise the trunk to a sitting posture until the legs are passively flexed; noticed in epidemic poliomyelitis.

Moschcowitz's s., see under tests.

Mosler's s., sternal tenderness in acute myeloblastic anemia.

Moulage s., a waxy cast appearance of bowel segments, a roentgenographic sign of celiac disease.

Muller's s., a sign of aortic insufficiency consisting of pulsation of the uvula and redness of the tonsils and velum palati, occurring synchronously with the action of the heart.

Munson's s., abnormal bulging of the lower lid when the patient rolls his eyes downward, caused by abnormal curvature of the cornea (keratoconus).

Murat's s., in the tuberculous patient there is vibration of the affected side of the chest with a feeling of discomfort when speaking.

Murphy's s., a sign of gallbladder disease consisting of interruption of the patient's deep inspiration when the physician's fingers are pressed deeply beneath the right costal arch, below the hepatic margin.

Musset's s., rhythmical jerking movement of the head; seen in cases of aortic aneurysm and aortic insufficiency.

Myerson's s., ready induction of blepharospasm when the frontalis muscle is tapped, a sign of Parkinson's disease.

Neck s., see Brudzinski's s., def. 1.

Negro s., see cogwheel phenomenon.

Neri's s., 1. A sign of organic hemiplegia, consisting in the spontaneous bending of the knee of the affected side as the leg is passively lifted, the patient being in the dorsal position. 2. With the patient standing, forward bending of the trunk will cause flexion of the knee on the affected side in lumbosacral and iliosacral lesions.

Niche s., see Haudek's s.

Nicoladoni's s., see Branham's s.

Nikolsky's s., ready separation of the outer layer of the epidermis from the basal layer with sloughing of the skin produced by minor trauma, such as by exerting a sliding or rubbing pressure on the area involved, which may occur in pemphigus and in other conditions such as certain hereditary blistering skin diseases, scalded skin syndrome, adult toxic epidermal necrolysis, and thermal burns.

Ober's s., see under tests.

Objective s., one that can be seen, heard, or felt by the diagnostician; called also physical s.

Obturator s., 1. Hypogastric or adductor pain elicited by passive internal rotation of the flexed thigh, due to contact between an inflammatory process and the internal obturator muscle; a sign of appendicitis. 2. See Hefke-Turner s.

Oliver's s., tracheal tugging—a pulling senation in the trachea, due to aneurysm of the arch of the aorta; it is most apparent when the head is extended and the finger is placed on the thyroid cartilage.

Ophthalmoscopic s., as death approaches, the blood in the retinal vessels gradually ceases to move and the column of blood splits into fragments.

Oppenheim's s., dorsiflexion of the big toe on stroking downward the medial side of the tibia; seen in pyramidal tract disease.

Orbicularis s., in hemiplegia, inability to close the eye on the paralyzed side without closing the other.

Ortolani's s., the presence of a palpable click in and out as the hip is reduced by abduction and dislocated by adduction in congenital dislocation of the hip; called also Ortolani's click.

Osler's s., small, painful, erythematous swellings in the skin of the hands and feet in malignant endocarditis; Osler's nodes.

Palmoplantar s., see Filipovitch's s.

Parkinson's s., a stolid mask like expression of the face, with infrequent blinking, pathognomonic of parkinsonism.

Parrot's s., 1. Dilatation of the pupil on pinching the skin of the neck; seen in meningitis. 2. Bony nodes on the outer table of the skull of infants with congenital syphilis, giving it a buttock shape; called also Parrot's nodes.

Pastia's s., linear striations of hyperpigmentation produced by confluent petechiae in body creases, such as anticubital fossae and inguinal regions, that occur at the onset of the rash of scarlet fever and persist after desquamation.

Patent bronchus s., the radiologic finding of an unobstructed bronchus supplying a collapsed lung, lobe, or segment.

Patrick's s., see under tests.

Pende's s., see Andre Thomas s.

Perez's s., a friction sound heard over the sternum when the patient raises and drops his arms; a sign of mediastinal tumor or of aneurysm of the arch of the aorta.

Peroneal s., dorsal flexion and abduction of the foot, a sign of latent tetany elicited by tapping the peroneal nerve just below the head of the fibula, while the knee is relaxed and slightly flexed.

Pfuhl's s., inspiration increases the force of flow in paracentesis in the case of subphrenic abscess, but lessens it in the case of pyopneumothorax. This distinction is lost when the diaphragm is paralyzed.

Pfuhl-Jaffe s., in pyopneumothorax, the liquid issues from the exploratory puncture or incision with considerable force during inspiration; in true pneumothorax, during expiration.

Physical s., see objective s.

Piltz's s., 1. Attention reflex of pupil—alteration of size in the pupil when the attention is suddenly fixed. 2. Orbicularis pupillary reflex—unilateral contraction of the pupil, followed by dilatation after closure or attempted closure of eyelids that are forcibly held apart.

Pins' s., see Ewart's s., def. 2.

Piotrowski's s., percussion of the anterior tibialis muscle produces dorsal flexion and supination of the foot. When this reflex is excessive it indicates organic disease of the central nervous system. Called also anticus s. or reflex.

Piskacek's s., asymmetrical enlargement of the corpus uteri, a sign of pregnancy.

Pitres' s., 1. Hyperesthesia of the scrotum and testes in tabes dorsalis 2. Anterior deviation of the sternum in pleuritic effusion.

Placental s., implantation bleeding.

Plumb-line s., the estimation in sternal displacement by a plumb-line in the diagnosis of pleuritic effusion.

Plummer's s., inability to step up onto a chair or to walk up steps, in Graves' disease.

Pneumatic s., see Hennebert's s.

Pool-Schlesinger s., see Schlesinger's s.

Porter's s., see Oliver's sign.

Potain's s., 1. Extension of percussion dullness over the arch of the aorta, in dilatation of the aorta, from the manubrium to the third costal cartilage on the right-hand side. 2. Timbre metallique—a high-pitched tympanic sound heard in dilatation of the aorta. When heard in persons under fifty five years of age it has been considered suggestive of syphilitic aortitis.

Pottenger's s., 1. Intercostal muscle rigidity on palpation in pulmonary and pleural inflammatory conditions. 2. Different degrees of resistance on light touch palpation, noted (i) over solid organs when compared with hollow organs; (ii) over foci of disease in the lungs and pleura when compared with that over normal organs.

Prehn's s., elevation and support of the scrotum will relieve the pain in epididymo-orchitis, but not in torsion of the testicle.

Prevost's s., conjugate deviation of the head and eyes, the eyes looking toward the affected hemisphere and away from the palsied extremities; seen in hemiplegia.

Pronation s., 1. See Babinski's s. (def. 5). 2. See Strumpell's s. (def. 3).

Pseudo-Babinski's s., in poliomyelitis the Babinski reflex is modified so that only the big toe is extended, because all the foot muscles except the dorsiflexors of the big toe are paralyzed.

Pseudo-Graefe's s., slow descent of the upper lid on looking down, and quick ascent on looking up; seen in conditions other than Graves' disease.

Psoas s., flexion of or pain on hyperextension of the hip due to contact between an inflammatory process and the psoas muscle; a sign often seen in appendicitis. Called also Cope's s.

Puddle s., in examination for ascites, a method for detecting free fluid in the abdominal cavity. The patient lies prone for five minutes, then rises to his hands and knees. While the examiner lightly flicks a finger against one flank, a Bowles stethoscope is moved slowly from the most dependent part of the abdomen to the flank. That part of the ventral abdomen containing the fluid "puddle" shows a loss of high-frequency vibration, which will be detected as soon as the edge of the fluid is reached, indicating the amount of fluid.

Pyramid s., pyramidal s., any sign pointing to disease of the pyramidal tract.

Quant's s; a T-shaped depression in the occipital bone, sometimes seen in rickets.

Queckenstedt's s., when the veins in the neck are compressed on one or both sides, there is a rapid rise in the pressure of the cerebrospinal fluid of healthy persons, and this rise quickly disappears when pressure is taken off the neck. But when there is a block in the vertebral canal the pressure of the cerebrospinal fluid is little or not at all affected by this maneuver.

Quenu-Muret s., in aneurysm, the main artery of the limb is compressed and then a puncture is made at the periphery; if blood flows, the collateral circulation is probably established.

Quincke's s., alternate blanching and flushing of the skin that may be elicited in several ways, e.g., by observing the nailbed or skin at the root of the nail while pressing on the end of the nail. Caused by pulsation of subpapillary arteriolar and venous plexuses, it is sometimes seen in aortic insufficiency and other disorders, but may occur in normal persons under certain conditions. It was originally thought to be due to pulsations of the capillaries.

Radialis s., see Strumpell's s., def. 2.

Radovici's s., see palm-chin reflex.*

Raimiste's s., the patient's hand and arm are held upright by the examiner: if the hand is sound, it remains upright on being released; if paretic the hand flexes abruptly at the wrist.

Ramond's s., rigidity of the erector spinae muscle indicative of pleurisy with effusion; the rigidity relaxes when the effusion becomes purulent.

Rasin's s., see Jellinek's s.

Raynaud's s., a condition marked by symmetrical cyanosis of the extremities with persistent, uneven, mottled blue or red discoloration of the skin of the digits, wrists and ankles and with profuse sweating and coldness of the digits.

Remak's s., polyesthesia; also a prolongation of the lapse of time before a painful impression is perceived; both are noted in tabes dorsalis.

---

* See Appendix

Revilliod's s., see orbicularis s.

Richardson's s., the application of a tight fillet to the arm as a test of death: if life is present, the veins on the distal side of the fillet become more or less distended.

Riesman's s., 1. A bruit heard with the stethoscope over the closed eye in Graves' disease. 2. Softening of the eyeball in diabetic coma.

Ripault's s., external pressure upon the eye during life causes only a temporary change in the normal roundness of the pupil; but after death the change so caused may be permanent.

Ritter-Rollet s; see under phenomenon.

Riviere's s., an area of change in percussion note denoting a band of increased density across the back at the plane of the spinous processes of the fifth, sixth, and seventh dorsal vertebrae: a sign of pulmonary tuberculosis.

Robertson's s., 1. Fibrillary contraction of the pectoralis muscle over the cardiac area in approaching death from heart disease. 2. Absence of pupillary dilatation on pressure over alleged painful areas in malingering. 3. In ascites, fullness and tension in the patient's flanks, felt by the examiner with the patient supine.

Roche's s., in torsion of the testis, the epididymis cannot be distinguished from the body of the testis, whereas in epididymitis the body of the testis can be felt in the enlarged crescent of the epididymis.

Romana's s., unilateral ophthalmia with palpebral edema, conjunctivitis, and swelling of regional lymph glands as a sign of Chagas' disease.

Romberg's s., swaying of the body or falling when standing with the feet close together and the eyes closed; observed in tabes dorsalis.

Rommelaere's s., an abnormally small proportion of normal phosphates and of sodium chloride in the urine in cancerous cachexia.

Rope s., acute angulation between chin and larynx, due to weakness of hyoid muscles, noted in bulbar poliomyelitis.

Rosenbach's s., 1. Absence of the abdominal skin reflex in inflammatory disease of the intestines. 2. Absence of the abdominal skin reflex in pinching the skin of the abdomen on the paralyzed side in hemiplegia. 3. A fine rapid tremor of the closed eyelids in Graves' disease.

Roser's s., Roser-Braun s., absence of dural pulsation, a sign of cerebral tumor or abscess.

Rossolimo's s., on tapping the plantar surface of the toes, plantar flexion of the toes occurs when there are lesions of the pyramidal tract.

Rotch's s., dullness on percussion of the right fifth intercostal space, a sign of pericardial effusion.

Rothschild's s., 1. Preternatural flattening and mobility of the sternal angle; seen in tuberculosis. 2. Loss of hair from the outer third of the eyebrows in hypothyroidism.

Rovighi's s., a fremitus felt on percussion and palpation of a superficial hepatic hydatid cyst.

Rovsing's s., pressure on the left side over the point corresponding to McBurney's point will elicit the typical pain at McBurney's point in appendicitis.

Ruggeri's s., acceleration of the pulse following strong convergence of the eyeballs toward something very close to the eyes. It indicates sympathetic excitability.

Rumpel-Leede s., see under phenomenon.

Rust's s., see under phenomenon.

Saenger's s., a light reflex of the pupil that has ceased returns after a short stay in the dark; Observed in cerebral syphilis but not in tabes dorsalis.

Salisbury and Melvin's s., see Ophthalmoscopic s.

Sansom's s., 1. Marked increase of the area of dullness in the second and third intercostal spaces, due to pericardial effusion. 2. A rhythmical murmur heard with a stethoscope applied to the lips in aneurysm of the thoracic aorta.

Sarbo's s., analgesia of the peroneal nerve; sometimes noticed in tabes dorsalis.

Saunders' s., on wide opening of the mouth there take place in children associated movements of the hand consisting of opening of the hand and extension and separation of the fingers; called also mouth-and-hand synkinesia.

Schepelmann's s., in dry pleurisy, the pain is increased when the patient bends his body toward the normal side, whereas in intercostal neuralgia it is increased by bending toward the affected side.

Schick's s., stridor heard on expiration in an infant with tuberculosis of the bronchial glands.

Schlesinger's s., in tetany, if the patient's leg is held at the knee joint and flexed strongly at the hip joint, there will follow within a short time an extensor spasm at the knee joint, with extreme supination of the foot. Called also Pool's phenomenon.

Schultze's s., 1. see Chvostek's sign. 2. see tongue phenomenon.

Schultze-Chvostek s., see Chvotek's s.

Seeligmuller's s., mydriasis on the side of the face affected with neuralgia.

Seguin's s., the involuntary contraction of the muscles just before an epileptic attack, a sensation, aura, or other subjective experience that gives warning of the approach of an epileptic or other seizure.

Seidel's s., a further development of an arcuate scotoma (a scotoma arising at or near the blind spot and arcing inferiorly or superiorly toward the nasal field, following the paths of the retinal nerve fibers, which extends or either or both ends, the concavity of the prolongation always being directed toward the fixation point.

Seitz's s., bronchial inspiration which begins harshly and then becomes faint; indicative of a cavity in the lung.

Semon's s., impairment of the mobility of the vocal cords in malignant disease of the larynx.

Setting-sun s., downward deviation of the eyes, so that each iris appears to "set" beneath the lower lid, with white sclera exposed between it and the upper lid; indicative of intracranial pressure (hemorrhage or meningoependymitis) or irritation of the brain stem (as in kernicterus).

Shibley's s., in the presence of consolidation of the lung or a collection of fluid in the pleural cavity, all spoken vowels are heard through the stethoscope as "ah."

Sicar's s., a metallic resonance on percussion with two coins on the front of the chest and auscultation at the back; observed in some cases of effusion within the pleura.

Siegert's s., in Down's syndrome, the little fingers are short and curved inward.

Sieur's s., see coin test under tests.

Signorelli's s., extreme tenderness on pressure on the retromandibular point in meningitis.

Silex's s., furrows radiating from the mouth in congenital syphilis.

Simon's s., 1. (CE Simon) Retraction or fixation of the umbilicus during inspiration. 2. (J. Simon) Absence of the usual correlation between the movements of the diaphragm and thorax; seen in beginning meningitis.

Sisto's s., constant crying as a sign of congenital syphilis in infancy.

Skoda's s., a tympanitic sound heard on percussing the chest above a large pleural effusion or above a consolidation in pneumonia.

Smith's s., a murmur heard in cases of enlarged bronchial glands on auscultation over the manubrium with the patient's head thrown back.

Snellen's s., the bruit heard with a stethoscope over the closed eye in Graves' disease.

Soto-Hall s., with the patient flat on his back, on flexion of the spine beginning at the neck and going downward, pain will be felt at the site of the lesion in back abnormalities.

Souques' s., 1. When the patient seated in a chair is suddenly thrown back, the lower extremities do not extend normally or otherwise attempt to counteract the loss of balance; it indicates advanced striatal disease. 2. See Souques' phenomenon.

Spalding's s., in the X-ray film of the fetus *in utero*, overriding of the bones of the vault of the skull indicates death of the fetus.

Spinal s., tonic contraction of the spinal muscles on the diseased side in pleurisy.

Spine s., disinclination to flex the spine anteriorly on account of pain; seen in poliomyelitis.

Squire's s., alternate contraction and dilatation of the pupil, indicative, of basilar meningitis.

Stairs s., difficulty in descending a stairway in tabes dorsalis.

Stellwag's s., retraction of the upper eyelids producing apparent widening of the palpebral opening with which is associated infrequent and incomplete blinking; seen in Graves' disease.

Sterles's., increased pulsation over the cardiac region in intrathoracic tumors.

Sternberg's s., sensitiveness to palpation of the muscles of the shoulder girdle in pleurisy.

Stewart-Holmes s., see rebound phenomenon.

Stierlin's s., indurating and ulcerative processes, especially tuberculosis of the cecum and ascending colon, are shown in the roentgen plate by absence of the normal shadow following a contrast meal.

Stocker's s., in typhoid fever, if the bed clothes are pulled down, the patient takes no notice, but in tuberculous meningitis the patient resents the interference and immediately draws the clothes up again.

Strauss' s., increase of fat following the use of fatty foods in chylous ascites.

String s., 1. See Kantor's s. 2. The stringing out of tubules, observed on pulling the tissues of an intact testis or one in which there is active spermatogenesis, a phenomenon which is prevented by the fibrosis and hyalinization about the tubules when the testis is atrophic.

Strumpell's s., 1. Dorsal flexion of the foot when the thigh is drawn up toward the body; seen in spastic paralysis of the lower limb. Called also tibialis s. 2. Inability to close the fist without marked dorsal extension of the wrist; called also radialis s. 3. Pronation sign: passive flexion of the forearm caused by pronation; seen in hemiplegia.

Strunsky's s., a sign for detecting lesions of the anterior arch of the foot. The examiner grasps the toes and flexes them suddenly. This procedure is painless in the normal foot, but causes pain if there is inflammation of the anterior arch.

Suker's s., deficient complementary fixation in lateral eye rotation; seen in Graves' disease.

Summer's s., on gentle palpation of the iliac fossa, a slight increase in tonus of the abdominal muscles may indicate appendicitis, stone in the ureter or kidney, or a twisted pedicle of an ovarian cyst.

Swinging flashlight s., with the patient's eyes fixed at a distance and a strong light shining before the intact eye, a crisp bilateral contraction of the pupil is noted. On moving the light to the affected eye, both pupils dilate for a short period. Then on return of the light to the intact eye, both pupils contract promptly and remain contracted. Indicative of minimal damage to the optic nerve. Called also Marcus Gunn pupillary phenomenon or sign.

Tay's s., a red circular area (the choroid) surrounded by a gray-white retina, seen though fovea centralis of the eye in the infantile and sometimes in the late infantile form of amaurotic familial idiocy.

Testivin's s., the formation of a collodion -like pellicle on the urine after removing the albumin and treating with acid and then with one-third of its volume of ether, said to occur during the incubation of infectious diseases.

Theimich's lip s., a protrusion or pouting of the lips elicited by tapping the orbicularis oris muscle.

Thermic s., see Kashida's s.

Thomas' s., 1. Flexion of the hip joint can be compensated by lordosis. 2. Pinching of the trapezius muscle causes goose flesh above the level of a spinal cord lesion.

Thomson's s., see Pastia's s.

Thornton's s., severe pain in the region of the flanks in nephrolithiasis.

Tibialis s., see Strumpell's s., def. 1.

Tinel's s., a tingling sensation in the distal end of a limb when percussion is made over the site of a divided nerve. It indicates a partial lesion or the beginning regeneration of the nerve. Called also formication s. and distal tingling on percussion.

Toe s., see Babinski's s.

Tournay's s., unilateral dilatation of the pupil of the abducting eye on extreme lateral fixation.

Traube's s., a loud 'pistol-shot' sound heard in auscultation over the femoral arteries in aortic regurgitation.

Trendelenburg's s., see under tests.

Trepidation s., rhythmic jerking movement of the patella produced by grasping the patella between the thumb and forefinger and pushing it forcibly toward the foot one or more times; an abnormal reflex with alternate contraction and relaxation of the puadriceps muscle.

Tresilian's s., a reddish appearance in Stensen's duct in mumps.

Trimadeau's s., if the dilatation above an esophageal stricture is conic, the stricture is fcbrous; if cup shaped, the stricture is malignant.

Troisier's s., enlargement of the lymph nodes above the clavicle; a sign of intra-abodominal malignant disease or of retrosternal tumor.

Tromner's s., see Hoffmann's s., def. 2.

Trousseau's s. 1. See under phenomenon. 2. Tache cerebrale—a congested streak produced by drawing the nail across the skin: a concomitant of various nervous or cerebral diseases.

Turner's s., discoloration (bruising) of the skin of the loin in acute hemorrhagic pancreatitis.

Turyn's s., in sciatica, if the patient's great toe is bent dorsally, pain will be felt in the gluteal region.

Uhthoff's s., nystagmus occurring in multiple cerebrospinal sclerosis.

Unschuld's s., a tendency to cramp in the calves of the legs; a nonspecific early indication of diabetes.

Vanzetti's s., in sciatia the pelvis is always horizontal in spite of scoliosis, but in other lesions with scoliosis the pelvis is inclined.

Vedder's s., (of beriberi), slight pressure on muscles of calf causes pain; ascertain the presence of anesthesia with a pin over anterior surface of leg; note any changes in patellar reflexes; when patient squats upon heels, note the inability to rise without use of hands.

Vein s., a bluish cord along the midaxillary line formed by the swollen junction of the thoracic and superficial epigastric vein; seen in tuberculosis of the bronchial glands in superior vena cava obstruction.

Vital s' s., the pulse, respiration, and temperature.

Voltolini's s., see Heryng's s.

von Graefe's s., see Graefe's s.

Wartenberg's s., 1. A sign of ulnar palsy, consisting of a position of abduction assumed by the little finger. 2. Reduction or absence of the pendulum movements of the arm in walking; seen in patients with cerebellar disease.

Weber's s., paralysis of the oculomotor nerve of one side and hemiplegia of the opposite side. See syndrome of Weber.

Wegner's s., a broadened, discolored apperance of the epiphyseal line in infants dying from hereditary syphilis.

Weill's s., absence of expansion in the subclavicular region of the affected side in infantile pneumonia.

Weiss's s., see Chvostek's s.

Wernicke's s., hemiopic pupillary reaction—reaction in certain cases of hemianopia in which the stimulus of light thrown upon one side of the retina causes the iris to contract, while light thrown on the other side arouses no response.

Westermark's s., transient clearing (avascularity) of the normal radiologic shadow of pulmonary tissue distal to a pulmonary embolism.

Westphal's s., loss of the knee jerk in tabes dorsalis.

Widowwitz's s., protusion of the eyeballs and sluggish movement of the eyeballs and eyelids seen in diphtheritic paralysis.

Wilder's s., an early sign of Grave's disease consisting in a slight twitch of the eyeball when it changes its movement from adduction to abduction or vice versa.

Williams s., a dull tympanitic resonance heard in the second intercostal space in severe pleural effusion.

Williamsons' s., markedly diminished blood pressure in the leg as compared with that in the arm on the same side; seen in pneumothorax and pleural effusion.

Winterbottom's s., enlargement of posterior cervical lymph nodes in African trypanosomiasis.

Wintrich's s., a change in the pitch of the percussion note when the mouth is open and closed; it indicates a cavity in the lung.

Wood's s., relaxation of the orbicularis muscle, fixation of the eyeball, and divergent strabismus, indicative of profound anesthesia.

Wreden's s., a presence of a gelatinous matter in the external auditory meatus in children who are born dead.

Zaufal's s., saddle nose—concavity of the contour of the bridge of the nose due to collapse of cartilaginous or bony support, or both; it was once most often due to congenital syphilis, but is now more commonly the result of congenital epidermal defect or of leprosy.

5
Tests

Abortus Bang ring (ABR) t., a screening test for brucellosis in cattle; since Brucella agglutinins, as well as the organism, are shed in the milk of infected cattle, a drop of hematoxylin-stained brucellae are mixed in a sample of pooled milk from the herd. After incubation, agglutinated bacteria are adsorbed by the globules of fat that rise to the surface to form a colored ring. Also called milk-ring t. and ring t. ABR t., abortus Bang ring t.

Acetoacetic acid t., see specific tests, including Gerhardt's t., Harding and Ruttan's t., Hartley's t., Lindemann's t., and Nobel's t. (1). See also acetoacetic acid, methods for, under method.

Acid elution t., (for fetal hemoglobin), air-dried blood smears on a glass slide are fixed in 80 percent methanol and immersed in a buffer at pH 3.3 (citric acid and sodium phosphate); all hemoglobulins are eluted except fetal hemoglobulin, which remains fixed in the red cells and can be detected after staining.

Acidified serum t., (for paroxysmal nocturnal hemoglobinuria) the patient's washed red cells are incubated at 37°C in acidified normal serum or the patient's acidified serum; after centrifugation, the supernatant is examined colorimetrically for hemolysis. In PNH red cells are abnormally susceptible to lysis by complement, which is activated by the alternate pathway in acidified serum, and hemolysis is observed in normal serum and to a lesser degree in the patient's serum. No hemolysis is observed when normal red cells or heat-inactivated serum are used as controls. Also called Ham's t.

Acid-lability t., a test to distinguish rhinoviruses from enteroviruses on the basis of their activity at various pH levels, rhinoviruses being inactivated by incubation at pH 3 to 5 for one to three hours.

Acoustic reflex t., measurement of the acoustic reflex threshold; used to differentiate between conductive and sensorineural deafness and to diagnose acoustic neuroma.

Addis' t., after the patient is given a dry diet for 24 hours, the specific gravity of the urine is determined; also called Addis' method.

Adler's t., see benzidine t.

Adson's t., (for thoracic outlet syndrome), with the patient in a sitting position, his hands resting on thighs, the examiner palpates both radial pulses as the patient rapidly fills his lungs by deep inspiration and, holding his breath, hyperextends his neck and turns his head toward the affected side. If the radial pulse on that side is decidedly or completely obliterated, the result is considered positive. Also called Adson's maneuver.

Alkali denaturation t., a moderately sensitive spectrophotometric method for determining the concentration of fetal (F) hemoglobin, which depends on the resistance of the hemoglobin molecule to denaturation of its globin moiety when exposed to alkali.

Allen's t., (for glucose in the urine) add urine to boiling Fehling's solution, and allow it to cool; turbidity will be seen if dextrose is present. (Alfred Henry Alien) 2. (for phenol) to 2 drops of the suspected liquid, add 5 drops of hydrochloric acid and 1 of nitric acid. Phenol, if present, will produce a cherry-red color (Alfred Henry Alien) 3. (for strychnine) extract with ether, concentrate by letting drops fall into a warmed porcelain capsule, cool the residue, and treat with sulfuric acid and manganese dioxide. Strychnine gives a violet color. 4. (for occlusion of ulnar or radial arteries) the patient makes a tight fist so as to express the blood from the skin of the palm and fingers; the examiner makes digital compression on either the radial or the ulnar artery. If on opening the hand blood fails to return to the palm and fingers, there is indicated obstruction to the blood flow, in the artery that has not been compressed (Edgar V Allen).

Allen-Doisy t., (for estrogenic substance in laboratory animals), a positive test is the presence in the vaginal secretion of cornified epithelial cells; a negative test shows only leukocytes in the secretion.

Alpha t., a test of intelligence administered by the US Army in the World War 1 to persons who could read.

Alternate binaural loudness balance (ABLE) t., comparison of the intensity levels at which a given pure tone sounds equally loud to the normal ear and the ear with hearing lose; done to determine recruitment with unilateral sensorineural loss.

Alternate cover t., a test for determining the type of tropia and/or phoria done by alternately covering each eye and noting the movement of the uncovered eye.

Alternate loudness balance t., a hearing test done with pure tones that compares the loudness perceived in one ear with that perceived in the other, with the frequency kept constant.

Ames t., (for carcinogenicity), a mutant stain of *Salmonella typhimurium* that lacks the ability to synthesize histidine is inoculated into a medium deficient in histidine but containing the test compound. If the compound causes DNA damage resulting in mutations, some of the bacteria will regain the ability to synthesize histidine and will proliferate to form colonies. The ability to cause mutations indicates that the substance is carcinogenic.

Antiglobulin t. (AGT)., a test for the presence of nonagglutinating antibodies against red cells that use antihuman globulin antibody to agglutinate red cells coated with the nonagglutinating antibody. The *direct antiglobulin test* detects antibodies bound to circulating red cells *in vivo*. It is used in the evaluation of autoimmune and drug-induced hemolytic anemia and hemolytic disease of the newborn. *The indirect antiglobulin test* detects serum antibodies that bind to red cells in an *in vitro* incubation step. It is used in typing of erythrocyte antigens and in compatibility testing (cross-match). Also called *Coombs' test*.

Antiglobulin consumption t., a test for serum antibodies against cellular antigens. Cells are incubated with the serum sample and then with antiglobulin; any serum antibody that binds to the cells will take up antiglobulin. The amount of antiglobulin consumed is determined by testing the supernatant with antibody-coated red cells; the amount of agglutination is inversely proportional to the antiglobulin consumption.

Apt t., (for differentiating fetal from adult hemoglobin), mix the infant's specimen (vomitus or stool) with 5 volumes of water, centrifuge the mixture, and separate the clear pink supernatant. Add 1 ml 1 percent sodium hydroxide to 5 ml of the supernatant. If hemoglobin F is present, the pink color persists for more than 2 minutes (indicating fetal blood). If hemoglobin A is present, it turns from pink to yellow within 2 minutes (indicating swallowed maternal blood).

Aptitude t., tests given to determine aptitude or ability to undertake study or training in a particular field.

Army General Classification t., an intelligence test whose results are used for placement in the military.

Arylsulfatase t., (for differentiating species of rapid-growing mycobacteria), a sample from a tween-albumin broth culture of the suspected organism is incubated with tripotassium phenolphthalein disulfate for three days and then alkalinized. Those species producing arylsulfatase (*Mycobacterium fortuitum* and *M. chelonei*) show a pink to red positive reaction; a colorless reaction is negative.

Aschheim-Zondek t., (for pregnancy), the subcutaneous injection of the urine of pregnant women into immature female mice is followed by swelling, congestion, and hemorrhages of the ovaries and premature maturation of the ovarian follicles. Abbreviated AST and A-Z t.

Aschner's t., Aschner-Danini t., Aschner's phenomenon—slowing of pulse following pressure on the eyeball; it is indicative of cardiac vagus irritability.

Association t., a test based on associative reaction. It is usually performed by mentioning words to a subject and noting what other words he will give as the ones called up in his mind. The reaction time is also noted.

Augmented histamine t., (of gastric function), after a 12-hour fast, the residual gastric contents are aspirated. Basal gastric secretion is then collected for 1 hour in divided 15-minute aliquots. Thirty minutes before completion of collection, a suitable dose of antihistamine is given intramuscularly. At conclusion of basal secretion collection, histamine acid phosphate (0.04 mg per kg body weight) is given subcutaneously, and gastric contents collected in 15-minute aliquots for 1 hour. Volume, pH, and titratable acidity are measured for each aliquot. When Histalog (1.7 mg. per kg of body sweight) is used in place of histamine, the antihistamine injection is omitted and 8 (rather than 4) 15-minute aliquots are taken after its injection.

Autohemolysis t., one performed in investigation of certain hemolytic states, particularly the congenital, nonspherocytic hemolytic anemias. Defibrinated blood is incubated at 37°C, under sterile conditions, for 24 and 48 hours, and the amount of spontaneous hemolysis is quantitated.

Automated reagin t. (ART), a modification of the rapid plasma reagin (RPR) test for use with automated analyzers used in clinical chemistry.

Ayer's t., (for spinal block), with a spinal manometer, the pressure in lumbar puncture and that in a cisterna magna puncture should be identical in the normal subject.

Ayer-Tobey t., see Tobey-Ayer t.

Babinski's t., see under sign.

Babinski-Weil t., the patient, with his eyes shut, is made to walk forward and backward ten times in a clear space. A person with labyrinthine disease deviates from the straight path, bends to one side when walking forward and to the other side when walking backward.

Bacteriolytic t., the lysis of *Vibrio cholerae* when injected into the peritoneal cavity of an immunized guinea pig; the term is also used to describe the *in vitro* lysis of cholera vibrios or other bacteria when incubated with specific antibody and complement.

Baermann's t., (for extraction of soil nematodes from earth and detecting larvae of *Strongyloides stercoralis* in feces), a specimen of soil or feces is suspended over gauze or wire mesh in a water-filled funnel to which a piece of rubber tubing is attached; larval nematodes migrate from the specimen to the water, and collect in the rubber tubing.

Bang's t., see milk ring t.

Barany's t., see caioric t.

Bárány's pointing t., have the patient point at a fixed object alternately with the eyes open and closed; a constant error with the eyes closed indicates a brain lesion.

Bar-reading t., a test for binocular and stereoscopic vision, which consists of holding a ruler midway between the eyes and the printed page. It is also used as an exercise to develop stereoscopic vision; also called Welland's t.

Becker's t., 1. (for picrotoxin) Fehling's solution is added and the mixture is warmed; if the alkaloid is present, the solution is reduced. 2. (for astigmatism) the patient looks at a test card containing lines radiating in sets of three and points out which seem blurred.

Bekhterev's t., the patient seated in bed is directed to stretch out both legs; in sciatica he cannot do this, but can stretch out each leg in turn.

Bender's Gestalt t., Bender's Visual-Motor Gestalt t., a psychological test used for evaluating perceptual-motor coordination, for assessing personality dynamics, as a test of organic brain impairment, and for measuring neurological maturation. The subject is asked to make free-hand copies of nine simple geometric designs presented separately on cards or sometimes to reproduce the design from memory.

Benedict's t., 1. (for dextrose) 200 gm of sodium or potassium citrate and 200 gm crystallized sodium carbonate and 125 gm of potassium sulfocyanate are dissolved in 800 ml of boiling water. This is cooled and filtered and 18 gm copper sulfate dissolved in 100 ml water are added and the whole diluted to make 1 liter. To 5 ml of this reagent, in a test tube, 8 or 10 drops of the solution to be tested are added. Boil for one or two minutes and allow to cool slowly. If dextrose is present, the solution will be filled with a precipitate red, yellow, or green in color. 2. (for urea) the urea is hydrolyzed to ammonium carbonate by $KHSO$ and $ZNSO.$, made alkaline, and distilled as usual.

Bentonite flocculation t., any agglutination test using antigen adsorbed on particles of bentonite when the antigen is added to serum containing specific antibodies, flocculation occurs.

Benzidine t. (for occult blood in urine or feces), benzidine, acetic acid, and hydrogen peroxide are added to the specimen; hemoglobin catalyzes the oxidation of benzidine by hydrogen peroxide, giving a blue color. This is the most sensitive screening test for occult blood, but it is seldom used because benzidine is a carcinogen, and its use is restricted.

Bernstein's t., esophageal acid infusion test.

Beta t., a test of intelligence administered by the US Army in the World War1 to persons who could not read or did not speak English.

Bial's t., (for pentose in urine), make a reagent consisting of orcinol 1.5 gm., fuming hydrochloric acid 500 gm, and ferric chloride (10 percent) 20 to 30 drops. Five ml of this reagent is boiled in a test tube, and after removal from the flame, several drops of urine are added. A green color appearing at once indicates pentose.

Bielschowsky's head-tilting t., tilting the head to the right and the left shoulder with the patient looking at a distance fixation device permits distinction between superior rectus paresis and contralateral superior oblique paresis.

Bile solubility t., (for differentiation of pneumococci from other streptococci), a sample of a broth culture is incubated at pH 7.4 to 7.6 with sodium deoxycholate. A decrease in turbidity (positive test) indicates lysing of the cells. Pneumococci give a positive result, whereas other viridans streptococci give a negative one.

Bilirubin t., see specific tests, including Fouchet's t., Harrison's spot t.

Binaural distorted speech t., tests of the capacity of the central nervous system to coordinate two incoming speech patterns, each of which is incomplete.

Binet's t., a method of testing the mental capacity of children and youth by asking a series of questions adapted to, and standardized on the capacity of normal children at various ages. According to the answers given, the mental age of the subject is ascertained.

Binet-Simon t., see Binet's t.

Bing's t., a vibrating tuning fork is held to the mastoid process and the auditory meatus is alternately occluded and left open: an increase and decrease in loudness (positive Bing) is perceived by the normal ear and in sensorineural hearing impairment, but in conductive hearing impairment no difference in loudness is perceived (negative Bing).

Biuret t., 1. (For proteins) in 2 ml of unknown solution, add 2 ml of 2N sodium hydroxide solution and then a few drops of 1 percent copper sulfate solution. A pinkish-violet color indicates the presence of biuret or of a similar double—CO-NH—grouping. 2. (For urea) melt the substance in a dry test tube and gently heat it. Cool, and dissolve in 2 ml of water. Add 2 ml of 2N sodium hydroxide solution, and mix drop by drop with a 1 percent copper sulfate solution. A pink and finally a bluish color is produced.

Bodal's t., test of color perception by the use of colored blocks.

Bone conduction t., if a vibrating tuning fork, when the handle is placed against the skull, is heard more distinctly than when held near the ear, it indicates loss in conduction through the middle ear.

Bozicevich's t., a serologic test for the detection of trichinosis.

Bracelet t., the production of pain on moderate lateral compression of the lower ends of the radius and ulna; observed in rheumatoid arthritis.

Brenner's t., with the cathode in the external meatus of ear, a loud sound is heard on closing the circuit, intensity is diminised during closure, and the sound ceases when the circuit is broken with the anode in the meatus, no sound is heard on closing or during closure; a weak sound is heard at the break.

Broadbent's t., (for cerebral dominance of language function), different numbers (or words) are presented simultaneously to the two ears; right-handed persons tend to report first the words going into the right ear.

Burchard-Liebermann t., see Liebermann's t.

Butyric acid t., see pineapple t.

Calcium t., see Sulkowitch's t. See also calcium, methods for, under method.

California mastitis t. (CMT), (for subclinical mastitis in cows), equal amounts of milk, bromcresol purple, and an anionic surface-active substance are mixed in four separate cups within a plastic paddle by rapidly rotating the paddle horizontally; a positive reaction is indicated by various degrees of gel formation, according to the degree of abnormality of the milk. Also called Schalm's t.

Calmette's t. (obs), a tuberculin test in which tuberculin is instilled into the conjunctival sac; a positive response is development of conjunctivitis. Also called Calmette's ophthalmic reaction and Calmette's conjunctival reaction.

Caloric t., irrigation of the normal ear with warm water produces a rotatory nystagmus toward the side of the irrigated ear; irrigation with cold water produces a rotatory nystagmus away from the irrigated side. There is no nystagmus in vestibular disease.

CAMP t., [Christie, Atkins, and Munch-Petersen, discoverers of the phenomenon] (for the presumptive identification of Group B beta-hemolytic streptococci), a culture of *Streptococcus* is streaked on a blood agar plate near a streak of beta-lysin-producing *Staphylococcus aureus*. Group B streptococci produce a substance (CAMP factor) that enlarges the zone of lysis formed by the staphylococcal beta-hemolysin.

Cannabis indica t., see Gayer's t.

Capillary fragility t., capillary resistance, apply blood pressure cuff for five minutes tightly enough to obstruct venous return only, or apply a cupping glass, and note the number of petechiae thus produced.

Carbohydrate t., see Moore's t., Schiff's t. (1).

Carbohydrate tolerance t., see Killian's t.

Carbon monoxide t., see specific tests, including Dejust's t., Hoppe-Seyler t. (1), Katayama's t., Preyer's t., Rubner's t. (1), Salkowski's t. (1), Wetzel's t., Zaleski's t.

Carotid sinus t., (for angina pectoris), on slowing of the heart rate by massage over the right (or left) carotid sinus, the pain of an attack of angina pectoris will lessen or disappear.

Casoni's intradermal t., (for hydatid disease), injection into the skin of hydatid fluid followed by the immediate or delayed production of a wheal-and-flare reaction denotes hydatid infection.

Catalase t., (for the production of catalase by bacteria), a slant culture is treated with hydrogen peroxide. The presence of gas bubbles indicates positive reaction. Micrococci, staphylococci, most species of

Bacillus and anaerobic *Diphtheroids* are catalase positive; streptococci, pneumococci, and most *Actinomyces* are catalase negative.

Catoptric t., a test for cataract made by observing the reflections from the cornea and from the surfaces of the crystalline lens.

Cephalin-cholesterol flocculation t., a flocculation test formerly used as a test of liver function; a positive result (flocculation when a cephalin-cholesterol emulsion is added to serum) reflects serum protein abnormalities, chiefly, hypergammaglobulinemia or hypoalbuminemia. Also called Hanger's t.

Chemiluminescence t., a sensitive test of neutrophil microbicidal function that involves detection of the chemiluminescent energy emitted by unstable and highly reactive oxygen metabolites, e.g. singlet oxygen, produced during the respiratory burst following phagocytosis. It is able to detect heterozygous carriers of chronic granulomatous disease as well as homozygotes and also patients with myeloperoxidase deficiency.

Chick-Martin t., a test for the efficiency of disinfectants in the presence of organic matter; see under method.

Chimani-Moos t., a test for detecting simulated deafness.

Chi-squared (χ^2) t., any statistical hypothesis test that employs the χ^2 distribution (qv) especially two tests applied to categorical data: the χ^2 test of goodness of fit, which tests whether an observed frequency distribution fits a specified theoretical model, and the χ^2 test of independence or homogeneity, which tests whether two or more series of frequencies (the rows and columns of a contingency table) are independent. In both cases, the test statistic is the sum over all cate-gories, of the squared difference between the observed and expected frequencies divided by the expected frequency. The sampling distribution of this χ^2 statistic approaches the χ^2 distribution as the sample size increases.

Cholesterol t., see Liebermann-Burchard t., Obermiller's t., Salkowski's (2), Schiff's t. (2), (3), Schultze's t. (2), and Zwenger's t. (1). See also cholesterol, methods for, under method.

Chromatin t., (for determination of genetic sex), examination of somatic cells for presence of the sex chromatin situated at the periphery of the nucleus in normal females but not in normal males; an index of the presence of XX chromosomal constitution.

Chvostek's t., see under sign.

Cis-trans t., in microbial genetics, a test to determine whether two mutations that have the same phenotypic effect (in a haploid cell or a cell with single phage infection) are located in the same gene (resulting in noncomplementation) or in different genes (resulting in complementation and hence in loss of the mutant defect). The test depends on the independent behavior of two alleles of a gene in a diploid cell or in a cell infected with two phages carrying different alleles.

Citrate t., (for differentiation of organisms of the *Enterobacter* group of bacteria), the test organism is grown on a medium containing citrate as its sole carbon source (Simmon's citrate agar). The metabolism of citrate (positive reaction) turns the medium from green to blue. The Enterobacteriaceae are mostly positive; *Edwardsiella, Escherichia, Morganella, Shigella,* and *Yersinia* are negative.

Clauberg's t., a formerly used biological assay method for the standardi-zation of corpus luteum preparations or progesterone. Immature rabbits are primed with estrogen and the degree of secretory endometrial development is the end-point.

CMT., see California mastitis t.

Coagulase t., a test for coagulase activity in which bacteria are added to citrated or oxalated (human or rabbit) blood plasma; in the presence of coagulase, the plasma gels within three hours. Coagulase activity is also demonstrable by mixing bacteria with blood plasma on a slide; if positive, clumping occurs, with fibrin formation.

Cocaine t., after instillation of a cocaine solution in each eye, the pupil of an eye affected by Horner's syndrome remains smaller than that of the normal eye.

Coccidioidin t., an intracutaneous test for coccidioidomycosis—a skin test antigen prepared from mycelial phase *Coccidioides immitis* organisms, because most individuals in endemic areas are skin test positive, it is not useful in diagnosis. A negative skin test (cutaneous energy) occurs in many patients with disseminated disease and indicates a poor prognosis.

Conn's t., a test for color perception by the use of variously colored embroidery patterns.

Colchicin t., see Zeiscl's t.

Cold pressor t., see Hines-Brown t.

Collateral circulation t., see specific tests, including Henle-Coenen t., Korotkoff's t., Pachon's t., tourniquet t. (2), (3), Tuffier's t., von Frisch t.

Colloidal gold t., (for protein-globulin in the cerebrospinal fluid and thus for the diagnosis of certain central nervous system disorders such as neurosyphilis, multiple sclerosis, poliomyetitis and encephalitis), progressive dilutions of cerebrospinal fluid are added to ten test tubes containing colloidal gold solution. The extent of precipitation is indicative of various diseases, and the results are interpreted according to the color changes that result. When no color change occurs, the reaction is negative, i.e., the deep red colloidal gold color remains unchanged, and is recorded as 0. The appearance of the solution in the tube depends upon the amount of gold precipitated and is scored as 1+ (reddish blue), 2+ (lilac to purple), 3+ (deep blue), 4+ (pale blue), and 5+ (colorless, due to complete precipitation of the gold). Also called Lange's t. or Lange's colloidal gold t.

Color perception t., see specific tests, including Bodal's t., Cohn's t, Donders' t., Holmgren's t., Ishihara's t., Jennings' t., Lantern t. Mauthner's t., Nagel's t.

Complement fixation t., the consumption of complement upon reaction with immune complexes containing complement-fixing antibodies. The basis of complement fixation tests widely used procedures for the detection of antigens or antibodies. These are two stage procedures in which heat inactivated antiserum (or antigen) is reacted with the test material in the presence of a known amount of complement. If the homologous antigen (or antibody) is present in the test material in the presence of a known amount of complement. If the homologous antigen (or antibody) is present in the test material, complement is fixed. Then sheep red blood cells and antisheep erythrocyte antibody are added; lack of hemolysis indicate complement fixation, i.e. a positive best result. Quantitative results are obtained by determining the highest dilution of antiserum or test material that gives a positive reaction.

Concentration t., (for renal function), the patient is placed under conditions which cause the normal person to elaborate urine containing one or more constituents in high concentration and the results are observed to see whether the patient is able to attain this concentration, as in the urea concentration t., xylose concentration t.

Conglutinating complement absorption t. (CCAT), a test resembling the complement fixation test, using as the indicator of antigen-antibody reaction the disappearance of conglutinin (qv) activity.

Congo red t., (for amyloidosis), congo red is injected intravenously, if more than 60 percent of the dye disappears after one hour, amyloidosis is indicated.

Conjunctiva t., the local reaction which occurs when a pollen or an extract of the pollen is instilled into the conjunctival sac of a person sensitive to that pollen.

Contact t., see patch t.

Coombs' t., see antiglobulin t.

Copper t., see Schonbein's t. (2).

Corner-Allen t., a biological method of assay for progesterone or corpus luteum preparations containing it. The rabbits are mated, the ovaries removed eighteen hours later, and the material to be assayed injected. The results are read according to the intensity of the endometrial changes.

Cover t., see alternate cover t. and cover-uncover t.

Cover-uncover t., a test for determining the type of phoria, by covering one eye and noting its movement as it is uncovered.

Crafts' t., in organic disease of the pyramidal tract, stroking with a blunt point upward over the dorsal surface of the ankle the leg being extended and the muscles relaxed, produces dorsal extension of the great toe.

Crampton's t., a test for physical resistance and condition based on the difference between the pulse and blood pressure in the recumbent position and in the standing position. A difference of 75 or more indicates good condition; one of 65 or less shows a poor condition.

Creatinine t., see specific tests, including Jaffe's t. (1), Kerner's t., Salkowshi's t. (5), Thuducgyn's t., Maschke's t., Weyl's t. (1) See also creatinine, methods for, under method.

Cuff t., a test for angina pectoris by producing ischemia in the left arm for five minutes by raising the pressure in a blood-pressure cuff on the arm to 50 mm above the usual systolic pressure. This may produce an anginal attack in persons with coronary disease.

Cuignet's t., (for simulated unilaterat blindness), the bar-reading test used to detect simulated unilateral blindness or malingering.

Cysteine t., see specific tests, including nitroprusside t. (1), Sullivan's t.

Cystine t., see Liebig's t.

Cytosine t., see Wheeler and Johnson's t.

Dark-adaptation t., (for vitamin A deficiency), a test based on the fact that with a deficient intake of vitamin A the ability to see a dimly illuminated object in a darkroom is diminished.

Darkroom t., a test to determine the tendency to develop acute angle glaucoma—ocular pressure is measured by the applanation tonometer, the subject is placed in a darkroom of one hour and applanation tonometry is then repeated.

Davidsohn's t. (differential test for infectious mononucleosis), the determination of the agglutination of sheep erythrocytes by the patient's serum after absorption with Forssman's antigen (guinea pig kidney or horse kidney) and beef antigen respectively.

Davidsohn differential absorption t., Paul Bunnell-Davidsohn t.

Dehio's t., if bradycardia is relieved by injection of atrophine, the condition is caused by increased vagal tone; but if the bradycardia is not relieved, the cause is some affection of the heart muscle.

Dehydrocholate t., (for the speed of blood circulation), sodium dehydrocholate solution is injected intravenously; the usual time elapsing until a bitter taste in the mouth occurs is between 10 and 14 seconds.

Denver Developmental screening t., a test for identification of infants and preschool children with developmental delay.

Deoxyribonuclease (DNase) t., (for the presence of deoxyribonuclease in bacteria), a nutrient agar plate containing deoxyribonucleic acid and toluidine blue is inoculated from a young agar slant; after incubation, a red zone around the inoculum indicates the presence of deoxyribonuclease.

Deoxyuridine suppression t., a test for folate or cobalamin deficiency, in which lack of 5, 10-methylene tetrahydrofolate inhibits incorporation of deoxyuridine into DNA so that deoxyuridine fails to inhibit incorporation of H-thymidine.

Dexamethasone suppression t., a test of hypothalamic-pituitary-adrenocortical function; oral administration of dexamethasone causes suppresion of adrenal cortisol secretion in normal persons but not in those with Cushing's disease.

Dextrose t., see specific tests, including Allen's t. (1), Benedict's., Gerrard's t., Hager's t., Haines' t., Heller's t. (3), Horsley's t., hydroxylamine t., Maumené's t., Molisch's t. (1), (2), Moore's t., Mulder's t., (1), nitropropiol t., Oliver's t. (2), Pavy's t., Pelouse-Moore t., Pezoldt's t. (2), Purdy's t. (1), Riegler's t. (3), Roberts' t. (2), Rubner's t. (2), Saccharimeter t., Sachsse's t., Salkowski's t. (4), silver t., Soldaini's t., Toller's t. (2), Trommer's t., von Jacksch's t. (2), Wender's t., Womi-Miller t. See also glucose (dextrose), methods for, under method.

Diabetes t., see specific tests, including Bremer's t., Hickey-Hare t., Kowarsky's t. (2), Loewi's t., Williamson's blood t.

Diacetyl t., (for urea), the solution to be tested is mixed with concentrated hydrochloric acid and diacetyl monoxime; a yellow color develops on boiling if urea is present.

Dick t., (for susceptibility to scarlet fever), purified erythrogenic toxin from group A streptococci is injected intradermally; appearance within 24 to 48 hours of a small area of reddening of the skin indicates susceptibility of the subject.

Differential t., (for infectious mononucleosis), a test based on the fact that antisheep agglutinins in infectious mononucleosis are not absorbed by Forssman's antigen (whereas as those in serum disease and of normal persons are), but are absorbed by beef cells (whereas those in conditions other than infections mononucleosis may or may not be).

Dilution t. (for antibiotic sensitivity in bacteria), serial dilutions of an antibacterial agent in an agar or broth medium are inoculated with a suspension of a known concentration of a microorganism. Following incubation, the lowest concentration at which there is no visible growth is referred to as the minimum inhibitory concentration of the specific antibiotic.

Diphtheria t., see specific test, including Schick's t. and tellurite t.

Disk diffusion t., (for antibiotic sensitivity in bacteria), agar plates are inoculated with a standardized suspension of a microorganism. Antibiotic-containing disks are applied to the agar surface. Following overnight incubation, the diameters of the zones of inhibition or clearing surrounding the disks are measured. Zone diameters are interpreted as sensitive (susceptible), indeterminate (or intermediate), or resistant.

Dolman's t., (for ocular dominance), the patient holds in both hands a card with a hole in it through which to sight at a light.

Donath-Landsteiner t., (for paroxysmal cold hemoglobinuria), a test based on the fact that the blood of patients with this disease contains complement dependent iso-and autohemolysin which unites with red cells only at low temperatures (2 to 10°C). Hemolysis occurring only after warming to 37°C.

Donders' t., a color vision test performed by lanterns with sides of colored glass.

Double glucagon t., (for deficiency of amylo-1-6-glucosidase), glucagon is administered after a twelve-hour fast and again shortly after a meal; if the blood sugar fails to rise after the first administration but has a normal rise after the second, the test is positive.

Drinking t., (for glaucoma), one quart of water is ingested as rapidly as possible before breakfast. The intraocular pressure is measured every fifteen minutes. A rise of from 8 to 15 mm Hg is less than one-half hour indicates glaucoma. Also called water provocative t.

Duane's t., the employment of a candle flame and prisms to measure the degree of ocular heterophoria.

Dugas' t., a test for the existence of dislocation of the shoulder, made by placing the hand of the affected side on the opposite shoulder and bringing the elbow to the side of the chest. If this cannot be accomplished (Dugas' sign), dislocation of the shoulder exists.

Dukes' t., a test which measures bleeding time.

Dye exclusion t., the determination of cell viability *in vitro*. Following exposure of a cell preparaton to trypan blue or eosin, dead cells take up the dye from the medium, whereas living cells remain unstained.

Early pregnancy t., a do-it-yourself immunological test for pregnancy performed in the home as early as nine days after menstruation was expected (missed period). The test materials consist of mixture of human chorionic gonadotropin (hCG) antiserum and hCG-coated red blood cells in a glass test tube, a vial of water, and a medical dropper. Three drops of urine are placed in the test tube and the vial of water is added. The tube is shaken for 10 seconds and placed in a holder for 2 hours. A brown ring of nonagglutinated red 'blood cells' is positive (indicates pregnancy).

Ehrlich's t., 1. A reaction of a pure pink or red color resulting from the action of diazotised sulfanilic acid and ammonia upon certain aromatic substances, e.g., urobilinogen, found in the urine in some conditions. This reaction has diagnostic value in hepatic disease, typhoid fever, and measles and pronostic value in tuberculosis. 2. The benzaldehyde test for urobilinogen.

Ehrmann's t., (for mydriatic substances), the suspected substance is applied to an enucleated frog's eye, dilatation indicating the presence of a mydriatic substance.

Einhorn's string t., a test for determining whether the site of bleeding is in the low esophagus, stomach, or duodenum.

Elek t., see toxigenicity t. (*in vitro*).

Elsberg's t., a method of testing the sense of smell for determining the existence of a brain tumor.

Ely's t., with the patient prone, if flexion of the leg on the thigh causes the buttocks to arch away from the table and the leg to abduct at the hip joint, there is contracture of the lateral fascia of the thigh.

Erhard's t., a test for detecting simulated deafness.

Erichsen's t., See under sign

Erythrocyte protoporphyrin (EP) t., a screening test for lead toxicity, in which erthrocyte protoprophyrin levels are determined by direct flurometry of whole blood or fluorescence analysis of whole blood extracts; levels are increased in lead poisoning and iron deficiency.

Esophageal acid infusion t., (for diagnosis of gastroesophageal reflux), 0.1 N hydrogen chloride infused at a rate of 120 drops per minute produces pain and other symptoms.

Euglobulin lysis t., a test for the presence of palsminogen activator, done by determining the time required to dissolve an incubated clot composed of precipitated plasma euglobulin and exogenous thrombin.

Exercise t's., tests for detecting previously undetected coronary artery disease; they are graded tests for coronary fitness in which the subject exercise, as by walking a treadmill or pedaling a stationary bicycle, while under continuous electrocardiographic monitoring, usually by means by an oscilloscope, before, during, and after the exercise. Also called stress t's. See also Master 2-step exercise t.

Fantus t., (for differentiating between predominant water or salt depletion), place 10 drops of urine in a test tube with 1 drop of 20 percent potassium chromate, then add 2.9 percent silver nitrate 1 drop at a time, all the while agitating the tube, until there is a sudden color change from yellow to brick red. The number of drops of silver nitrate required to attain this change is the number of grams of chloride per liter in the urine; thus, the addition of 4 drops to elicit the end point indicates a urine chloride concentration of 400 mg 100 ml (4 gm/l).

Farber's t., presence of swallowed vernix cells in the meconium of a newborn baby indicates partial intestinal stenosis; their absence indicates intestinal atresia.

Farr's t., a radioimmunoassay for measuring absolute amounts of antibody—antibody is reacted with radiolabeled antigen and precipitated with ammonium sulfate; bound antigen or hapten is precipitated while free antigen remains in solution. This test is based on the capacity of antibody to combine with antigen rather than on such secondary properties as precipitation and, therefore, measures all immunoglobulin classes and subclasses.

Fat t., see specific tests, including Leffmann-Beam t., Meigs' t., Soathoff's t. Volenta's t.

FE$_{Na}$ t., excreted fraction of filtered sodium test, a measure of renal tubular reabsorption of sodium, calculated as follows: (U/P) Na/(U/P) Cr × 100, where U and P represent concentrations of sodium and creatinine in urine and plasma, respectively.

Femoral nerve stretch t., (for lesions of third or fourth lumbar disk), passive knee flexion in the prone position causes pain in the back or thighs.

Fermentation t., (for dextrose), fill a graduated fermentation tube with the urine or unknown solution, add a small portion of compressed yeast, and incubate for twelve hours; the amounts of gas that accumulates in the closed arm indicates the amounts of dextrose present.

Fern t., (for estrogen), the appearance of a fernlike pattern in dried smears of uterine cervical mucus indicates the presence of estrogen; the level of secretion is determined by the extent of ferning.

Ferric chloride t., 1. (for thiocyanates in saliva), add a few drops of dilute ferric chloride to saliva and acidify with hydrochloric acid; red ferric thiocyanate forms, which is decolorized by adding mercury bichloride. 2. (for salicylic acid) see Remont's t.

Finger-to-finger t., similar to finger-nose test, for testing coordinated movements of the extremities.

Finger-nose t., (for coordinated movements of the extremities), with arm extended to one side the patient is asked to slowly try to touch the end of his nose with the point of his index finger.

Fishberg's concentration t., (for renal function), the patient is given supper with not more than 200 ml of fluid and nothing thereafter. Urine voided during the night is discarded. The morning urine is saved, the patient kept in bed, and the urine of one hour later and of two hours later is saved. If the specific gravity of any of these three specimens is less than 1.024 there is impairment of renal function.

Fisher exact t., a statistical hypothesis test of independence of rows and columns in a 2 × 2 contingency table based on the exact sampling distribution of the observed frequencies.

Fishman-Doubilet t., (for quick differential diagnosis of acute pancreatitis), a minute amount of starch is incubated with serum for 5 minutes. A normal concentration of amylase will leave some of the starch undigested and give a blue color with iodine; a high serum amylase digests all the starch, and the addition of iodine will give only the yellow color of iodine. When the reaction color is yellow, the diagnosis of acute pancreatitis is strongly indicated. Also called rapid serum amylase t.

Fistula t., the air in the external auditory canal is compressed or rarefied if there is erosion of the inner osseous wall of the tympanum exposing the mebranous labyrinth, nystagmus will be produced, provided the labyrinth still functions. The site of the fistula is usually in the bony lateral semicircular canal.

Flack's t., (of physical efficiency), after a full inspiration the subject blows as long as he can into a mercury manometer with a force of 40 mm mercury.

Flicker t., the visual sensation produced by regular flashes of light. The flashes may appear to flutter or to be be steady according to rate of interruption (flicker phenomenon). The number of flashes per second at which the light just appears to be continuous is known as flicker fusion threshold (fusion frequency; critical fusion frequency). The Flicker test, an application of the flicker fusion threshold, has been used to diagnose hypertension and angina pectoris, to determine vessel spasms, or to indicate conditions of fatigue or anoxemia. A low threshold indicates disease.

Flocculation t., 1. Any of variety of nonspecific tests of liver function, now obsolete, in which a precipitating reagent is added to serum, e.g., the cephalin-cholesterol flocculation test or the thymol turbity test; positive results generally reflect increased gamma and beta globulin and lipoproteins or decreased albumin. 2. Any serologic test in which a flocculent agglomerate is formed; usually the term is applied to a variant form of the precipitin reaction, rarely to agglutination reactions.

Fluhmann's t., a modification of the Allen-Doisy test for estrogenic substance in the body, using mice in which a positive reaction is the mucinification of the vaginal mucosa.

Fluorescent treponemal antibody absorption (FTA-ABS) t., the standard treponemal antigen serologic test for syphilis; patient serum is diluted with an extract of Reiter treponemes to remove nonspecific antibodies, then reacted with the Nichol's stain of *Treponema pallidum* fixed to a glass slide; specific antibodies adhering to the treponemes with fluorescein-labeled antihuman globulin. Positive tests are seen in about 85 percent of cases of primary syphilis, 100 percent in secondary syphilis, and 98 percent in late syphilis.

Formaldehyde t., see specific test, including Burnam's t., Jorissen's t., Kentmann's t., Leach's t., Schiff's t. (6).

Foshay's t., (for tularemia), a suspension of *Pasteurella tularensis* is injected into the skin; a positive reaction resembles that in a positive tuberculin test.

Fouchet's t., (for bilirubin in blood), to a sample of the blood serum there is added an equal part of a reagent consisting of 5 gm trichloracetic acid, 20 ml water, and 2 ml ferric chloride; a green color is produced, if bilirubin is present.

Fournier's t., the patient is asked to rise on command from a sitting position; he is asked to rise and walk, then stop quickly on command; he is asked to walk and turn around quickly on command. The ataxic gait is thus brought out.

Francis' t., 1. (for bile acids in urine) in a test tube is placed 2 gm of dextrose in 15 gm of sulfuric acid and the urine is placed on top of this; a purple color forms if bile acids are present. 2. An intracutaneous test in pneumonia for ascertaining the body response to the infection and whether the specific antibodies are present after treatment with antipneumococcus serum. The homologous pneumococcus polysaccharide is used in the skin test.

Frankel's t., examination of the nasal cavity with the patient's head bent down between his knees and rotated so that the side to be examined is turned upward. If pus is seen in the middle meatus, suppuration in some of the anterior accessory sinuses is indicated.

Frei's t., a skin test for lymphogranuloma venereum using material prepared from lymphogranuloma venereum organisms grown in chick embryo yolk sacs; the test is both insensitive and nonspecific and is now rarely used.

Friderichsen's t., (for vitamin A deficiency), determination of the weakest light stimulus which will give rise to an oculomotor reflex. A variation from normal indicates vitamin A deficiency.

Friedman's t., Friedman-Lapham t., (for pregnancy), the injection of the urine of a pregnant woman into female rabbits will cause the formation of corpora lutea and corpora haemorrhagica in the rabbits.

Frohn's t., the use of the double iodide of bismuth and potassium as a test for alkaloids.

Fructose t., see levulose t.

FTA-ABS t., fluorescent treponemal antibody absorption t.

Fundus reflex t., retinoscopy.

Funkenstein's t., an index of central autonomic reactivity, consisting of observing the response in systolic blood pressure after intramuscular injection of 10 mg of acetylcholine.

Furfurol t., (for proteins), heat the suspected substance with sulfuric acid; if proteins are present, furfurol is formed.

Gaenslen's t., see under sign.

Galli Mainini t., (for pregnancy), 10 ml of urine from the patient is injected into a normal male batrachian (frog or toad); the presence of spermatozoa in a drop of the batrachian's urine indicates the existence of pregnancy.

Gastric function t., see specific tests, including augmented histamine t., chlorophyll t., Rehfuss's t., Sahli's t., Sahli's glutoid t., Schwarz's t. (2).

Gault's t., (for simulated deafness), the patient's good ear is closed and a sound is made near the supposed bad ear; a winking motion of the lid on the tested side indicates hearing.

Gel diffusion t., any technique involving diffusion of antigen or antibody through a semisolid medium, usually agar or agarose gel resulting in a precipitin reaction. Precipitin lines or bands from where the concentration of an antigen and antibody are seroligically equivalent.

Gerhardt's t., 1. (for acetone in the urine) add a solution of ferric chloride and a red color is produced. This test is not reliable (Carl J Gerhardt). 2. (for acetoacetic acid in the urine) filter, in order to remove the phosphates, and add a few drops of a solution of ferric chloride, which produces a deep red color, which disappears when sulfuric acid is added. 3. (for bile pigments in the urine) shake urine with an equal measure of chloroform and then add tincture of iodine and potassium hydroxide to the separated chloroform; a yellowish brown color is produced (Charles Frederic Gerhardt).

Gerrard's t., (for destrose in the urine), Fehling's solution is treated with a 5 percent solution of potassium cyanide until the blue color begins to disappear. The suspected liquid is heated with this mixture, and if there is dextrose present, more or less discoloration takes place.

Gibbon-Landis t., (for peripheral circulation), a pair of extremities (the hands, if the feet are to be tested; the feet, if the hands are to be tested) are immersed in a bath of 43°-45°C. If the temperature in the unimmersed extremities rises, the circulation is normal.

Gies' biuret t., (for proteins), Gies uses the following reagent in making the test: mix 25 ml of a 3 percent solution of cupric sulfate and 975 ml of a 10 percent solution of potassium hydroxide.

Globulin t., see specific tests, including ammonium sulfate t. (1), Gordon's t., Hammarslen's t., Kaplan's t., colloidal gold t., Mayerhofer's t., Noguchi's t. (2), Nonne-Apelt t., Pondy's t., Pohl's t., Ross-Jones t., Weichbrodt's t.

Glucagon stimulation t., (for deficiency of growth hormone), blood samples are taken immediately and at intervals of 1, 2, 2½, and 3 hours after subcutaneous or intramuscular injection of glucagon, radiommunoassay of the serum is then done by enzyme partition.

Glucose t., see dextrose t.

Glucose tolerance t., a metabolic test of carbohydrate tolerance; it measures active insulin, a hepatic function based on the power of the normal liver to absorb and store large quantities of glucose, and the effectiveness of intestinal absorption of glucose. Blood sugar should return to normal in two and one-half hours after ingesting 100 gm of glucose into a fasting stomach.

Glutoid t., see Sahil's glutoid t.

Gluzinski's t., 1. (for bile pigments) boil the solution with solution of formaldehyde until it becomes green; adding a little hydrochloric acid changes the tint to an amethyst violet. 2. (for differentiation between ulcer and cancer of stomach) examination of the gastric contents recovered from a fasting patient: (a) after a test breakfast consisting of the white of boiled egg and 200 ml of water, which is recovered after three quarters of an hour. (b) after a test and three-quarters hours. In ulcer, both the breakfast and the dinner give the reaction of free HCl in beginning cancer, the first meal will give reaction of free HCl, whereas the second meal will show only a slight trace or none at all.

Glycerol t., see specific tests, including hypochlorite-orcinol t.

Glycerophosphate t., (for renal function), 500 mg of sodium glycerophosphate is injected intravenously, and then the free and total phosphorus in the urine collected during the following hour is determined.

Glycosylated hemoglobin t., measurement of the percentage of hemoglobin A molecules that have formed a stable ketoamine linkage between their terminal amino acid position of the beta-3-chains and a glucose group; in normal persons, this amounts to about .7 percent of the total, in diabetics about 14.5 percent.

Glycuronates t., see specific tests, including Tollens' t. (4) and Tollens, Neuberg and Schwket t.

Glycyltryptophan t., (for carcinoma of stomach), filtered gastric contents and glycyltryptophan are placed in a test tube and kept at body temperature for twenty-four hours; if on the addition of a few drops of bromine, a reddish violet color is formed, carcinoma is indicated.

Glyoxylic acid t., see Hopkins-Cole test.

Gmelin's t., (for bile pigments), fuming nitric acid is so added to the suspected urine that it forms a layer under it. Near the junction of the two liquids, rings are formed—a green ring above, and under it a blue, violet-red, and reddish yellow. If the green and violet-red rings are absent, the reaction shows the probable presence of lutein.

Gold number t., see colloidal gold t.

Goldscheider's t. (for cutaneous thermal sensibility) (obs), consists in touching the skin with the slightly pointed end of a metallic cylinder varyingly heated.

Gold-sol t., see colloidal gold t.

Goodenough draw-a-man t., Goodenough draw-a-person t., a method of testing the general intelligence of children by asking the subject to draw a picture of a man to the best of his ability.

Goodenough-Harris drawing t., a revision of the Goodenough draw-a-man test, in which scoring emphasizes the presence or absence of body and clothing detail rather than artistic skill.

Gordon's t., (for the presence of globulin-albumin in the spinal fluid), one ml of spinal fluid is placed in a small test tube and 0.1 ml of 1 percent solution of corrosive mercuric chloride in distilled water; the formation of cloud or precipitate after standing an hour indicates a positive reaction.

Gordon's biological t., (for Hodgkin's disease), lymphadenomatous tissue injected intracerebrally into rabbits causes the development of a characteristic lesion in the rabbits nervous tissues, accompanied by ataxia, spasm, and paralysis.

Göthlin's t., a test for capillary fragility, done by testing the capillary resistance in the arm.

Graefe's t., (for heterophoria), on holding a prism of 10 degrees before one eye, base up or down, two images are formed; one of these images is displaced laterally in heterophoria.

Graham's t., the intravenous or oral administration of tetriaodophthalein sodium prior to roentgenologic examination of the gallbladder.

Gregerson-Boas t., (for blood), a modification of the benzidine test to make it less sensitive for use in testing feces. Use a 0.5 percent solution of benzidine instead of saturated solution and barium peroxide instead of hydrogen peroxide.

Gries' t., (for nitrites in the saliva), mix it with 5 parts of water; add a few drops of dilute solution of sulfuric acid and a few drops of metadiamidobenzene; this produces a strong yellow color if nitrites are present.

Grigg's t., (for protiens), metaphosphoric acid precipitates all proteins except the peptones.

Grocco's t. (obs), in slight cases of purpura rheumatica, if an elastic ligature is placed around the forearm, punctiform hemorrhages will appear in the bend of the elbow.

Gross' t., 1. (for trypsin in feces) in a mortar, thoroughly rub up a portion of the fecal mass with three times its bulk of 0.1 percent sodium carbonate solution Filter. Mix 10 ml of the filtrate with 100 ml of fresh solution consisting of 0.5 gm Grubler's pure casein, 1 gm sodium carbonate, and 1000 ml distilled water. Add a little toluol to prevent bacterial activity and place in an incubator at about 38°C. At intervals, remove a few cubic centimeters and test for casein by adding a few drops of acetic acid of about 1 percent strength. A white appears as long as any casein remains undigested. With the patient on a protein diet, there is normally a sufficient amount of trypsin to digest all the casein in from ten to fifteen hours. Delay or complete failure of digestion shows diminution or absence of trypsin. 2. A color reaction for the diagnosis of carcinoma.

Group t., a test of intelligence or aptitude given to a number of persons at one time.

Guaiac t., (for occult blood), glacial acetic acid and a solution of gum guaiac are mixed with the specimen; on addition of hydrogen peroxide, the presence of blood is indicated by a blue tint.

Gunning's t., (for acetone in urine), to a few milliliters of urine or distillate in a test tube, add a few drops of tincture of iodine and of ammonia alternately until a heavy black cloud appears. This cloud will gradually clear up and, if acetone is present, iodoform, usually crystalline, will separate out. The iodoform can be recognized by its odor or by detection of the crystals microscopically. Iodoform crystals are yellowish six-pointed stars or six-sided plates.

Gunning-Lieben t., see Gunning's t.,

Günzberg's t., (for hydrochloric acid in the stomach contents), dissolve 2 gm of phloroglucin and 1 gm of vanillin in 30 ml of alcohol; of this, mix 2 drops with 2 drops of filtered gastric juice; heat it slowly in procelain cell. Free HCl produces a bright-red color; it is not present if the color is brownish red or brown.

Guthrie's t., (for phenylketonuria) in the presence of blood containing phenylalanine, β-2-thienylalanine does not inhibit growth of *Bacillus subtilis*.

Gutzeit's t., (for arsenic), a paper is moistened with an acidulated silver nitrate solution and exposed to the fumes from the suspected liquid, which is mixed with zinc and dilute sulfuric acid. The formation of a yellow spot on the paper indicates the presence of inorganic arsenic compounds.

Haagensen's t., observation of the contour of the breasts when the patient leans forward as a means of detecting malignant changes in the mammae.

Hager's t., cephalin-cholesterol flocculation t.

Haines' t., (for destrose), copper sulfate, 30 grains; glycerin, 1/2 fl. oz; liquor potassae, 5 fl.oz; water, sufficient to make 6 fl.oz when boiled and a little urine added, and again boiled, a yellowish or reddish yellow precipitate is produced.

Hallion's t., see Tuffier's t.

Ham's t., acidified serum t.

Hamel's t., (for slight jaundice), a little blood is drawn by punture from the lobe of the ear into a capillary tube and the tube is allowed to stand for a few hours; the serum which collects in the upper part of the tube will be yellow if jaundice is present.

Hamilton's t., when the shoulder joint is luxated, a rule or straight rod applied to the humerus can be made to touch the outer condyle and the acromion at the same time.

Hammarsten's t., 1. (for globulin) in a neutral solution suspected to contain globulin, dissolve magnesium sulfate to saturation; the globulin will be precipitated and may be filtered out. 2. (for bile pigment) to one volume of acid mixture 1 part HNO, and 19 parts HCl (each 25 percent) add four volumes of alcohol, then a few drops of the unknown, a green color indicates biliverdin.

Hammerschlag's t., see under method.

Hanger's t., (for liver cell disease), see cephalin-cholesterol flocculation t.

Hanke-Koessler t., (for phenols, hydroxyaromatic acids, and imidazoles), to 5 ml of 1.1 percent sodium carbonate solution, add 2 ml of para-diazobenzene sulfonic acid reagent. Then add 1 ml of solution to be tested.

Hapten inhibition t., serological characterization of antigenic determinant by employing known haptens to mask the antigen-binding site of antibody specific for it.

Harding-Ruttan t., (for acetoacetic acid), acidify the urine with acetic acid, add 0.5 ml of N/10 sodium nitroprusside, and then overlay the solution with concentrated aqueous NH_4OH; a violet ring is produced.

Harris-Ray t., a microtitration for vitamin C in the urine.

Harrison's spot t., (for bilirubin in urine), add to 10 ml of urine, 5 ml of a 10 percent solution of barium chloride, mix, and filter. Spread filter paper on dry filter paper. Add one to two drops of Fouchet's reagent (trichloroacetic acid 25 gm, water 100 ml and 10 percent solution of ferric chloride 10 ml); a positive reaction gives a blue to green color (Godfried).

Hart's t., (for oxybutyric acid in urine), remove acetone and diacetic acid by diluting 20 ml urine with 20 ml of water, adding a few drops of acetic acid, and boiling down to 10 ml. To this add 10 ml of water, mix, and divide between two test tubes. To one tube add 1 ml of hydrogen peroxide, warm gently, and cool. This transforms β-hydroxybutyric acid to acetone. Now apply Lange's test for acetone to each tube. A positive reaction in the tube to which hydrogen peroxide has been added shows the presence of β-oxybutyric acid in the original sample of urine.

Hatching t., a test for the detection of live schistosome eggs in urine or feces, dependent upon the eggs hatching to produce miracidia when placed in water; the miracidia are attracted to light and can readily be identified.

Hay's t., (for bile salts), a pinch of sublimated sulfur is dropped in the urine; the sulfur sinks if bile is present, but floats if it is absent.

Heaf's t., see tuberculin t.

Heel-knee t., (for coordinated movements of the extremities), the patient lying on his back, is asked to touch the knee of one leg with the heel of the other and then to pass the heel slowly down the front of the shin to the ankle.

Heel-tap t., see heel tap, under tap.

Heller's t., 1. (for albumin in urine) stratify cold nitric acid below the urine in a test tube; albumin will form a white coagulum between the urine and the acid. 2. (for blood in the urine) add potassium hydroxide solution and heat; the earthy phosphates are precipitated, and if blood is present, they are stained red by hematic. 3. (for dextrose in urine) add a solution of potassium hydroxide; sugar will cause a brownish or reddish precipitate.

Hemadsorption t., an *in vitro* test for detecting hemagglutinating viruses based on the adherence of red blood cells to cells of the infected tissue in the presence of hemagglutinin.

Hemagglutination inhibition t., (HI, HAI) 1. A highly sensitive procedure for the measurement of soluble antigens in biologic specimens in which the specimen is first incubated with homologous antibody and then incubated with antigen-coated red cells; the amount of hemagglutination reflects the amount of free antibody present after reaction with the specimen and thus varies inversely with the amount of antigen in the specimen. 2. A procedure for the measurement of serum antibodies directed against a hemagglutinating virus; the highest dilution of serum that completely inhibits hemagglutination by a standardized viral preparation is reported as the hemagglutination titer.

Hematein t., (for blood), to 5 ml of the unknown, add 5 ml of sodium hydroxide, 2 drops of hematein solution, and 10 drops of hydrogen peroxide. If blood is present the contents will turn rapidly to violet red, then to clear brown, and then to pale yellow. Without blood, these changes occur more slowly.

Hematin t., see Schumm's t. (2).

Heme t., see Schumm's t.,

Hemin t., (for blood), see Teuchmann's t.

Hemoglobin t., see specific tests, including alkali denaturation t., Heller's t. (2), Kalayama's t., Kobert's t., sand t. See also hemoglobin, methods for, under method.

Hemosiderin t., see specific tests, including Perls' t. and Rous' t.

Hench-Aldrich t., (for the mercury-combining power of saliva), titrate 5 ml of saliva with a 5 percent solution of bichloride of mercury until a drop gives a reddish brown color with a saturated solution of sodium carbonate.

Henle-Coenen t., the amount of retrograde flow of blood which is obtained from the open end of the distal stump of divided artery, while the proximal portion is being compressed with a clamp, is a measure (or index) of the adequacy of the collateral circulation.

Hennebert's t., see under sign.

Henry's t., Henry's melanoflocculation t., (for malaria), an obsolete flocculation test for malaria using melanin from ox eyes as the antigen.

Henshaw's t., a test to aid in the selection of the appropriate homeopathic remedy in a given case of disease. A visible flocculation zone develops in the patient's blood serum when brought into contact with a potentized remedy homeopathically indicated in the case.

Hepatic function t., see liver function t.

Hering's t., the subject looks with both eyes through a tube blackened within and having a thread running vertically across the farther end, and a small round body is placed either before or behind the thread—if vision is binocular, the subject is able at once to tell whether the ball is nearer to him than the thread or farther off; but if vision is monocular, he cannot tell whether it is nearer or farther than the thread.

Herter's t., 1. (for indole) to the unknown, add 1 drop of a 2 percent solution of betanaphtha-quinone-sodium-mono-sulfonate and then a drop of a 10 percent solution of potassium hydroxide; a blue or bluish green color indicates indole. 2. (for skatole) to the unknown, add 1 ml of an acid solution of para-dimethyl-amino-benzaldehyde and heat to boiling. The purplish blue color is intensified by the addition of hydro-chloric acid.

Herzberg's t., (for free hydrochloric acid in the gastric juice), moisten a paper with a solution of congo red and dry it; free HCl colors it blue or bluish black.

Hess' capillary t., (for condition of the capillary walls), see tourniquet t., def 1.

Heterophile antibody t., see horse cell t., Paul-Bunnell t., and Paul-Bunnell-Davidsohn t.

Heynsius' t., (for albumin), to a suspected liquid, add enough acetic acid to render acidulous, and then boil with a saturated solution of sodium chloride; albumin will form a flocculent precipitate.

Hickey-Hare t., (for diabetes insipidus), intravenous infusion of hypertonic saline after establishment of water diuresis induces antidiuresis in normal subjects but not in patients with diabetes insipidus.

Hildebrandt's t., (for urobilin in urine), the reagent consists of an unfiltered solution of 10 parts of zinc acetate and 90 parts of absolute alcohol. The reagent is shaken before using, and equal parts of reagent and urine are mixed. The precipitate which forms being filtered off. With increase of urobilin, the filtrate shows a distinct green fluorescence, either directly or after the addition of ammonia.

Hindenlang's t., (for albumin), to the liquid to be tested add solid metaphosphoric acid; albumin, if present, form a precipitate.

Hines-Brown t., cold pressor test; a test which measures the response of the blood pressure to the immersion of one hand in ice water and excessive increase in pressure (hyperreaction) is said to identify a latent hypertensive state.

Hinton t., (obs), a nontreponemal antigen serologic test for syphilis.

Hippuric acid t., see specific tests, including Lucke's t., Quick's t. (1), Spire's, (2). See also hippuric acid, methods for, under method.

Histalog t., see augmented histamine t.

Histamine t., 1. One ml of a 0.1 percent solution of histamine is injected subcutaneously as a stimulant of gastric secretion; see also augmented histamine t. 2. (for lesion of the sympathetic nervous system) a small area of skin on the wrist, ankle, or knee is cleansed with alcohol, which is allowed to dry. A drop of 1:1000 solution of histamine phosphate is placed on it and introduced into the epidermis by multiple needle punctures in a manner similar to that used for cowpox vaccination. The excess histamine is gently removed: (a) a reddish purple spot appears as the result of local capillary dilatation, (b) a local wheal succeeds, because of transudation of serum from increased permeability of the capillaries, (c) a flare results as the effect of dilatation of the arteries by the reflex of a local axon. The flare being dependent on the integrity of the peripheral nerve, it therefore occurs in hysterical anesthesia and malingering but not in neural lesion. 3. (for pheochro-mocytoma) following rapid intravenous injection of histamine phosphate administered in a standardized dosage of 0.010 to 0.50 mg of histamine base, normal individuals experience transient headache, flush, and a brief fall in blood pressure, but those with pheochro-mocytoma, after a fall in blood pressure, experience a marked rise in blood pressure, fear, excitability, etc.

Histamine flare t., (for leprosy and postherpetic neuralgia), a drop of 1:1000 histamine acid phosphate solution is placed on the skin and a needle puncture is made through it; the test is positive if there is no erythema flare when the puncture is made within the suspected lesion area, or if the flare stops at the border of the lesion when it is made slightly to the outside of it.

Histidine loading t., (for folic acid deficiency), a loading dose of histidine is given, and the resultant urinary excretion of excess formiminoglutamic acid (FIGLU) secondary to decreased amounts of tetrahydrofolic acid, is measured. Also called FIGLU excretion t.

Hitzig's t., (for vestibular apparatus), the positive electrode of a galvanic current is applied just in front of the ear being examined while the negative electrode is held in the patient's hand, the patient standing with feet together and eyes closed. A current of 5 milliamperes causes a leaning toward the positive pole in normal persons.

Hock t., see., spavin t.

Hoffmann's t., (for tyrosine), add mercuric nitrate to the suspected liquid and boil it; then add nitric acid with a little nitrous acid. A red color is produced if tyrosine is present, and a red precipitate is seen.

Hofmeister's t., 1. (for leucine) warm the suspected liquid with mercurous nitrate; if leucine is present, metallic mercury is deposited. 2. (for peptones) mix phosphotungstic and hydrochloric acids; let the mixture stand twenty-four hours, and filter. WIth this reagent, a solution containing peptones with no albumin will afford a precipitate..

Hogben t., see Xenopus t.

Holmgren's t., the use of skeins of colored worsted as a test of the perception of colors; a skein is given to the subject of the test, and he is asked to match it out of a set of a variously colored skeins.

Holten's t., a creatinine clearance test for renal efficiency.

Hopkin's thiophene t., (for lactic acid), add a few drops of stomach contents to 5 ml of concentrated sulfuric acid containing a little cupric sulfate and heat two minutes. Cool and add a very little thiophene. A cherry-red color indicates lactic acid.

Hopkins-Cole t., (for protein), glyoxylic acid is prepared by the action of sodium amalgam on a solution of oxalic acid. A few drops of this solution are added to the protein solution and strong sulfuric acid is poured down the side of the tube. A bluish violet color is produced at the junction of the two fluid due to the presence of tryptophan.

Hoppe Seyler's t., 1. (for carbon monoxide in the blood) add to blood twice its volume of a solution of sodium hydroxide of 1.3 specific gravity: normal blood will form a dingy brown mass with a green shade if spread thin on a white surface; but if carbon monoxide is present, the mass is red, and so is the thin layer. 2. (for xanthine) add the substance to be tested to a mixture of chlorinated lime in a porcelain dish; a dark-green ring is formed at first.

Hormone t., see specific tests, including Aschheim-Zondek t. and Siddall t.

Horse cell t., a modification of the Paul-Bunnell-Davidsohn test (qv) for heterophile antibodies associated with infectious mononucleosis that uses horse erythrocytes instead of sheep erythrocytes. No centrifugation step is needed and the whole test is performed in minutes.

Horsley's t., (for dextrose), the solution is boiled with potassium hydroxide and potassium chromate; if dextrose is present, a green color is produced.

Hotis' t., (for garget or mastitis in cows), fresh milk containing bromcresol purple is incubated for twenty-four hours; a positive reaction is the formation of yellow flakes on the sides of the test tube.

Howard's t., (for renal function); both ureters are catheterized and urine collected separately from each kidney; the quantity of urine in each collection and its sodium and creatinine concentrations are then determined. Also called split-renal function t.

Howell's t., (for prothrombin), a test for the amount of prothrombin in the blood depending on the clotting time of the oxalated plasma treated with calcium chloride and thromboplastin.

Huddleson's t., an agglutination test for brucellosis in man.

Huhner's t., examination of the secretions aspirated from the vaginal fornix and the endocervical canal after coitus, to determine the number and condition of spermatozoa present and the extent to which they have penetrated the cervical mucus.

Huppert's t., (for bile pigments), the suspected solution is treated with lime water or calcium chloride solution and then with a solution of ammonium or sodium carbonate. The precipitate of bile pigments may be removed by shaking with chloroform after washing with water and acidulating with acetic acid. Bilirubin colors the chloroform yellow and the acetic acid solution green.

Huppert-Cole t., (for bile pigments), to 50 ml of the unknown, add an excess of baryta water or lime water. To the precipitate, add 5 ml of 95 percent alcohol, 2 drops of strong sulfuric acid, and 2 drops of a 5 percent solution of potassium chlorate. Boil, and the supernatant liquid will be emerald or bluish green if bile is present.

Hurtley's t., (for acetoacetic acid), to 10 ml of the unknown, add 2 ml of strong hydrochloric acid and 1 ml of fresh 1 percent sodium nitrite solution. Shake and add 15 ml of concentrated ammonium hydroxide and 5 ml of 10 percent ferrous sulfate. A violet or purple color develops slowly if acetoacetic acid is present.

Hydrochloric acid t., see specific tests, including dimethylaminoazobenze t. (1). Gimberg's t., Herzberg's t., Leo's t., Littke's t., Maly's t. (1), (2), Mohr's t., Rabuteau's t. (1), (2), Riggler's t. (2), Scivoletto's t., Szabo's t., Topfer's t., Uffelmann's t., von Jacksch's t. (1), (2), Winckler's t. (2), Witz's t.

Hydrogen peroxide t., (for blood), a 20 percent solution of hydrogen peroxide is added to the suspected fluid; if blood is present even in minute proportion, bubbles will rise, forming foam on the surface of the fluid.

Hydrostatic t., floating of the lungs of a dead infant when placed in water indicates that the child was born alive; also called Raygat's t.

Hydroxyaromatic acid t., see Hanke-Koessler t.

Hydroxylamine t., (for dextrose), see Bang's method, under method.

Hyperemia t., see see Moschcowitz's t.

Hypochlorite-orcinol t., (for glycerin), to 3 ml of the unknown, add 3 drops of N/1 sodium hypochlorite solution and boil for one minute to drive off chlorine. Then add an equal volume of strong hydrochloric acid and a little orcinol. Boil, and a violet or greenish blue color indicates glycerine or a sugar, or some substance that can be oxidized to a sugar.

Hypothesis t., an abstract procedure for determining whether a set of observations is consistent with a hypothesis under consideration; it is the theoretical basis of most statistical tests. A hypothesis test decides between two hypotheses, one stating that the effect under investigation does not exist (the null hypothesis H_0), and the other that some specified effect does exist (the alternative hypothesis H_1), based on the observed value of a test statistic whose sampling distribution is completely determined by H_0. When the test statistic falls in a set of values known as the critical region, H_0 is rejected. The level of probability of incorrectly rejecting H_0, may be set before the data are collected, usually at 0.05 or 0.01; this is called the significance level or alpha level. It is now more common to report the smallest alpha at which the null hypothesis can be rejected; this is called the significance probability or P value.

Hypoxanthine t., see Kossel's t.

Ilimow's t., (for albumin), acidulate with acid sodium phosphate. Filter and add a solution of phenol (1:20); a cloudy precipitate indicates albumin.

Ilosvay's t., (for nitrites), see under reagent.

Imidazole t., see Hanke-Koessler t.

Immobilization t., detection of antibody based on its ability to inhibit the motility of a bacterial cell or protozoon.

IMViC t., (modified acronym from indole, methyl red, Voges-Proskauer citrate), a series of metabolic tests used as standard procedure to differentiate genera of the Enterobacterioaceae. See also the individual tests.

Indican t., see specific tests, including Jaffe's t. (2), Jotles't. (2), MacMunn's t., Obermayer's t., Porter's (2), Wang's t., Weber's t., (2), See also iredican, methods for, under method.

Indigo carmine t., (for renal permeability), a solution of indigo carmine is injected intramuscularly and the time of its appearance in the urine is noted. Normally, it begins to appear in about five minutes. Delay beyond this, points to defective renal adequacy.

Indigo red t., see Rosin's t.

Indole t., see specific tests, including Baeyer's t. (2), Herter's t. (1), Kondo's t., Legal's t. (2), Nencki's t., nitroso-indole-nitrate t., pine wood t., Salkowski's t. (3). See also indole, methods for, under method.

Indophenol t., (for the presence of oxidizing enzymes in cells and for detecting the presence of myelobasts, etc), cover glass films of the cells are fixed in alcohol. Float for ten to twenty minutes, face down, upon a freshly prepared solution of equal parts of 1 percent aqueous solutions of dimethyl paraphenylenediamine and of alpha naphthol (Nadi's reagent). Rinse and mount in glycerin. The cytoplasm of cells containing oxidase (myeloblasts, myelocytes, polymorphonuclears, and large mononuclears) will be colored blue by indophenol.

Inkblot t., see Rorschach t.

Inoculation t., (for acute anterior poliomyelitis), the cerebrospinal fluid of the suspected patient (i.e., before the appearance of paralytic symptoms) is injected into a monkey. Paralysis will appear in the monkey within seven days if the patient is affected.

Inosite t., see specific tests, including Scherer's t. (1) and Seidel's t.

Intelligence t., a set of problems or tasks posed to assess an individual's innate ability to judge, comprehend, and reason.

Intracutaneous t., see intradermal t.

Intracutaneous tuberculin t., see Mantoux t.

Intradermal t., a skin test in which the antigen is injected intradermally.

Inulin clearance t., Inulin It's a vegetable starch, an indigestible polysaccharide occurring in the rhizome of certain plants. It is a polymer of fructofuranose, yields fructose on hydrolysis and is used in a test for determining renal function.

Iodine t., 1. (for starch) when a compound solution of iodine is added to starch, and especially to an acid or neutral solution of cooked starch paste, a deep-blue color is produced which disappears on heating and reappears on cooling. Erythrodextrin and glycogen give a red color with iodine. 2. See specific tests, including Lessor's t., Winckler's t. (3).

Iodoform t., 1. (for acetone) see Gunning's t. 2. (for alcohol) make the unknown alkaline, and add a few drops of iodine solution. Heat gently, and yellow iodoform crystals indicate alcohol or some similar body.

Iowa pressure articulation t., a test of the ability to produce the consonant sounds in isolated words, particularly the pressure sounds.

Irresistible impulse t., an impulse to commit a criminal act that cannot be resisted because mental disease has destroyed the person's freedom of will and power to choose between right and wrong. The irresistible impulse test that a person is not criminally responsible if the act was due to an irresistible impulse is still used in some states.

Irrigation t., the patient is examined with the bladder full. The anterior urethra is washed out with a warm solution of boric acid (3 percent), the perineum being compressed to prevent the entrance of the fluid into the posterior urethra. When the washings are perfectly clear, the patient voids his urine and any turbidity must come from the posterior urethra.

Ishihara's t., a test for color vision made by the use of a series of plates composed of round dots of various sizes and colors.

Ito-Reenstierna t., **(obs)**, intracutaneous injection of a vaccine of killed *Haemophilus ducreyi* elicits a positive skin reaction in persons who have been infected with chancroid.

Jacoby's t., (for pepsin), the greatest dilution of gastric juice which will clarify an acid solution of ricin in three hours at 38°C gives the number of peptic units in the juice.

Jacquemin's t., (for phenol), add to the suspected liquid an equal quantity of aniline and some sodium hypochlorite in solution; a blue color is produced.

Jadassohn's t., see irrigation t.

Jaffé's t., 1. (for creatinine and dextrose) to the liquid, add trinitrophenol and then make alkaline with sodium hydroxide. A red color without heating indicates creatinine; a red color after heating indicates dextrose. 2. (for indican) to the suspected liquid are added an equal amount of concentrated hydrochloric acid, 1 ml of chloroform, and a few drops of a strong solution of chlorinated soda. The chloroform is colored blue if indican is present.

Jaksch's t., see von Jaksch's t.

Janet's t., (for differentiating between functional and organic anesthesia), the patient is instructed to say "yes" or "no" according as he does or does not feel the examiner's touch. He may say "no" in functional anesthesia, but he will say nothing in cases of organic anesthesia.

Jansen's t., (for osteoarthritis deformans of the hip), the patient is told to cross his legs with a point just above the ankle resting on the opposite knee; this motion is impossible when the disease exists.

Javorski's t., Jaworski's t., in hourglass stomach a splashing sound will be heard on succussion of the pyloric portion after siphonage.

Jennings' t., a modification of Holmgren's test for color perception. Small patches of colored worsted are placed so as to be protected from light and dust. The person to be exmined indicates his color selection by pricking the record sheet with a pointed pencil.

Jochmann's t., 1. Muller-Jochmann t. 2. antitrypsin t.

Johnson's t., (for albumin), put the urine in a test tube and carefully pour upon it a strong solution of trinitrophenol. A white coagulum of albumin appears at the junction of the liquids, which heating augments.

Jolles' t., 1. (for bile pigments in urine) the urine is shaken with barium chloride solution, chloroform, and a few drops of hydrochloric acid. The precipitate is removed and partially dried. Treatment with 2 drops of strong sulfuric acid will bring out the characteristic colors of the bile pigments. 2. (for indican) to the urine, add a little alcholic solution of thymol and fuming hydrochloric acid containing 0.5 percent of ferric chloride; chloroform shaken with this mixture becomes violet in color.

Jones-Cantarow t., see urea concentration t.

Jorissen's t., (for formaldehyde), add 0.5 ml of a 1 percent solution of phoroglucinol in 10 percent sodium hydroxide to 1 ml of the urine; a bright red color indicates free formaldehyde.

Kantor-Gies t., (for proteins), test papers, made by dipping them in Gies' reagent (see under Gies' t.), drying, and cutting into strips, are used in making biuret test.

Kaplan's t., (for globulin-albumin in spinal fluid), to 0.2 ml of the fluid in a test tube is added 0.3 ml of distilled water. This is boiled up twice. Three drops of a 5 percent solution of butyric acid in physiologic salt solution are added and the mixture carefully underlaid with 0.5 ml of a saturated aqueous solution of ammonium sulfate. After twenty minutes a definite ring will form at the point of contact if globulin-albumin is present.

Kapsinow's t., (for bile pigments), add Obermayer's reagent to the urine and heat; a green color indicates bile pigments.

Kashiwado's t., (for pancreatic disease), the patient swallows stained nuclei from a calf's thymus mixed with lycopodium grains; these later serve to indicate the portion of the feces which is to be examined.

Kastle's t., (for raw milk), to 5 ml of milk, add 0.3 ml of N/10 hydrogen peroxide solution and 1 ml of a 1 percent solution of tricresol; raw milk will give a slight yellow color, boiled milk will not.

Kastle-Meyer t., see phenolphthalein t.

Katayama's t., (for carbonyl-hemoglobin), to 5 drops of blood, add 10 ml of water, 5 drops of orange-colored ammonium sulfide, and enough acetic acid to make the mixture acidic. CO causes a rose-red color; normal blood, a dirty greenish gray.

Kathrein's t., see Maréchal's t.

Kato's t., a technique for the quantitative estimation of the worm burden of an individual, based on estimation of standard 50 mg sample for fresh feces cleared with glycerine.

Kelling's t., 1. (for lactic acid in the stomach) the stomach contents are diluted with water, and to them are added one or two drops of a 5 percent watery solution of ferric chloride. A greenish yellow color is formed when lectic acid is present. 2. A test for the presence and location of an esophageal diverticulum by the sound of swallowing. 3. (for gastric carcinoma) a test based on the fact that the serum of cancer patients will dissolve the red corpuscles of the hen.

Kentmann's t., (for formaldehyde), dissolve in a test tube 0.1 gm of morphine in 1 ml of sulfuric acid; add, without mixing, an equal volume of the liquid to be tested: in a short time the latter will take on a reddish violet color if any formaldehyde is present.

Kerner's t., (for creatinine), acidify the suspected solution and add phosphomolybdic or phosphotungstic acid in solution; if creatinine is present, it will form a crystalline precipitate.

Kidney function t., see specific tests, including amylase t. (1), blood-urea clearance t., concentration t., Fishberg's concentration t., glycerophosphate t., Holten's t., Howard t., indigo carmine t., inulin clearance t., lactose t. (1), Mosenthal's t., Nyiri's t., phenolsulfonphthalein t., phlorhizin t., potassiumiodide t., Pregl's t., radioactive renogram t., radioisotope renal excretion t., Rehberg's t., Simonelli's t. (2), (4), urea concentration (urine concentration t., xylose absorption or tolerance t.).

Killian's t., (for carbohydrate tolerance), two hours after a standard breakfast, give the patient 200 ml of water. One hour later, give 1.75 gm of dextrose per kilogram of body weight. Determine amount of dextrose in blood specimens taken at hourly and in the twenty-four hour specimen of urine.

Kinberg's t., (for live function), after a low nitrogen content diet for several days, 50 gm of gelatin dissolved in hot chocolate is taken fasting; in liver disease, there is an increase in the output of amino acids, except in congestion of the liver and catarrhal jaundice.

Kitzmiller's t., see antithrombin t.

Kjeldahl's t., (for nitrogen), see under method.

Klein's t., a modification of Freund's reaction for cancer, using for carcinolysis is a cell suspension from an adenocarcinoma of the mouse.

Klimow's t., (for blood in urine), to a specimen of urine is added an equal quantity of H_2O_2 and a little powdered aloin; formation of a purple color indicates the presence of blood.

Kline's t., (obs), a nontreponemal antigen serologic test for syphilis.

Knapp's t., 1. (for sugar in the urine) ten gm of mercuric cyanide is dissolved in 100 ml of a solution of caustic soda and diluted; heated with diabetic urine, metalic mercury is precipitated. 2. (for organic acids in stomach) stomach contents are filtered and 1 ml treated with 5 ml of either; the extract is floated on diluted iron solution in test tubes, and the various colored rings formed will indicate the presence of the various acids.

Knott's t., a test for nicrofilariae or worm larvae in the blood by lysis of the blood in a dilute (2 percent) formalin solution, centrifugation, and examination of the stained sediment for microfilariae or larvae.

Kober's t., (for estrogens), when estrogens are treated with a mixture of sulfuric acid and phenolsulfonic acid and then diluted with water, a clear pink color is formed; suitable for qualitative analysis.

Kobert's t., (for hemoglobin), the suspected liquid is treated with zinc powder or a solution of zinc sulfate; the resulting precipitate is stained red by alkalis.

Kolmer's t., a modification of the Wassermann's test, introduced in 1922, or any of its subsequent improvements; these tests used complement fixation rather than flocculation as the indicator reaction and were once the standard confirmatory tests for syphilis; they are now little used.

Komolgorov-Smirnov t., a statistical test of goodness of fit of a sample to a specified theoretical distribution function, or of whether two samples are drawn from the same population, based on the size of the maximum difference between the cumulative distribution function of the sample and theoretical distributions, or of the two samples, and using the exact sampling distribution of this difference to determine the significance level.

Kondo's t., (for indole or skatole), to 1 ml of the unknown, add 3 drops of solution of formaldehyde and 1 ml of concentrated sulfuric acid; a violet-red color indicates indole, a yellow or brown color skatole.

Korotkoff's t., in aneurysm, if the blood pressure in the peripheral circulation remains fairly high while that artery above the aneurysm is compressed, the collateral circulation is good.

Kossel's t., (for hypoxanthine), the liquid to be tested is treated with zinc and hydrochloric acid with sodium hydroxide in excess; if hypoxanthine is present, a ruby-red color is produced.

Kowarsky's t., 1. (for dextrose in urine) in a test tube place 5 drops of pure phenylhydrazine, 10 drops of glacial acetic acid, and 1 ml of saturated solution of sodium chloride. To the mass which results add 2 or 3 ml of urine; boil for two minutes, and cool. If dextrose is present, crystals of phenylglucosazone will be seen with the microscope. 2. (blood test for diabetes) test of the patient's blood based on the reduction of a copper solution by the sugar in the blood to cuprous oxide, and the dissolving of the latter in an acid solution of ferrous sulphate, which causes the separation of an equal amount of ferrous oxide, which is measured by titration with potassium permanganate.

Krokiewicz's t., (for bile pigment in urine), 1 ml of a 1 percent solution of sodium nitrate and 1 ml of a 1 percent solution of sulfanilic acid are mixed and added drop by drop to 0.5 ml of urine. The amount added must not exceed 10 drops. The nixture becomes bright red, changing to amethyst on the addition of 1 or 2 drops of concentrated hydrochloric acid and a large amount of water.

Kuhlmann's t., a modification of Binet's test for use in infants.

Külz's t., (for β-hydroxybutyric acid), 1. The fermented urine is evaporated to a syrupy consistence, strong sulfuric acid in equal volume is added, and the mixture is distilled. If hydroxybutyric acid is present, α-crotonic acid will be formed, which will crystallize. 2. If after fermentation, the urine shows dextrorotatory properties, β-hydroxybutyric acid is present.

Kurzrok-Miller t., an *in vitro* test of compatibility of cervical mucus and spermatozoa, involving observation, under the microscope, of the behavior of sperm placed beside a sample of mucus taken from the cervical canal at the time of ovulation.

Kveim t., (for sarcoidosis), a skin test using antigen from human sarcoid tissue injected intradermally; any palpable nodule developing at the inoculation site within 6 weeks is biopsied, and histopathologic evidene of epithelioid cell granulomas constitutes a positive reaction. The test is positive in about 60 to 80 percent of patients.

Laborde's t., (for death), see Cloquet's needle sign.

Lactic acid t., see specific tests, including Hopkin's thiophene t., MacLean t., Uffelmann's t. See also lactic acid, methods for, under method.

Lactose t., 1. (for renal function) 20 gm of lactose dissolved in 20 ml of distilled water is injected under aseptic precautions into a vein at the bend of the elbow. The urine is collected hourly and testes (Nylander's test) until the sugar reaction ceases to be positive. If lactose secretion continues for more than five hours, renal disease is indicated. 2. See specific tests, including Mathews' t., Rubner's t. (2).

Ladendorff's t., (for blood), treat the suspected liquid with tincture of guaiacum, and afterward with eucalyptus oil; the upper stratum of the mixture is turned violet and the lower blue if blood is present.

Lancefield's precipitation t., a ring precipitation test used to classify and identify streptococci. Group specific antibody reacts *in vitro* with group specific polysaccharide to produce a ring precipitation where the two reagents react at the interface.

Lang's t., (for tauring), the solution to be tested is boiled with freshly prepared mercuric oxide; taurine will cause a white precipitate to appear.

Lange's t., 1. See colloidal gold t. 2. (for acetone in urine) 15 ml of urine are mixed with 0.5 to 1 ml of acetic acid, and a few drops of a freshly prepared concentrated solution of sodium nitroprusside added. The mixture is overlaid with ammonia. At the point of junction a characteristic violet ring is formed.

Lantern t., a test for color blindness made with a set of specially devised lanterns.

Latex agglutination t., latex fixation t., a type of agglutination test using latex particles as passive carriers of adsorbed antigens. The particles agglutinate following the addition of specific antibody. This test has been used extensively for the detection of rheumatoid factor and for the detection of urine human chorionic gonadotropin (hCG) in pregnancy testing.

Leach's t., (for formaldehyde), to 10 ml of milk, add 10 ml of concentrated hydrochloric acid containing 0.02 percent of ferric chloride. Heat, and if formaldehyde is present a violet color will be produced.

Lebbin's t., (for formaldehyde in milk), a small amount of milk is boiled with a mixture of 0.05 gm of resorcinol and the same quantity of a 5 percent solution of sodium hydroxide. Change from a yellow to a red color indicates the presence of formaldehyde.

Lechini's t., (for blood in urine), 10 ml of urine are treated with 1 drop of acetic acid and 3 ml of chloroform; with blood, the chloroform layer becomes red.

Lee's t., (for rennin), add 5 drops of gastric juice to 5 ml of milk; coagulation should take place in twenty minutes in the incubator.

Legal's t., 1. (for acetone) render the urine acid with HCl and distill it. Solution of sodium hydroxide and sodium nitroprusside added to the distillate produce a ruby-red tint, which acetic acid changes to purple. Creatinine will also produce a red color, but this color disappears when acetic acid is put in. 2. (for indole) to the unknown, add a few drops of sodium nitroprusside; make alkaline with potassium hydroxide. The violet color changes to blue on the addition of acetic acid.

Leishmanin t., intradermal injection of leishmanin (*Leishmania promastigote* antigens); a positive reaction consists of palpable nodule developing in 48 to 72 hours and indicates delayed hypersensitivity, but not necessarily immunity, to *Leishmania* organisms. The test is not species-specific. It becomes positive early in the course of cutaneous or mucocutaneous leishmaniasis, particularly the New World forms, except in diffuse cutaneous lesihmaniasis, it becomes positive only after recovery from visceral leishmaniasis. Also called Montenegro t.

Le Nobel's t., see Nobel's t.

Lentochol t., see Sachs-Georgi t.

Leo's t., (for free hydrochloric acid): calcium carbonate is added to the solution, which is neutralized if the acidity is due to free acid, but not if due to acid salts.

Lepromin t., intradermal injection of lepromin (a suspension of heat-killed *Mycobacterium leprae*); a positive reaction consists of tuberculin-type reaction at 48 to 72 hours (Fernandez reaction) or a nodular, occasionally ulcerated lesion at 3 to 4 weeks (Mitsuda reaction). The test is not diagnostic; a large fraction of the normal population exhibits lepromin reactivity owing to sensitivity to cross-reacting antigens. In individuals known to have leprosy, lepromin reactivity is indicative of tuberculoid leprosy or borderline leprosy near the tuberculoid end of the spectrum, whereas lepromin anergy is indicative of lepromatous or near-lepromatous disease.

Lesser's t., any iodine-containing secretion turns yellow when treated with calomel.

Leucine t., see specific tests, including Hofmeister's t. (1), Scherer's (2).

Levinson's t., (for tuberculous meningitis and other intracranial conditions), one ml of spinal fluid is placed in each of the two test tubes 8 mm in diamter. To one is added 1 ml of a 1 percent solution of mercuric chloride and, to the other, 1 ml of a 3 percent solution of sulfosalicylic acid. The tubes are well shaken, stoppered, and allowed to stand at room temperature for forty-eight hours. At the end of twenty-four and forty-eight hours, the column of precipitate in each tube is measured in millimeters. When the height of precipitate in the first test tubes is seen to be twice that of the precipitate in the second tube, the result of the test is positive.

Levulose t., see Borchard's t., methylphenylhydrazine t., Rubner's t. (2), Selivanoff's t.

Levulose tolerance t., a test of hepatic function based on the power of the liver to absorb and store large quantities of levulose.

Lewis-Pickering t., the employment of a rapid rise of temperature to produce vasodilatation in the part to be tested for the state of the peripheral circulation.

Lichtheim's t., if a patient is able to indicate the number of syllables in a word which he cannot utter, it indicates that the cortex is less involved than the association fibers.

Lieben's t., (for acetone in urine), acidulate and distill it, and treat with ammonia and tincture of iodine; if acetone is present, a yellow precipitate of iodoform is produced.

Lieben-Ralfe t., (for acetone), boil 1.3 gm of potassium iodide in 3.75 ml of solution of potassium hydroxide; float the urine on the surface of the reagent in a test tube a precipitate of phosphate is formed at the upper surface of the reagent, which, if acetone is present will be rendered yellow by iodoform.

Liebermann's t., (for proteins), a precipitate is made from the urine with either and heat with strong hydrochloric acid this produces a fine violet-blue color if proteins are present.

Liebermann-Burchard t., (for cholesterol), dissolve the suspected substance in chloroform, add acetic anhydride, and treat with strong sulfuric acid; if cholesterol is present, a violet color is produced, which soon changes to green.

Liebig's t., (for cystine), boil the suspected substance with a sodium hydroxide solution and a little lead sulfide; if cystine is present, the lead sulfide will form a black precipitate.

Ligat's t., (for cutaneous hyperesthesia in abdominal disease), the skin is pinched between the thumb and forefinger and lifted up from the parts below.

Limulus t., an extract of blood cells from the horseshoe crab (*Limulus polyphemus*) is exposed to a blood sample from a patient; if gram-negative endotoxin is present in the sample, it will produce gelation of the extract of blood cells.

Lindemann's t., (for acetoacetic acid in urine), to about 10 ml of urine, add 5 drops of 30 percent acetic acid, 5 drops Lugol's solution, and 2 or 3 ml chloroform, and shake. The chloroform does not change color if diacetic acid is present, but becomes reddish violet in its absence. Uric acid also decolorizes iodine, and if much is present double the amount of Lugol's solution should be used.

Lindner's t., see under sign.

Lipase t., 1. (for liver function) a test based on the fact that lipase is present in the blood plasma of normal persons in a constant amount. Liver injury will cause a rise in the lipase of the blood plasma as measured by the power of the blood to split ethyl butyrate. 2. See specific tests, including copper soap t., litmus milk t.

Lipps' t., see sand t.

Litmus milk t., (for pancreatic lipase), add pancreatic lipase to litmus milk, incubate, and note change of color; pancreatic lipase is indicated by a pink coloration.

Liver function t., see specific tests, including Kinberg's t., levulose tolerance t., lipase t., Macdonald's t., nitrogen partition t., phenolterrachlorophthalein t., Quick's t. (1), rose bengal t., Rosenthal's t. (2), santonin t., Zappacosta's t.

Loewe's t., (for dextrose in urine), treat the urine with a solution of sodium carbonate containing bismuth subnitrate and glycerine; sugar gives a dark precipitate.

Loewi's t., three drops of epinephrine chloride solution 1:1000 are instilled into the conjunctival sac, followed in five minutes by 3 more drops. This produces dilatation of the pupil in pancreatic insufficiency, diabetes, and hyperthyroidism.

Lombard's t., a test for simulated deafness using a noise apparatus.

Löwenthal's t., (for dextrose not in urine), boil the suspected substance with a solution of ferric chloride, tartaric acid and sodium carbonate; if dextrose is present, the liquid becomes dark, and iron oxide is freely precipitated.

Lucké's t., (for hippuric acid), add boiling hot nitric acid evaporate, and heat the dry residue; a strong odor of nitrobenzene proves the presence of hippuric acid.

Luebert's t., (for formaldehyde in milk), 5 gm of coarsely powdered potassium sulfate is placed in a 100 ml flask; 5 ml of suspected milk is put over it by a pipet, and 10 ml of sulfuric acid (specific gravity, 1.84) is run down the side of the flask. If formaldehyde is present, a violet coloration soon occurs; if none is present, the fluid becomes brown or black.

Lupus band t., an immunofluorescence test to determine the presence and extent of immunoglobulin and complement deposits at the dermal-epidermal junction of skin specimens from patients with systemic lupus erythematosus.

Lüttke's t., (for free hydrochloric acid in gastric juice), a quantitative determination in succession of the total chlorides. The chlorine in the fixed chlorides, and then the combined and free HCl.

Lyle-Curtman t., (for blood), boil the stool with acetic acid, extract it with ether, and to the ethereal extract add a little guaiaconic acid in 95 percent alcohol; a decided green, light-blue, or purple color indicates the presence of blood.

Lymphocyte proliferation t., a functional test of the ability of lymphocytes to respond to mitogens, specific antigens, or allogenic cells. Lymphocytes are cultured both with and without the stimulant for several days and then are cultured for several hours with ^{3}H-labeled thymidine. The ratio of the thymidine uptake in the stimulated and control cultures is reported as the "stimulation index" (SI) or "stimulation ratio" (SR). The test with allogenic cells, called a mixed lymphocyte culture (MLC), is commonly performed for transplantation tissue typing; all three types of stimulants are used in investigation of immunodeficiency. Commonly used mitogens are phytohemagglutinin (PHA), concanavalin A (ConA), and pokeweed mitogen (PWN); commonly used antigens are PPD (tuberculin), *Candida* antigen, and streptokinase-streptodornase. Also called blastogenesis assay and lymphocyte proliferation assay.

Lyon's t., see Meltzer-Lyon t.

Macdonald's d., (for liver function), inject 2 mg per kilogram of sodium sulfobromophthalein (Bromsulphalein) and take food specimens every five minutes for thirty minutes after the injection.

Machado's t., Machodo-Guerreiro t., (for Chagas' disease), a complement-fixation test, using as antigen an extract of the spleen of puppies severely infected with *Trypanosoma cruzi*.

Maclagan's t., see thymol turbidity t.

MacLean's t., (for lactic acid in gastric juice), to 5 ml of gastric juice, add 5 drops of the following reagent: ferric chloride, 5 gm; concentrated hydrochloric acid, 1.5 ml; saturated solution of mercury bichloride, 100 ml. Lactic acid is indicated by a yellow coloration.

MacLean-de Wesselow t., see urea concentration t.

MacMunn's t., (for indican), boil the urine in an equal quantity of hydrochloric acid and a little nitric acid; cool and shake with chloroform, which becomes violet, and shows one absorption band due to indigo blue and one due to indigo red.

MacWilliam's t., (for albumin), take 20 ml of urine and add 2 drops of a saturated solution of salicylsulfonic acid if albumin is present, cloudiness or precipitate will be seen; if albumoses or peptones are present, this precipitate will disappear on boiling, but appear again on cooling.

Magnesionitric t., (for albumin in urine), mix 1 part of nitric acid and 1 part magnesium sulfate; turbidity indicates the presence of albumin.

Magpie's t., (for salts of mercury), stannous chloride is added to the suspected solution; a white and gray precipitate is formed, consisting of metabolic mercury and mild mercurous chloride.

Male frog t., male toad t., (for pregnancy), urine or serum of a woman suspected of being pregnant is injected into the dorsal lymph sac of two male frogs (*Rana pipiens*) or male toads (*Bufo marinus*). The presence of spermatozoa in the cloacal fluid of both animals is positive; in one animal, inconclusive: in neither animal, negative.

Malerba's t., (for acetone), add a solution of dimethyl-para-phenylenediamine: a fine red or reddish color is seen.

Mallein t., a concentrate prepared from cultures or extracts of the glanders bacillus, *Pseudomonas mallei*, used in skin test analogous to the tuberculin test for the diagnosis of glanders.

Malot's t., a test for the quantitative determination of phosphoric acid in urine by the reaction with cochineal and a uranium salt.

Maltose t., see Rubner's t. (2).

Maly's t., 1. (for free hydrochloric acid in the gastric juice), a solution of methylene blue is added; the free acid will turn it from a violet to a green or blue tint. 2. (for free hydrochloric acid in stomach contents), filter into a glass dish and stain blue with ultramarine; place a piece of lead paper over it and cover, warm the mixture. The free acid will turn the blue to brown and darken the lead paper.

Mann-Whitney t., Mann-Whitney-Wilcoxon t., see rank sum t.

Mantoux's t., intracutaneous tuberculin test; the now standard type of tuberculin test in which tuberculin is administered intradermally using a needle and syringe.

Maréchal's t., (for bile pigments in urine), drop tincture of iodine carefully into the tube; when the drops touch the urine, a green color is seen.

Maréchal-Rosin t., see Maréchal's t.

Marlow's t., (for heterophoria), one eye is occluded by a bandage for some time; after the bandage is removed, measurements for heterophoria are made.

Marquardt's t., (for fusel oil), add a few drops of dilute potassium permanganate until the light pink color persists. Cork for twenty-four hours. Add more permanganate if necessary to keep the pink color. Note the sickening odor of valeric acid.

Marquis' t., (for morphine), evaporate the unknown to dryness on a white porcelain plate and touch with a mixture of 3 ml of concentrated sulfuric acid and 2 drops of formalin. A purple-red color changing to violet and then to blue indicates morphine.

Marshall's t., (for urea), treat the specimen with urease and titrate the ammonia so formed; see under method.

Maschke's t., see von Maschke's t.

Masset's t., (for bile pigments in urine), add 2 or 3 drops of sulfuric acid and a crystal of potassium nitrite; a grass-green color shows the presence of bile pigments.

Master's "2-step" exercise t., (for coronary insufficiency), an electrocardiographic test, the tracings being recorded while the subject repeatedly ascends and descends two steps, each 9 inches high, immediately after cessation of the climbs, and then 2 and 6 minutes later. The amount of work (number of trips) is standardized for age, weight, and sex.

Matas' t., see tourniquet t., def. 2.

Match t., a screening test of expiration in which a match is held 3 inches from the subject's wide open mouth and several attempts are made to blow it out. Failure after six attempts indicates a maximal breathing capacity below 40 liters per minute and a maximal midexpiratory flow rate below 0.6 liter per second.

Mathews' t., (for lactose and dextrose), if both dextrose and lactose are suspected, make a total quantitative test by Benedict's method. Add yeast to the urine and ferment out the dextrose, then make a second quatitative determination. The second determination is or may be lactose; confirm with the osazone test. The difference between the two determinations is dextrose.

Maumené's t., (for dextrose), heat the urine with a little stannous chloride; if sugar is present, a dark-brown precipitate will be formed.

Mauthner's t., a method of testing color blindness by the use of small bottles filled with different pigments, some with one only and some with two, the latter containing either pseudoisochromatic or isochromatic solutions.

Mayer's t., (for alkaloids), mercuric chloride, 13-1/2 gm, and potassium iodide, 50 gm, are dissolved in 1000 ml of water: this is used as a test for alkaloid, with which it gives a white precipitate.

Mayerhofer's t., the reduction of a decinormal solution of potassium permanganate solution by 1 ml of spinal fluid in an acid medium as an index of the amount of protein substance present in the fluid; used as an indication of the existence of tuberculous meningitis.

McMurray's t., (for torn meniscus), as the patient lies supine with knee fully flexed, the examiner rotates the patient's foot fully outward and the knee is slowly extended; a painful "click" indicates a tear of the medial meniscus of the knee joint. If the click occurs when the foot is rotated inward, the tear is in the lateral meniscus.

Méhu's t., (for albumin in urine), add a little nitric acid, and mix with 10 volumes of a solution of 2 parts of alcohol, 1 part of phenol, and 1 part of acetic acid; shake it and a white precipitate appears. This test is said not to be entirely trustworthy.

Meigs' t., (for fat in milk), to 10 ml of milk in a special apparatus, add 20 ml of water; 20 ml of ethyl either, and shake. Then add 20 ml of percent alcohol. Remove the ethereal layer, evaporate, and weigh.

Meinické's t., (obs), any of several nontreponemal antigen serologic tests for syphilis.

Melanin t., see specific tests, including Thormählen's t., von Jaksch's t. (3), Zeller's t. (1).

Mendel's t., see Mantoux's t.

Mendelsohn's t., a test for efficiency of the heart muscle based on the rapidity of the recovery of the pulse from its acceleration produced by exertion.

Meningitis t., see specific tests, including Levinson's t., Mayerhofer's t., Takata-Ara t., tryptophan t. (2).

Mercury t., see specific tests, including Magpie's t., Reinsch's t. (2), Vogel-Lee t.

Mester's t., (for rheumatic disease), blood is withdrawn from the middle finger of the right hand of a fasting patient before and again thirty and sixty minutes after administration of two or three intracutaneous injection of 0.2 ml each of a sterile 0.1 percent aqueous solution of salicylic acid and the number of leukocytes is determined after each withdrawal. The injections are made at the flexor aspect of the right forearm at a distance of about 5 cm from each other. They are followed by severe pain and burning sensation of short duration and by the formation at the points of the injections, of wheals which disappear in a few hours. Positive results are shown by transient leukopenia within the first thirty minutes after administration of the injections.

Methylphenylhydrazine t., (for levulose), add 4 gm of methylphenylhydrazine to 10 ml of unknown (containing about 2 gm of levulose) and enough alcohol to clarify the solution; add 4 ml of 50 percent acetic acid and heat for five to ten minutes. Reddish yellow needles of methylphenyllevulosazone indicate levulose.

Methyl red t., (for differentiation of Enterobacteriaceae), the organism is inoculated into a buffered glucose-peptone broth containing methyl red. In a positive reaction, the medium remains red after incubation owing to acid metabolic products. Most enterobacteriaceae are positive; the klebsielleae are negative and erwinieae are variable.

Mett's t., (for estimating pepsin), tubes (Mett's tubes) of coagulated albumin are introduced into the unknown and into a standard pepsin HCl mixture and the amount of digestion occurring in a given time is noted.

Michailow's t., (for proteins), add ferrous sulfate to the solution, underlay it with strong sulfuric acid and a drop or so of nitric acid; a brown ring and red coloration indicate the presence of proteins.

Microprecipitation t., a precipitation test in which a minute quantity of the serum is employed.

MIF t., see migration inhibitory factor t.

Migration inhibitory factor (MIF) t., an *in vitro* test for the production of MIF by lymphocytes in response to specific antigens; used for evaluation of cell-mediated immunity. MIF production is absent in certain immunodeficiency disorders, e.g., DiGeorge's syndrome, Wiskott-Aldrich syndrome, Hodgkin's disease.

Milk t., see specific tests, including Babcock's t., Bauer's t. (3), benzidine peroxidase t., dirt t., Kastle's t., Kober t. (2), methylene blue t. (2), phosphatase t. (1), Store's t., Wilkinson-Peter t.

Milk ring t., see abortus Bang ring t.

Millard's t., (for albumin), make a reagent of 2 parts of liquefied carbolic acid, 6 parts of glacial acetic acid, and 22 parts of a solution of potassium hydroxide; this precipitates albumin.

Miller-Kurzrok t., a laboratory procedure to test the ability of sperm to penetrate the mucus plug in a woman's cervix.

40 millimeter t., (for athletic efficiency), the subject sits with nasal respiration occluded with a clamp, and by expiring through a mouthpiece, sustains a column of mercury at the height of 40 mm as long as he can. The pulse rate is taken meanwhile, every five seconds. In a satisfactory test the pulse rate is unaltered for a minute or more.

Millon's t., (for proteins and nitrogenous compounds), a solution is made of 10 gm of mercury and 20 gm of nitric add; this is diluted with an equal volume of water and decanted after standing twenty-four hours. This reagent gives a red color with proteins and other substances, such as tyrosine, phenol, and thymol, which contain the hydroxyphenyl group.

Mills t., (for tennis elbow), with the wrist and fingers fully flexed and the forearm pronated, complete extension of the elbow is painful.

Mirror t., a mirror is held horizontally above the larynx and the patient instructed to cough. The mirror is thus sprayed with bronchial secretion. Small flecks of secretion of the mirror indicate the nature of the expectoration.

Mitscherlich's t., (for phosphorus in the stomach), the contents of the stomach are made acid and distilled in the dark. The condenser will contain a luminous ring. Small amounts of alcohol, ether, or turpentine will prevent the reaction.

Mitsuda's t., see lepromin t.

Mittelmeyer's t., the patient is directed to take marching steps on one spot without progressing: in vestibular disorder he will turn to the side ipsilateral to vestibular loss, or contralateral to vestibular excitation.

Mixed lymphocyte culture t., see lymphocyte proliferation t.

Moerner-Sjöqvist t., see Sjöqvist method.

Mohr's t., (for hydrochloric acid in the stomach contents), dilute to a light-yellow color a solution of iron acetate, free from alkaline acetates; add a few drops of a solution of potassium thiocyanate, and then the filtered contents of the stomach: if they contain the acid, a red coloring ensues, which is destroyed by sodium acetate.

Molisch's t., 1. (for dextrose in urine) add 2 ml of urine, 2 drops of a 15 percent solution of thymol, and an equal volume of strong sulfuric acid; a deep-red color results. 2. (for dextrose in urine) to 1 ml of urine, add 2 or 3 drops of a 5 percent solution of alphanaphthol in alcohol, then add 2 ml of strong sulfuric add; a deep-violet color is produced, and a violet precipitate follows if water is added. 3. (for proteins) the substance is treated with a 15 percent alcoholic solution of alphanaphthol and then with concentrated sulfuric acid; a violet color is formed if proteins are present.

Moloney's t., (for delayed sensitivity to diphtheria toxoid), 0.1 ml of 1:10 dilution of fluid toxoid is injected intradermally on the flexor surface of the forearm: the appearance in 12 to 24 hours of an area of redness with induration of more than 12 mm in diameter is a positive reaction. Also called Moloney's reaction.

Monaural loudness balance (MLB) t., a test to determine recruitment in bilateral sensorineural hearing loss; the loudness sensation at impaired frequencies is compared with that at normal frequencies.

Montenegro t., see Leishmanin t.

Montigne's t., heat an alcoholic solution of a sterol with silicotungstic acid; a red-brown color appears.

Moore's t., (for dextrose or any carbohydrate), boil the suspected solution with sodium or potassium hydroxide; if dextrose or lactose is present, a yellow or brown color is produced.

Morelli's t., (to differentiate between an exudate and a transudate), add a few drops of the suspected fluid to a saturated solution of mercuric chloride in a test tube; a flaky precipitate indicates a transudate, a clot indicates an exudate.

Moretti's t., (for typhoid fever), 25 ml of urine is saturated with 20 gm of crystallized ammonium sulfate. After a quarter of an hour the urine is filtered and diluted to about one third. To 10 ml of the filtrate one fifth of its volume of a 10 percent of sodium hydroxide is added, and then a drop of 5 percent tincture of iodine. The solution is shaken, and if the reaction is positive a persistent golden-yellow color is produced.

Moritz's t., a reaction for distinguishing fluids of transudation and exudation utilizing acetic acid.

Mörner's t., 1. (for tyrosine), to a small quantity of the crystals in a test tube, add a few milliliters of Mörner's reagent (solution of formaldehyde, 1 nil distilled water 45 ml concentrated sulfuric acid, 55 ml). Heat gently to the boiling point. A green color shows the presence of tyrosine 2. See nitroprusside t. (1).

Moro's t., an obsolete tuberculin test in which tuberculin was applied to the skin in a lanolin-based ointment.

Morphine t., see specific test, including Deniges't. (3), Marquis' t., Oliver's t. (3), Weppen's t.

Morton's t., in metatarsalgia, transverse pressure across the heads of the metatarsals causes a sharp pain, especially between the second and third metatarsals.

Moschowitz's t., a test for arteriosclerosis made by rendering the lower limb bloodless by means of an Esmarch bandage. This is removed after five minutes have elapsed, when, in a normal limb, the color will return in a few seconds, but in one affected by arteriosclerosis the return of color takes place much more slowly. Also called hyperemia t.

Mosenthal's t., (for kidney function), with the patient on a prescribed general diet, take samples of urine in two-hour periods during the day and once at night. Examine them for volume, specific gravity, total nitrogen, and chlorides, and compare with normal.

Moynihan's t., (for hourglass stomach), the two parts of Seidlitz's powder are given separately, in hourglass stomach two separated protrusions on the abdomial wall can be observed.

Mulder's t., 1. (for dextrose) alkalinize the solution with sodium carbonate; on adding a solution of indigo-carmine and heating, the mixture is decolorized, but becomes blue again when shaken with air. 2. (for proteins) treat the suspected substance with nitric acid: proteins are turned yellow by it; alkalinize the substance and it becomes an orange yellow, due to the presence of the phenyl group. Also called xanthroproteic reaction.

Multiple-puncture t., an intracutaneous test in which the material used (e.g., tuberculin) is introduced into the skin by pressure of several needles or pointed tines or prongs. See also tine t. and tuberculin t., Sterneedle.

Mumps skin t., (for immunity to mumps), an unreliable and little used test consisting of intradermal injection of killed mumps virus, a positive response being development of a tuberculin-type delayed hypersensitivity reaction.

Murexide t., see Weidel's t. (1).

Murphy's t., the patient sits with his arms folded in front of him; the examiner's thumb is placed under the twelfth rib and short jabbing movements are made. Thus deep-seated tenderness and muscular rigidity are determined. Also called Murphy's kidney punch.

Mycobiologic t., see mycologic test.

Mycologic t., (for sugar in urine), to the specimen of urine, an equal quantity of 1 percent peptone solution is added; this mixture is sown with some species of *Candida*. If sugar is present, gas is developed. Also called mycobiologic t.

Myers-Fine t., (for amyloytic activity), add decreasing amounts of stomach contents to constant amounts of starch solution and note by means of iodine the amount required to completely hydrolyze the starch.

Mylius' t., (for bile acids), to each milliliter of the solution of bile acids, add 1 ml of strong sulfuric acid and 1 drop of furfurol solution; if bile acids are present, a red color is produced, which turns to a bluish violet in the the course of a day or so.

Naffziger's t., (for nerve root compression), increase or aggravation of pain or sensory disturbance over the distribution of the involved nerve root upon manual compression of the jugular veins bilaterally confirms the presence of an extruded intervertebral disk or other mass.

Nagel's t., a test for color vision in which one-half of the field of an anomaloscope is illuminated with standard yellow and the other half is matched to the yellow by the subject who mixes red and green.

Nagler's t., the formation of an opaque zone around colonies of *Clostridium perfringens* on egg yolk agar, produce by the action of diffusible lecithinase (α-toxin).

Nakayama's t., (for bile pigments), add 5 ml of acid urine to the same amount of 10 percent barium chloride solution and centrifugalize. To the precipitate is added 2 ml of a reagent consisting of 99 parts of 95 percent alcohol, 1 part of fuming hydrochloric acid to a liter of which 4 gm of ferric chloride has been added. The fluid is boiled; a green color obtained, which, on the addition of yellow nitric acid, becomes violet or red.

NBT t., see nitroblue tetrazolium t.

Nencki's t., (for indole), treat the suspected material with nitric acid and a little nitrous acid; a red color follows, and in concentrated solution a red precipitate may appear.

Nessler's t., an aqueous solution of 5 percent of potassium iodide, 2.5 percent of mercuric chloride, and 16 percent of potassium hydroxide used as a test for ammonia.

Neubauer-Fischer t., the glycyltryptophan test.

Neufeld's t., when pneumococci and other capsulated microorganisms are mixed with specific immune serum, there occurs in addition to agglutination a swelling (quellung) of the capsules of the organisms, owing to the binding of antibody with the capsular polysaccharide; also called capsular swelling and quellung reaction.

Neukomm's t., (for bile acids), a drop of the suspected substance is placed on a small white procelain cover with a drop of dilute cane sugar solution and one of dilute sulfuric acid. The mixture is carefully evaporated over a flame, a violet stain being left if bile acids are present.

Neutralization t., a test for the power of an antiserum or other substance to antagonize the pathogenic properties of a microorganism, toxin, virus, bacteriophage, or toxic substance.

Niacin t., (for *Mycobacterium tuberculosis*), in a chemical hood, add 0.1 ml of heavy growth from a 10-day old culture organisms in Dubos' liquid Tween-albumin medium to 3 ml of the same medium in a screw-cap tube. Add 1 ml of 4 percent aniline in 95 percent ethanol and 1 ml of 10 percent aqueous cyanogen bromide. A distinct yellow color indicates the presene of niacin, a characteristic of human stains of M. *tuberculosis;* bovine stains are doubtful or negative; other stains are negative. Alternatively, add to the culture being tested, 0.5 to 0.1 ml sterile saline or water, place the tube so that the fluid layers over the colonies, and allow to stand for 15 minutes. Remove 0.5 ml of the aqueous extract to a test tube. Add equal quantities of 4 percent aniline in 95 percent ethanol and 10 percent aqueous cyanogen bromide. If niacin is present, a yellow color will appear.

Nickerson-Kveim t., see Kveim t.

Ninhydrin t., see tricetohydrindene hydrate t.

Nippe's t., (for blood), a modified form of Teichmann's test.

Nitrate reduction t., 1. (for the reduction of nitrate to nitrite by a bacterial culture) the organism is cultured in a broth containing nitrate. The medium is tested for nitrite by mixing with solutions containing sulfanilic acid and alpha-naphthylamine in 5 N acetic acid; a red color indicates the presence of nitrite. The test is useful in identifying doubtful stains of enterobacteriaceae, mucobacteria, and certain aerobic bacteria. 2. A reagent used as a test for nitrites. It is prepared by treating a mixture of 0.5 gm of sulfanilic acid and 150 ml of dilute acetic acid with 0.1 gm of naphthylamine and then with 20 ml of boiling water. The sediment produced by this reaction is dissolved in 150 ml of dilute acetic acid. The suspected substance is heated with this reagent to 80°C, when a red color is formed if nitrites are present.

Nitric acid t., 1. (for albumin), see Heller's t. (1), 2. See specific tests, including Weyl's t. (2).

Nitric acid-magnesium sulfate t., (for albumin), see Roberts't. (1).

Nitrites t., (in saliva), to the saliva add 1 or 2 drops of H_2SO_4, a few drops of KI solution, and some starch paste; a blue color indicates nitrites. See also Gries' t., Ilosvay's t., Schaffer's t.

Nitroblue tetrazolium (NBT) t., a test of neutrophil microbicidal function; neutrophils are incubated with latex particles and NBT. Normally, phagocytosis of the particles is accompanied by reduction of NBT to a blue formazan pigment; absence of NBT reduction indicates a defect in some of the metabolic pathways involved in intracellular microbial killing, as seen in chronic granulomatous disease.

Nitrogenous compounds t., see Million's t.

Nitrogen partition t., a test of hepatic function based on alterations in the distribution of nitrogen in the various nitrogenous bodies of the blood and urine.

Nitropropiol t., (for sugar in urine), the urine is mixed with an alkali and heated with orthonitrophenylpropiolic acid; the indigo blue to green (blue and yellow) color reaction will be seen.

Nitroprusside t., 1. (for cysteine), if a protein containing cysteine is dissolved in water and 2 to 4 drops of a 4 or 5 percent solution of sodium nitroprusside and then a few drops of ammonia are added, a deep purple-red color appears: also called Morner's t. 2. (for acetone) see Legal's t. (1). 3. (for indole) see Legal's t. (2). 4. (for creatinine) see Wey's t. (1).

Nitroso-indole-nitrate t., (for indole and skatole), acidify the unknown with nitric acid and add a few drops of potassium nitrite; a red color or a red precipitate indicates indole, a white turbidity indicates skatole.

Nobel's t., 1. (for aceto-acetic acid and acetone), stratify ammonium hydroxide on urine acidified with acetic acid and to which a little sodium nitroprusside has been added; a violet ring at the junction indicates acetoacetic acid or acetone. 2. (for bile pigments) add zinc chloride and a little of the tincture of iodine; a dichromic coloration follows.

Noguchi's t., (for globulin), to 0.5 ml of Noguchi's reagent, add 0.1 ml of spinal fluid; boil and add 0.1 ml of N/l sodium hydroxide. A flocculent precipitate indicates globulin.

Nonne's t., see Ross-Jones t.

Nonne-Apelt t., 2 ml of cerebrospinal fluid is mixed with an equal quantity of neutral saturated solution of ammonium sulfate and compared after 3 minutes with another tube containing spinal fluid only; if there is no difference or only faint opalescence, the reaction is said to be negative. If there is an opalescence or turbidity, the reaction is said to be positive phase 1, which indicates an excess of globulin in fluid and points to nervous disorder. A normal fluid treated with heat and acetic acid only beocmes turbid and is called positive phase 2.

Nucleoalbumin t., see Ott's t.

Nyiri's t., a concentration test for kidney function by the use of thiosulfate.

Nystagmus t., 1. In disturbance of equilibrium of the vestibular apparatus, the direction of fall is influenced by changing the position of patient's head 2. See caloric test.

Oakley-Fulthorpe t., double diffusion in one dimension-immunodiffusion in which both the antigen and antibody diffuse through the medium toward each other, antiserum is placed in a test tube and overlaid with agar, which is allowed to solidify, and antigen is layered over the agar precipitin line from where the concentrations of each antigen and antibody are equivalent.

Ober's t., the patient lies on the side opposite that to be tested, with the underneath hip and knee flexed; with the upper knee flexed to a right angle, the upper hip is flexed to 90 degrees, fully abducted, brought into full hyperextension, and allowed to adduct; the angle that the thigh makes above the horizontal is the degree of abduction contracture.

Obermayer's t., (for indican in urine), precipitate the urine with a 1:5 lead acetate solution with care, least an excess of the reagent be taken; filter and agitate the filtrate with an equal amount of fuming hydrochloric acid containing a little of the solution of ferric chloride; to this add chloroform, which is turned blue by indigo.

Obermüller's t., (for cholesterin), put the substance to be tested in a test tube and melt it with a drop or two of propionic anhydride over a small flame; on cooling, the mass becomes successively blue, green, orange, carmine, and copper colored.

Obturator t., see Cope's t.

Occult blood t., see tests listed under blood t.

Oliver's t., 1. (for albumin), underlay the urine with a 1:4 solution of sodium tungstate and a 10:6 solution of citric acid; a white coagulum at the junction of the two layers shows the presence of albumin. 2. (for sugar), boil the suspected liquid with indigo carmine; sugar will change the blue to a red or yellow. 3. (for morphine) if, to a solution of morphine, a few milliliters of hydrogen peroxide is added and the mixture is stirred with a piece of copper wire, the solution takes on a deep portwine color, with the evolution of gas. 4. (for bile acids), to 5 ml of the unknown, add to 2 to 3 drops of acetic acid and filter; an equal volume of 1 percent solution of peptone will produce a precipitate insoluble in excess of acetic acid if bile acids are present.

One-stage prothrombin time t., see Quick's t. (2).

One-tailed t., a hypothesis test (qv) in which the critical region is one tail of the distribution of the test statistic and the null hypothesis is tested against a one-sided alternative that includes deviations from the null hypothesis only in one direction, deviations in the other direction being of no consequence.

ONPG t., (for β-D-galactosidase in bacteria), the organism is grown in a buffered peptone medium containing D-nitrophenyl β-D-galactopyranoside (ONPG): production of β galactosidase is indicated by the appearance of a yellow color. Used to differentiate *Salmonella* (positive) from *Arizona* (negative), and *Neisseria lactamicus* (positive) from *N. meningitidis* (negative).

Orcinol t., (for pentose in urine), see Bial's t.

Organic acid t., see Knapp's t. (2).

Orientation t., see if the patient can give correctly the time of day, the day of the week, month, and year, and the place.

Orthotoluidine t., (for blood), see Ruttan-Hardisty t.

Osazone t., (for sugars), see Kowarsky's t. (1) and von Jaksch's t. (2).

Osgood-Haskins t., (for albumin), to 5 ml of urine, add 1 ml of 50 percent acetic acid; a precipitate at room temperature indicates bile salts, urates, or resin acids. Add 3 ml of a saturated solution of sodium chloride; a precipitate suggests Bence Jones protein or globulin. The Bence Jones protein will redissolve of heating.

Osterberg's t., (for beta-oxybutyric acid), to 800 mg of ammonium sulfate, add 0.15 ml of concentrated ammonium hydroxide solution, 2 drops of a 5 percent solution of nitroprusside, and 1 ml of the urine. Dilute to 50 ml and compare with a standard.

Ott's t., (for nucleoalbumin in urine), to the urine is added an equal volume of saturated solution of sodium chloride, and then Almen's reagent (dissolve 5 gm of tannic acid in 240 ml of 50 percent alcohol and add 100 ml of 25 percent acetic acid); a precipitate forms when nucleoalbumin is present.

Ouchterlony t., double diffusion in which antigen and antiserum are placed in wells cut in an agar plate; antigen solutions to be compared are placed in wells equidistant from the antiserum well. Three principal types of reaction may occur, reaction of identity, reaction of nonidentity, and reaction of partial identity, each identified by a characteristic pattern of precipitin lines, indicating the extent to which antigen samples share antigenic determinants.

Oudin t., a single diffusion (see under diffusion technique) in which agar-containing antiserum is placed in a test tube and antigen is layered over it; precipitin lines form where the concentrations of each antigen and antibody are equivalent.

Ovarian hyperemia t., (for pregnancy), the intraperitoneal injection of urine or blood serum of pregnant women into immature female mice produces a reddened appearance of the ovaries.

Oxyphenylsulfonic acid t., (for albumin in urine), dissolve in 20 parts of water 3 parts of oxyphenylsulfonic acid and 1 part of salicylsulfonic acid; add to 1 ml of urine a drop of the reagent: if albumin is present, a clear white precipitate appears.

Pachon's t., measuring of the blood pressure for the purpose of determining the state of the collateral circulation in aneurysm.

Paget's t., a solid tumor is most hard in its center, whereas a cyst is least hard in its center.

Palmin t., palmitin t., (for pancreatic efficiency), after a test meal containing palmitin, the contents of the stomach are examined for the presence of fatty acids. They will be found in cases in which the pancreas is normal, for the presence of fat in the stomach causes the pylorus to open and admit the pancreatic juice, which splits palmitin into fatty acids.

Pancreatic function t., see specific tests, including Kashiwado's t., litmus milk t., Loeive's t., palmin t., Sahli-Nencki t., secretin t.

Pandy's t., a test for globulin in the cerebrospinal fluid. Mix 80 to 100 ml pure phenol with distilled water, shake, and place in incubator several hours. After several days at room temperature, pour off the top watery part, which serves as the reagent. With a Pasteur pipet a drop (0.01 ml) of the fluid to be tested is deposited on the bottom of a watch crystal filled with the reagent. If no cloudy precipitate forms within five seconds, the reaction is negative.

Pap t., Papanicolaou's t., an exfoliative cytological staining procedure for the detection and diagnosis of various conditions, particularly malignant and premalignant conditions of the female genital tract (cancer of the vagina, cervix, and endometrium), in which cells which have been desquamated from the genital epithelium are obtained by smears, fixed and stained, and examined under the microscope for evidence of pathologic changes. Cytologic findings have commonly been expressed in terms of histologic lesions classified as class I to V, but preferably each examination should have an individual histologic description. The test is also used in evaluating endocrine function, and in the diagnosis of malignancies of other organs, as of the respiratory tract and lungs, gastrointestinal tract, urinary tract, and breast.

Paracasein t., see Leiner's t.

Parnum's t., (for albumin), filter the urine, add one-sixth volume of a saturated solution of magnesium or sodium sulfate, acidulate with acetic acid, and boil; if albumin is present, a white precipitate is formed.

Partial thromboplastin time t., a one-stage clotting test used clinically to detect deficiencies of the components of the intrinsic thromboplastin system; in reality, prolonged clotting time may reflect deficiency or absence of coagulation factors I, II, V and VIII through XII, separately or in combination.

Passive cutaneous anaphylaxis t., a passively transferred local anaphylactic reaction used in the study of reaginic antibodies; the skin of an animal is sensitized by intradermal injection of serum from a sensitized animal, and after a 24 to 72-hour latent period the antigen and Evans' blue dye are injected intravenously. Reaction of the antigen with skinfiked antibody causes the release of histamine, which increases vascular permeability, permits leakage of albumin bound dye, and produces a blue spot at the site of intradermal injection.

Passive protection t., a test in which antiserum is tested for protective antibody by parenteral inoculation of groups of animals with graded doses in constant volume.

Passive transfer t., an immediate hypersensitivity reaction produced in a nonatopic subject by intradermal injection of serum from an atopic subject followed 12 or more hours later by an injection of antigen into the same site; the presence of specific reaginic (IgE) antibody in the transferred serum results in a classic wheal and flare reaction to the antigen. Once the standard method of demonstrating reaginic antibody, this test is no longer used because of the risk of transmitting serum hepatitis and because serum IgE can now be measured by *in vitro* assays, e.g., RAST and RIST.

Patch t's, skin tests, used primarily in the diagnosis of allergies, in which small pieces of gauze of filter paper impregnated with suspected allergens are applied to the skin for a short time period; swelling or redness constitutes a positive reaction.

Patrick's t., with the patient supine, the thigh and knee are flexed and the external malleolus is placed over the patella of the opposite leg; the knee is depressed, and if pain is produced thereby arthritis of the hip is indicated. Patrick calls this test fabere sign, from the initial letters of movements that are necessary to elicit it, namely, flexion, abduction, external rotation, extension.

Patterson's t., a chemical spot test for the diagnosis of uremia. A drop of Ehrlich's reagent is applied to a drop of blood placed on a white filter paper; if there is greatly increased blood urea, the spot on the filter paper turns a greenish color.

Paul-Bunnell t., (for serum heterophile antibodies associated with infectious mononucleosis), determination of the highest dilution of the patient's serum capable of agglutinating sheep red blood cells.

Paul-Bunnell-Davidsohn t., a modification of the Paul-Bunnell test that differentiates among three types of heterophile sheep erythrocyte agglutinins: those associated with infectious mononucleosis, those associated with serum sickness, and natural antibodies against Forssman's antigen. The patient's serum is absorbed with guinea pig kidney cells or with beef erythrocytes and centrifuged. Unabsorbed serum has a high heterophile antibody titer in infectious mononucleosis and serum sickness; a low titer is seen in normal individuals. Absorption with guinea pig kidney removes Forssman's antibody and serum sickness heterophile antibody. Absorption with beef erythrocytes removes heterophile antibody associated with infectious mononucleosis or serum sickness. Also called Davidsohn's differential absorption t.

Pavy's t., (for dextrose in urine), prepare a reagent by mixing 120 ml of Fehling's solution with 200 ml of ammonia (specific gravity 0.88), 400 ml of a solution of sodium hydroxide (specific gravity 1.14) and 1000 ml of water; boil the suspected liquid with this solution: if dextrose is present, the reagent is decolorized.

PCA t., see passive cutaneous anaphylaxis test.

Pélouse-Moore t., (for sugar in urine), boil the urine with a solution of potassa, cool, and add 1 drop of concentrated sulfuric acid; the odor of burnt sugar will be given off.

Penzoldt's t., 1. (for acetone), to the suspected liquid, add a warm saturated solution of orthonitrobenzaldehyde, and render it alkaline with sodium hydroxide: if acetone is present, the mixture becomes yellow and then green; thereafter a precipitate forms which, on shaking with chloroform, gives a blue color. 2. (for dextrose in urine), add sodium hydroxide solution and a slightly alkaline solution of sodium diazobenzosulfonate; shake the mixture until it foams: a red or yellow-red color is produced, the foam also being red.

Penzoldt-Fisher t., (for phenol), alkalinize strongly the substance to be tested and dissolve in a solution of diazobenzolsulfonic acid; if present, produces a deep red color.

Peppermint t., (for pulmonary perforation), the pneumothorax cavity is filled with the vapor of essence of peppermint; if there is pulmonary perforation, the patient will recognize the characteristic smell.

Pepsin t., see specific tests, including Jacoby's t and Mett's t.

Peptide t., see triketohydrindene hydrate t.

Peptone t., see specific tests, including Hofmeister's t. (2), Ralfe's t. (2), Randolph's t., triketohydrindene hydrate t.

Perchloride t., a portwine colored reaction obtained by treating the urine of hyperemetic pregnant women with solution of ferric chloride; the intensity of the reaction indicates the gravity of the case.

Performance t., an intelligence test in which the subject is required to carry out certain actions rather than to answer questions.

Peria's t., (for tyrosine), see Piria's t.

Perls' t., a test for hemosiderin made by treating the substance with hydrochloric acid and potassium ferrocyanide; the Prussian blue reaction is produced if hemosiderin is present.

Permanganate t., see Weiss' t.

Peroxidase t., the appearance of deep blue granules in leukocytes of marrow origin when stained with Goodpasteure's stain, distinguishing them from cells of lymphatic origin.

Perthes' t., (for collateral circulation in varicose veins), see tourniquet t., def. 3.

Petri's t., (for proteins), add diazobenzolsulfonic acid and sodium hydroxide; an orange or brownish color is formed, and on shaking a red froth is produced.

Pettenkofer's t., (for bile acids in urine), drop a solution of the suspected material into a mixture of sugar and sulfuric acid; a purplish crimson color is produced. This test is also given by aminomyelin, cephalin, lecithin, and myelin.

Petzetakis' t., (for typhoid fever), 15 ml of urine is placed in a test tube and to this is added a little 5 percent alcoholic solution of iodine; if the upper part of the urine takes on a golden-yellow color, the test is positive.

Phenacetin t., (in urine), to the urine, add a little concentrated hydrochloric acid, a little 1 percent solution of sodium nitrate, and a little alkaline alphanaphthol solution; make the urine alkaline and a red color indicates phenacetin.

Phenol t., see specific tests, including Allen's t., Hanke-Koessler t., Jacquemin's t., Penzoldt-Fisher t., Plugge's. See also phenol, methods for, under method.

Phenolphthalein t., 1. (for blood) boil a thin fecal suspension, cool, and add it to half as much reagent (made by dissolving 1 to 2 gm of phenolphthalein and 25 gm of potassium hydroxide in water). Add 10 gm of metallic zinc and heat until decolorized. A pink color indicates the presence of blood. 2. (in urine) make the urine alkaline; a red color indicates phenolphthalein.

Phenolsulfonphthalein t., (for kidney function), inject 1 ml of 0.6 percent solution of the monosodium salt of phenosulfonphthalein intravenously or intramuscularly and collect the urine at hourly intervals. Make specimens alkaline with sodium hydroxide and match color in colorimeter with standard solution. Usually, 60 to 75 percent of the dye is excreted in two hours; 40 percent or less indicates impaired function.

Phenoltetrachlorphthalein t., (for liver function), phenoltetrachlorphthalein is injected intravenously, and normally it appears in the feces, being excreted by the liver with the bile, and giving a bright color to the feces. A decrease in the normal excretion of this substance points to liver injury.

Phenylhydrazine t., see specific tests, including Kowarsky's t. (1) and von Jaksch's t.

Phlorhizin t., phlorizin t., (for renal insufficiency), the bladder is emptied and a hypodermic injection given of a mixture of 5 to 10 each of sodium carbonate and phlorhizin. Sugar will appear in the urine within half an hour if the kidney is healthy. If only a small quantity of sugar appears, there is probably renal insufficiency; if none at all, then serious kidney disease probably exists.

Phosphoric acid t., see specific tests, including Malot's t. and Mitscherlich's t.

Phthalein t., see phenolsulfonphthalein t.

Picrotoxin t., see Becker's t. (1).

Pincus' t., typical colors are produced on heating 17-ketosteroids with concentrated antimony trichloride in glacial acetic acid.

Pineapple t., (for butyric acid in stomach), a few drops of sulfuric acid and alcohol are added to a dried ethereal extract of the gastric juice; if butyric acid is present, an odor of pineapple will be given off, caused by the formation of ethylbutyrate.

Pine wood t., (for indole), a pine splinter moistened with concentrated hydrochloric acid is turned cherry red by a solution of indole.

Piotrowski's t., see biuret t. (1).

Piria's t., (for tyrosine), moisten the suspected material with strong sulfuric acid and warm it; then dilute and warm it again; neutralize it with barium carbonate, filter, and add ferric chloride in dilute solution: if tyrosine is present, a violet color is seen, which is destroyed by an excess of ferric chloride.

Pirquet's t., (obs), a tuberculin test in which the tuberculin is applied by scarification.

P-K t., see passive transfer test.

Plantar ischemia t., test for circulatory disturbance in the legs and feet, in which the plantar surface of the patient's foot is checked for blanching after he extends and flexes his inclined leg.

Plesch's t., (for persistent ductus arteriosus), determination of the amount of oxygen and of carbonic acid in the blood.

Plugge's t., (for phenol), a dilute solution containing phenol becomes red on mixture with a mercuric nitrate solution containing a trace of nitrous acid; mercury is also precipitated and the odor of salicylol is given off.

Pneumatic t., see Hennerbert's sign.

Pohl's t., (for globulins), these substances are precipitated from solution by ammonium sulfate.

Pointing t., see Bérány's pointing t.

Politzer's t., (for deafness in one ear), when a tuning-fork is placed in front of the nares, it is heard only by an unaffected ear during deglutition.

Pollacci's t., (for albumin, in urine), dissolve in 100 ml of water 1 gm of tartaric acid, 5 gm of mercuric chloride, and 10 gm of sodium chloride, and add 5 ml of solution of formaldehyde; this solution added to urine will cause coagulation of albumin in a white zone.

Porges-Meier t., a nontreponemal antigen serologic test for syphilis.

Porphobilinogen t., see Watson-Schwartz t.

Porter's t., 1. (for excess of uric acid), the upper portion of the urine is boiled in a test tube and a few drops of 4 percent acetic acid added; in a few hours, crystals of uric acid will form just below the surface. 2. (for indican), 10 ml of urine is shaken with an equal amount of hydrochloric acid and 5 drops of a 0.5 percent solution of potassium permanganate; add 5 ml of chloroform and shake. A purple color with a deposit of blue matter indicates indican.

Porteus' maze t., a performance test in which the subject is required to trace with a pencil through printed mazes of increasing difficulty.

Posner's t., 1. (for the source of albumin in urine), a twenty-four-hour sample of urine is preserved with solution of formaldehyde, shaken, and the leukocytes counted in the blood-counting chamber-100,000 leukocytes per 2 ml, of urine indicates 0.1 percent of albumin. In this case, the albumin is probably due solely to the pus. If albumin is present in greater proportion than this, it is probably due to Bright's disease. 2. (for proteins), Posner makes a ring biuret test by mixing the potassium hydroxide solution and the unknown and then stratifying very dilute copper sulfate solution on top of the mixture.

Potassium iodide t., (for renal function), the patient receives 0.5 gm of potassium iodide in solution by mouth, and the urine is tested every two hours for iodine; if iodine secretion is prolonged beyond sixty hours, excretion through the renal tubules is indicated.

Prausnitz-Küstner (PK) t., see passive transfer test; P-K test.

Precipitin t., any serologic test based on a precipitin reaction (qv).

Pègl's t., (for kidney function) determine the specific gravity of the urine obtained by catheterization of the ureters. Using Haeser's coefficient, estimate the amount of solid substance excreted, and compare it with the weight of ash. The diseased kidney may excrete the same volume of water, but less solid material. A predominance of mineral substance (ash) over the organic also speaks for a lower function of the kidney.

Pregnancy t., see specific tests, including antitrypsin t., Friedman's t., Galli Mainini t., male frog or male toad t., ovarian hyperemia t., pregnanediol t., Prostigmin t., Venning Browne t., Visscher-Bowman t., Xenopus t.

Preyer's t., a spectroscopic test for carbon monoxide in the blood.

Proetz's t., (for acuity of sence of smell), use of a series of substance each in 10 different concentration in a liter of petroleum of specific gravity 0.880, to determine the least concentration at which the substance can be recognized; termed olfactory coefficient or minimal identifiable odor.

Projective t., any of various tests in which an individual interprets ambiguous stimulus situations, e.g. a series of inkblots (Rorschach t.), according to his own unconscious dispositions, thus yielding information about this personality structure and its underlying dynamics.

Protection t., see serum neutralization t.

Protein t., see specific tests, including biuret t. (1), colloidal gold t., Gies' biuret t., Grigg's t., Hopkins-Cole t., Kantor-Gies t., Liebermann's t., Michailow's t., Millon's t., Molisch's t. (3), Mulder's t., (2), Petri's t., Posner's t. (2) Reichl's t, Schulte's t., Schultze's t. (3), Sicard-Carateloubfe t., sulfur t., triketohydrindene hydrate t., von Aldor's t.

Proteose t., proteose does not coagulate on boiling; but gives a ring test with trichloroacetic acid. See also von Aldor's t.

Prothrombin t., a test for prothrombin based on clotting time; see under time, and see Quick's t. (2).

Prothrombin consumption t., a test used, for the most part, to measure the formation of intrinsic thromboplastin by determining the residual serum prothrombin after blood coagulation is complete. Because the test is made on whole blood, it also measures, indirectly, the thromboplastic function of platelets.

Prothrombin-proconvertin t., a test used in the control of coumarin-type anticoagulants similar to the quick method, except that it employs a saline extract of brain as a thromboplastin and requires the presence of excess blood coagulation factor V, usually derived from deprothrombinized ox plasma.

Psychological t., any test to measure one's development, achievement, personality, intelligence, thought processes, etc.

Psychomotor t., a test that assesses the subject's ability to perceive instructions and perform motor responses, often including measurement of the speed of the reaction.

Pulp t., a diagnostic test to determine tooth pulp vitality or abnormality, usually by means of electric pulp testers or by application of a hot or cold stimulus.

Purdy's t., (for albumin), fill a test tube two thirds full of clear urine, add one sixth of its volume of a saturated solution of sodium chloride and 5 to 10 drops of 50 percent acetic acid. Gently heat the upper part of the tube and look for a cloud.

Purine bodies t., see purine bodies, methods for, under method.

Pus t., see Vitati's t. (6).

Pyramidon t., (for occult blood in urine), to the urine, add tincture of iodine; a yellow ring indicates pyramidon.

Quadriceps t., (for hyperthyroidism), the patient sits well forward on the edge of a straight chair and holds the leg out at right angles to the body. Normal persons can hold this position for at least a minute; those with hyperthyroidism can maintain it for only a few seconds.

Queckenstedt's t., see under sign.

Quellung t., when pneumococci and other capsulated microorganisms are mixed with specific immune serum, there occurs in addition to agglutination a swelling (quellung) of the capsules of the organism, owing to the binding of antibody with the capsular polysaccharide.

Quick's t., 1. (for liver function), a test based on excretion of hippuric acid following the administration of sodium benzoate. 2. (one-stage prothrombin time), by adding an extrinsic thromboplastin such as dried rabbit brain and calcium to oxalated blood the integrity of the prothrombin complex, composed of factors II, V, VII, X, may be defined; used widely to control administration of coumarin-type anticoagulants.

Quick's tourniquet t., see tourniquet t. (1).

Quinlan's t., (for bile) a 3 mm layer of the suspected liquid is examined by the spectroscope; of the bile is present, some of the violet color of the spectrum will be absorbed.

Raabe's t., (for albumin), filter the urine into a test tube and drop a crystal of trichloracetic acid into it; albumin will form a white ring about the crystal; uric acid may form a similar ring, but it is not so well defined.

Rabuteau's t., 1. (for hydrochloric acid in urine), add a little indigosulfonic acid to color the urine, and sulfurous acid to decompose what hydrochloric acid may be present; the urine will be decolorized. 2. (for hydrochloric acid in stomach contents), one gm of potassium iodate and 0.5 gm of potassium iodide are added to 50 ml of starch mucilage; filtered stomach liquids are added to it; free hydrochloric acid will render the mixture blue.

Radioactive renogram t., an intravenous injection of radioisotopic material is given and its uptake and excretion is monitored by an external schintillation counter over the kidneys.

Radioallergosorbent t., (RAST), a test used to measure specific IgE antibodies in serum. Allergen extract is coupled to a solid matrix (paper, cellulose particles); this immunosorbent is reacted with serum and washed and then reacted with radiolabeled anti-human IgE antibody and washed. Uptake of the labeled antibody is proportional to the level of specific serum IgE antibodies to the allergen. RAST is used as an alternative to skin tests to detemine sensitivity to suspected allergens.

Radioimmunosorbent t., (RIST), a highly sensitive radioimmunoassay for measuring the total IgE antibody concentration in serum; the serum sample is reacted with dilutions of radiolabeled IgE and anti-human IgE antibody coupled to an insoluble support. The amount of labeled IgE bound to the immunosorbent varies inversely with the amount of (unlabeled) IgE present in the sample.

Radioisotope renal excretion t., (for study of renal function), radioisotopic material diluted with saline is rapidly injected into a well-hydrated patient; urine collected by an indwelling urethral catheter or a ureteral catheter previously inserted into the kidney is collected at known intervals and the radioactivity of each specimen is determined and recorded.

Ralfe's t., 1. (for acetone in urine) boil 4 ml of solution of potassium hydroxide with 1.5 gm of potassium iodide; overlay it with 4 ml of urine; a yellow ring with specks of iodoform appears at the plane of contact. 2. (for peptones in urine) put 4 ml of Fehling's solution in a test tube and overlay it with urine, a rose-colored ring shows the presence of peptones.

Ramon's flocculation t., to a series of tubes containing a constant amount of toxin, e.g. diphtheria toxin, antitoxin is added in increasing amounts; when a zone of flocculation appears, the tube showing it contains a completely neutralized mixture of toxin and antitoxin. The first tube in which flocculation occurs is taken as the end-point.

Randolph's t., (for peptones in urine), add 2 drops of a saturated solution of potassium iodide and 3 drops of Millon's reagent to 5 ml of cold and slightly acid urine; a yellow precipitate shows the presence of peptones.

Rank sum t., a nonparametric statistical test of the null hypothesis that two samples are drawn from the same population versus the alternative hypothesis that the two samples are drawn from two populations having probability distributions of the same shape but different liocations, based on the value of the rank sum statistic calculated as the sum of the ranks of one sample when the observations in both samples are jointly ranked in ascending order. Also called Mann-Whitney t., Mann-Whitney-Wilcoxon t., Wilcoxon's t., and Wilcoxon's rank sum t.

Rantzman's t., a modification of Lange's test for acetone in which ammonium nitrate is used as a preservative.

Rapid plasma reagin (RPR) t., a group of flocculation tests for syphilis using unheated serum and a modified VDRL antigen containing choline chloride and charcoal particles enabling macroscopic identification of the flocculation; widely used for screening.

Rapid serum amylase t., see Fishman-Doubilet t.

Raygat's t., see hydrostatic t.

Rebuck t., a technique used to study the inflammatory process; an area of skin is abraded until capillary bleeding occurs and a cover slip or chamber containing balanced salt solution is applied. This permits direct observation of inflammatory cells migrating into the site; polymorphonuclear leuckocytes predominate about 10 hours; macrophages predominate at about 4 hours.

Red t., see phenolsulfonphthalein t.

Red-glass t., a test for ocular deviation using a red glass over the right eye while the patient looks at a light; the position at which the patient sees the red image reveals the affected muscle.

Rees' t., (for albumin), small amounts of albumin are precipitated from solution by tannic acid in alcoholic solution.

Rehberg's t., a test of kidney function based on the excretion of creatinine administered 2 gm in 500 gm of water.

Rehfuss' t., (of gastric secretion), by means of specially devised tube (Rehfus's tube) inserted into the stomach immediately after an Ewald's test meal, a specimen of the contents is drawn off at fifteen-minute intervals until the close of digestion. Each specimen is examined and the results are plotted in a graphic curve, the abscissa of which is the number of minutes at which the gastric contents were removed, and the ordinate the number of milliliters of decinormal sodium hydroxide solution necessary to titrate the free acidity and the total acidity of the gastric contents.

Reichl's t., (for proteins), add 2 or 3 drops of an alcoholic solution of benzaldehyde and a quantity of sulfuric acid previously diluted to twice its volume with water; then add a few drops of ferric sulfate solution. The mixture will sooner or later take on a deep-blue color if proteins are present.

Reinsch's t., (for heavy metals, including arsenic, mercury, bismuth, antimony, and large amounts of selenium, tellurium, and sulfide), insert a strip of clean copper into the suspected acidified liquid or finely ground tissue, and boil; if one or more heavy metals are present, a coating will form on the copper strip.

Remont's t., (for salicylic acid), make the milk acid with sulfuric acid, extract the salicylic acid with ether, and identify it by the purple or violet color produced on the addition of ferric chloride.

Renal function t., see kidney function t.

Rennin t., see individual tests, including Lee's t. and Riegel's t.

Resorcinol-hydrochloric acid t., (for levulose), see Selivanoff's t.

Reuss' t., (for atropine), the substance examined is treated with sulfuric acid and oxidizing agents; if atropine is present, an odor of roses and orange-flowers is given off.

Reynold's t., (for acetone), to the liquid to be examined, add freshly prepared mercuric oxide, shake and filter, and overlay the filtrate with ammonium sulfide; the liquid turns black if acetone is present.

Rheumatoid arthritis t., see specific tests, including bentonite t., bracelet t., latex agglutination t., sheep cell agglutination t.

Rhubarb t., (in urine), make the urine alkaline; a red color indicates rhubarb.

Rideal-Walker t., a test for the bactericidal activity of disinfectant as compared with that of phenol; see under method.

Riegel's t., (for rennin), to 10 ml of milk, add 5 ml of neutral gastric juice and incubate for fifteen minutes; coagulation will occur if rennin is present.

Riegler's t., 1. (for albumin) 10 gm of betanaphtholsulfonic acid is dissolved in 200 ml of distilled water and filtered; 5 ml of urine is treated with 20 to 30 drops of solution. Turbidity shows the presence of albumin. 2. (for hydrochloric acid in the gastric juice) Congo red is changed to blue if hydrochloric acid is present. 3. (for dextrose) place in a test tube 0.1 gm of phenyl-hydrazine-hydrochloride, 0.25 gm of sodium acetate, and 20 drops of the urine. Heat to boiling. Add

10 ml of 3 percent solution of potassium hydroxide and gently shake the tube. A red color indicates sugar.

Ring t., 1. (for antibiotic acitivity), the solution is placed in a ring resting on the surface of seeded agar and the size of the surrounding clear ara of inhibition indicates the activity. 2. (for protein), see Heller's t. (1), Posner's t. (2), Roberts' t. (1).

Rinne's t., a hearing test made, with the opposite ear masked, with tuning forks of 256, 512, and 1024 Hz; by alternately placing the stem of the vibrating fork on the mastoid process of the temporal bone of the patient and holding it ½ inch from the external auditory meatus until it is no longer heard at one of these positions. When air conduction is greater than bone. Conduction, it indicates normal hearing or sensorineural hearing loss. When bone conduction is greater than air conduction, it indicates conductive hearing loss.

Rivalta's t., a reaction for distinguishing fluids of transudation and exudation, utilizing acetic acid.

Robert's t., 1. (for albumin) underlay the urine with a mixture containing 5 parts of saturated solution of magnesium sulfate and 1 part of nitric acid; a white ring or layer forms at the plane of junction. 2. (for dextrose) determine the specific gravity of the urine at a certain temperature; add a little tartaric acid and some yeast; after twenty-four hours filter and again find the specific gravity. Each degree of density lost represents a grain of dextrose in a fluidounce of the urine.

Robinson-Kepler t., (for adrenocortical insufficiency), a test based on the fact that patients with adrenocortical insufficiency are unable to excrete a large water load at a normal rate, as opposed to normal subjects who will, for example, excrete 50 percent of 1500 ml of ingested water within four hours.

Robinson-Kepler-Power water t., (for sprue), a test based upon the fact that in sprue there is increased nocturnal elimination of urine, perhaps due to decreased absorption of water.

Romberg's t., (for differentiating between peripheral and cerebellar ataxia), an increase in clumsiness in all movements and in the width and uncertainty of the gait when the patient's eyes are closed indicates peripheral ataxia; no change indicates the cerebellar type.

Ronchese's t., (for quantitative determination of ammonia in urine), one based on the action of solution of formaldehyde on the ammonia salts. A 10 percent solution of sodium cabonate is added, a drop at a time, to the urine until the reaction becomes neutral. The solution of formaldehyde (40 percent) is neutralized with a one-fourth normal soda solution against phenolphthalein until a slight pink tint develops. Then 25 ml of the neutral urine and 10 ml of the neutral solution of formaldehyde are mixed and titrated against decinormal sodium carbonate solution until a deep pink develops. The calculation is simple 1 ml of the decinormal sodium carbonate solution for 100 ml of urine corresponds to 0.017 gm ammonia in 1000 ml of urine.

Rorschach t., a projective test in which the subject is asked to relate his associations to a series of inkblot designs.

Rose's t., (for blood), the scrapings from a blood stain are boiled in dilute caustic potash: when examined, the liquid will show a greenish color in a thin layer and a red color in a thicker layer.

Rose bengal t., (for liver function), rose bengal (1 percent in sodium chloride solution) is injected into the bloodstream. Normally, it disappears from the blood rapidly; delay in normal disappearance time points to diminished activity of liver.

Rose-Waaler t., an agglutination test for rheumatoid for (RF) using tanned sheep red blood cells (SRBC) coated with subagglutinating amount of rabbit anti-SRBC IgG antibody. These cells agglutinate when exposed to RF (anti-IgG autoantibodies) owing to cross-reaction between human and rabbit IgG.

Rosenbach-Gmelin t., (for bile pigment), filter the urine through a very small filter, and put a drop of nitric acid with a trace of nitrous acid on the inside of the filtrate; a pale yellow spot will appear, surrounded with yellowish red, violet, blue, and green rings.

Rosenheim-Drummond's t., (for vitamin A), dissolve 1 or 2 drops of cod liver oil in about 5 ml of an anhydrous fat solvent. Add 1 drop of concentrated sulfuric acid. A temporary deep-violet color indicates vitamin A.

Rosenthal's t., 1. (for blood in urine), add potassium hydroxide solution to the urine, remove the precipitate and dry it; place a small amount on a slide with a crystal of sodium chloride; apply a cover glass and cause a few drops of glacial acetic acid to flow under it; warm the plate. When it is cool, hemin crystals will appear if blood is present. 2. (for liver function), a modification of the phenoltetrachlorophthalein test based on the amount of the dye which remains in the blood at definite periods after injection of 5 mg per kilogram of body weight. The normal liver will remove most of the dye from the blood in fifteen minutes and all of it within an hour.

Rosin's t., (for indigo red), render the suspected liquid alkaline with sodium carbonate and extract with ether; this is colored red.

Ross-Jones t., (for excess of globulin in cerebrospinal fluid), 1 ml of cerebrospinal fluid is floated over 2 ml of concentrated ammonium sulfate solution; excess of globulin produces a fine white ring at the line of junction.

Rothera's t., (for acetone), to 5 ml of urine, add a little solid ammonium sulfate and add 2 to 3 drops of a fresh 5 percent solution of sodium nitroprusside and 1 to 2 ml of ammonium hydroxide; a purple color forms if acetone is present.

Rotter's t., (for ascorbic acid in the body), cutaneous injection of 2,6-dichlorphenolindophenol produces colorization of the tissues; decolorization occurring in ten minutes indicates adequate ascorbic acid.

Rous' t., (for hemosiderin), centrifuge the urine; to the sediment add 5 ml of a 2 percent solution of potassium ferrocyanide and 5 ml of a 1 percent solution of hydrochloric acid. Hemosiderin granules stain blue.

Roussin's t., microscopic examination of suspected blood stains.

Rowntree-Geraghty t., see phenolsulfonphthalein t.

RPR t., see rapid plasma reagin t.

Rubin's t., 1. a test for patency of the uterine tubes made by transuterine insufflation with carbon dioxide. If the tubes are patent, the gas enters the peritoneal cavity and may be demonstrated by the fluoroscope or roentgenogram. This subphrenic pneumoperitoneum causes pain in one or both shoulders of the patient. If the manometer registers not over 100 mm Hg, the tubes are patent; if between 120 and 130, there may be stenosis or stricture, but not complete occlusion; if it rises to 200, the tubes are completely occluded. 2. A test to detect avian leukosis viruses in egg-culture vaccines; if the viruses are present, they induce a cellular resistance to Rous' viruses subsequently inoculated (resistance-inducing factor).

Rubner's t., 1. (for carbon monoxide in blood), shake the blood with 4 or 5 volumes of lead acetate in solution: if the blood contains CO, it will retain its bright color; if not, it becomes a chocolate brown. 2. (for lactose, dextrose, maltose, and levulose in urine), add lead acetate to the urine, boil, and then add an excess of ammonium hydroxide: lactose gives a brick-red color, dextrose a coffee-brown color, maltose a light-yellow color, and levulose no color at all.

Ruhemann's t., (for uric acid in urine), see under method.

Ruler t., see Hamilton's test.

Rumpel-Leede t., the appearance of minute subcutaneous hemorrhages below the area at which a rubber bandage is applied not too tightly for ten minutes upon the upper arm; characteristic of scarlet fever and hemorrhagic diasthesis.

Russo's t., a reaction of the urine of typhoid patients on adding 4 drops of a solution of methylene blue to 15 ml of urine in the first stage of typhoid, the urine becomes light green; at the height of disease, an emerald color; and during the decline, a bluish color.

Ruttan-Hardisty t., (for blood), blood in the presence of a 4 percent glacial acetic acid solution of orthotoluiduine and hydrogen peroxide gives a bluish color.

Saathoff's t., (for fat in stools), rub up the feces with Sudan and warm: fat droplets stain yellow to red.

Sabin-Feldman dye t., a serologic test for the diagnosis of toxoplasmosis, based on the failure of living *Toxoplasmas* in the presence in the presence of specific antibody and accessory factor, to take up methylene blue dye.

Saccharimeter t., dextrose in solution rotates the plane of polarized light to the right, while levulose turns it to the left.

Sachs-Georgi t., (obs), a nontreponemal antigen serologic test for syphilis.

Sachsse's t., (for sugar in the urine), a solution of 18 gm of red mercuric iodide, 25 gm of potassium iodide, 80 gm of potassium hydroxide, in water enough to make a liter; sugar, if present, causes a black precipitate.

Sahli's t., (for motive and digestive power of stomach), the patient is fed a soup made of definite amounts of water, flour, butter, and salt, and in an hour the stomach contents are removed. The amount of fat present shows how much of the meal has been digested, and the acidity indicates how much the stomach has secreted.

Sahli's glutoid t., (for digestive function), a glutoid capsule containing 0.15 gm of iodoform is taken with an Ewald's breakfast. The capsule is not digested by the stomach fluid, but is readily digested by pancreatic juice. Appearance of iodine in the saliva and urine within four to six hours indicates normal gastric motility, normal intestinal digestion, and normal absorption. Glutoid capsules are prepared by soaking gelatin capsules in solution of formaldehyde.

Sahli-Nencki t., (for lipolytic activity of the pancreas), phenyl salicylate (salol) is administered; it is excreted as salicylic acid when pancreatic activity is normal.

Sakaguchi's t., (for arginine), a reddish or wine color is produced in the presence of arginine when a tissue section is treated with an alkaline mixture of α-naphthol and sodium hypochlorite.

Salicylic acid t., see specific tests, including Remont's t., Siebold Bradbury t.

Salkowski's t., 1. (for CO in the blood), add to the blood 20 volumes of water and sodium hydroxide in solution (specific gravity, 1.34). If CO is present, it becomes cloudy and then red; flakes of red afterward float on the surface. 2. (for chloesterol), dossolve in chloroform and add an equal volume of strong sulfuric acid. If cholesterol is present, the solution becomes bluish red, and slowly changes to a violet red, the sulfuric acid becomes red, with a green fluorescence. 3. (for indole), to the solution to be tested, add a little nitric acid, and drop in slowly a solution of potassium nitrite (2 percent): a red color shows that indole is present, and a red precipitate is afterward formed.

4. (for dextrose), a modified form of Trommer's test. 5. (for creatinine), to the yellow solution obtained in Weyl's test, add an excess of acetic acid and heat; a green color results, which turns to blue.

Salkowski-Ludwig t., (for uric acid), a solution of silver ammonio-nitrate and ammonium and magnesium chlorides precipitates uric acid.

Salkowski-Schipper t., (for bile pigments), to 10 ml of the unknown, add 5 drops of 20 percent solution of sodium carbonate and 10 drops of a 20 percent of strong hydrochloric acid and a few drops of sodium nitrite. Heat. A green color indicates bile pigments.

Salol t., see Sahli-Nencki t.

Salomon's t., test the stomach washing by means of Esbach's reagent, after twenty-four hours without protein food; the presence of albumin indicates ulcerative cancer.

Sand t., (for bile and hemoglobin in urine), a layer of white sand is spread on a plate and on this is poured some of the urine; if the urine contains pigments, a spot is left on the sand, which is brown with hemoglobin and greenish with bile pigment. Also called Lipps' t.

Sandrock t., (for thrombosis), vigorous friction is applied to the part; the degree of hyperemia which follows is an indication of the condition of the circulation

Sanford's t., prepare a series of dilutions of salt from 0.28 to 0.5 percent; add 1 drop of blood to each diluton, mix, allow to settle, and note the tubes which show hemolysis.

Santonin t., 1. (for the antitoxic efficiency of the liver), the patient is given 0.02 gm of santonin on a fasting stomach; the urine is examined hourly for oxysantonin by treating it with a dilute sodium hydroxide solution which will produce a red color with oxysantonin. 2. See Daclin t.

Saundby' s t., (for blood in feces), to a small quantity of feces in a test tube 10 drops of a saturated benzidine solution is added; to this is added 30 drops of hydrogen peroxide solution. A dark blue color will develop if blood is present.

Scarification t., a skin test in which the antigen is introduced by scarification, e.g., the Pirquet's test.

Schäffer's t., (for nitrites in urine), decolorize 4 ml of urine with animal charcoal and add to it 4 ml of 10 percent acetic acid and 3 drops of 5 percent solution of potassium ferrocyanide; an intense yellow color indicates nitrites.

Schalfijew's t., (for blood), treat defibrinated blood with excess of glacial acetic acid, heat 80°C, cool, and examine for hemin crystals.

Schalm's t., see California mastitis t.

Scherer's t., 1. (for inosite), evaporate on platinum foil with nitric acid, add ammonia water and a single drop of calcium chloride in solution, and re-evaporate to dryness; a rose-red coloration indicates the presence of inosite. 2. (for pure leucine), a small portion of leucine with a few drops of nitric acid are evaporated on platinum foil. The transparent residue turns a brownish color on the addition of a sodium hydroxide solution. When the mixture is concentrated, an oil-like drop is obtained. 3. (for tyrosine), treat with nitric acid and dry with care on platinum foil; the formation of nitroturosine nitrate renders it yellow, and sodium hydroxide solution changes the color to reddish yellow.

Schick's t., intradermal injection of a quantity of diphtheria toxin equal to one-fiftieth of the guinea pig minimal lethal dose in one arm (the test site) and of an equal quantity of heat-inactivated diphtheria toxin in the other arm (the control site). A positive reaction, which consists of an area of redness that appears in 24 to 36 hours at the test site only and persists for 4 to 5 days, leaving an area of brownish pigmentation, indicates a lack of immunity to diphtheria. A pseudoreaction, which consists of an area of redness appearing at both sites and usually disappearting in 48 hours without residual pigmentation, or a negative reaction indicates immunity.

Schiff's t., 1. (for carbohydrates in urine), warm and add sulfuric acid; expose to the fumes of the urine a paper dipped in a mixture of equal volumes of xylidine and glacial acetic acid with alcohol and then dried: the paper becomes red if carbohydrates are present. 2. (for cholesterol), add a reagent composed of 2 parts of sulfuric acid with 1 part of dilute solution of ferric chloride; evaporate to dryness and a violet color is produced. 3. (for cholesterol), evaporate with nitric acid and add ammonia water; a red color not changed by alkalis is produced. 4. (for allantoin and urea), add a solution of furfurol in hydrochloric acid; a yellow color appears, turning to purple and then to a brownish black. 5. (for uric acid), treat silver nitrate paper with an alkaline solution of the suspected substance; a brown stain shows the presence of uric acid. 6. (for formaldehyde in milk), the solution consists of an aqueous solution of magenta. 40 ml distilled water, 250 ml aqueous solution of sodium bisulfite 10 ml and pure concentrated sulfuric acid, 10 ml which is allowed to stand until it is colorless; 2 ml of this solution is added to a test tube two thirds full of milk. If formaldehyde is present, a pink or lilac color will appear in from thirty to sixty seconds.

Schiller's t., (for cancer of cervix), a test for early squamous cell cancer by treating the tissue with a solution of 1 gm of pure iodine and 2 gm of potassium iodide in 300 ml of water if the cervix is healthy, the surface turns brown; if there is cancer, the treated area turns white in yellow, because cancer cells do not contain glycogen and, therefore, do not stain with iodine.

Schilling's t., (for gastrointestinal absorption of vitamin B_{12}), a measured amount of radioactive vitamin B_{12}, is given orally, followed by a parenteral flushing dose of the nonradioactive vitamin, and the percentage of radioactivity is determined in the urine excreted over a 24-hour period.

Schirmer's t., (for keratoconjunctivitis sicca), a test of tear production in which a piece of filter paper is inserted over the conjunctival sac of the lower lid, with the end of the paper hanging down on the outside. The range of normal wetting, determined by measuring the area of moisture on the projecting paper, depends on age and sex.

Schlesinger's t., (for urobilin), to about 5 ml of the urine in a test tube, add a few drops of Lugol's solution to transform the chromogen into the pigment. Now add 4 or 5 ml of a saturated solution of zinc chloride in absolute alcohol and filter. A greenish fluorescence, best seen when the tube is viewed against a black background and the light is concentrated upon it with a lens, shows the presence of urobilin. Bile pigment, if present, should be removed by adding about one fifth volume of 10 percent calcium chloride solution and filtering.

Schlichter's t., see serum bactericidal activity t.

Schönbein's t., 1. (for blood), blue coloration obtained by adding solution of hydrogen peroxide to tincture of guaiac mixed with suspected blood. 2. (for copper), a solution containing a copper salt becomes blue if potassium cyanide and tincture of guaiac are added.

Schopfer's t., minute amounts of vitamin B in the blood catalyze the mold *Phycomyces blaksleeanus.*

Schroeder's t., (for urea), add a crystal of the substance to a solution of bromine in chloroform; the urea will decompose and gas will be formed.

Schulte's t., (for proteins), remove all coagulable protein, precipitate with six volumes of absolute alcohol, dissolve the precipitate in water, and apply the biuret test.

Schültz-Charlton t., when scarlet fever antitoxin or scarlet fever convalescent serum is injected into an area of the skin showing a bright red rash, a blanching of the skin at the site of the injection occurs. Serum from scarlet fever paients do not produce this reaction.

Schultze's t., 1. (for cellulose), iodine is dissolved to saturation in a zinc chloride solution (specific gravity, 1.8), and 6 parts of potassium iodide are added: this reagent colors cellulose blue. 2. (for cholesterol), evaporate with nitric acid, using a porcelain dish and water bath; if cholesterol is present, a yellow deposit is formed, which changes to yellowish red when ammonia is added. 3. (for protein), to a suspected solution, add a very little of a dilute solution of cane sugar and concentrated sulfuric acid; keep it at 60°C, and a bluish red coloration is produced.

Schultze's indophenol oxydase t., see indophenol t.

Schumm's t., 1. See bemidine t. 2. (for hemein plasma), a given volume of plasma is covered with a layer of ether; one-tenth the volume of concentrated ammonium sulfide (analar) is then run in with a pipette and subsequently mixed by shaking. A positive reaction is indicated by the appearance of a hemochromogen with a sharply defined α band at 55 mμ in a depth up to 4 cm of plasma.

Schwabach's t., a hearing test made, with the opposite ear masked, with tuning forks of 256, 512, 1024, and 2048 Hz, alternately placing the stem of the vibrating fork on the mastoid process of the temporal bone of the patient and that of the examiner (whose hearing should be normal) until it is no longer heard by one of them. The result is expressed as "Schwabach prolonged" if heard longer by the patient (indicative of conductive hearing impairment), as "Schwabach shortened or diminished" if heard longer by the examiner (indicative sensorineural hearing impairment) and as "Schwabach normal" if heard for the same time by both.

Scivoletto's t., (for hydrochloric acid in urine), dip filter paper in starch paste and dry; sprinkle it with urine and dry; hang it in a flask containing strontium acetate in solution; a blue color indicates the presence of the acid.

Scleroscope t., a test to determine the hardness of material by dropping a steel ball of standard weight from a specific height onto the material being tested and measuring the height of rebound.

Scratch t., a skin test in which the antigen is applied on a superficial scratch.

Screen t., 1. Alternate cover t. 2. Cover-uncover t.

Screening t., any test used to eliminate those who are definitely not affected by the disease in question, the remainder (those with positive reactions) being subjected to more defined diagnostic tests.

Secretin t., a test for pancreatic function done by examining the pancreatic secretion produced by the intravenous injection of secretin.

Seidel's t., (for inosite), evaporate in a platinum crucible with nitric acid, and treat with ammonia and strontium acetate in solution; inosite, if present, causes a green coloration and a violet precipitate.

Seidlitz's powder t., (for diaphragmatic hernia), the stomach is distended by the administation of Seidlitz's powder, which will enable roentgen visualization of a herniated stomach loop.

Selivanoff's t., Seliwanow's t.,(for fructose in urine), to the urine is added an equal volume of hydrochloric acid containing resorcinol in the following proportion; 5 mg resorcinol, 5 ml water, and 5 ml 25 percent concentrated hydrochloric acid. Formation of burgundy-red color after boiling for 10 seconds indicates fructose.

Semen t., Huhner's t., serum t.

Senna t., (in urine), make the urine alkaline; a red color indicates senna.

Sereny t., (to dermine invasiveness of bacteria), the organism is inoculated into the eye of a guinea pig; invasiveness is determined by the organism's ability to produce conjunctivitis. The test is used particularly for dertermining the invasiveness of strains of *Escherichia coli* and *Listeria monocytogenes*.

Serologic t., any laboratory test involving serologic reactions (precipitin reaction, agglutination, complement fixation, etc), especially any such test measuring serum antibody titer.

Serologic t., [for syphilis (STS)], any test for serum antibodies indicative of *Treponema pallidum* infection. There are two types: Nontreponemal antigen tests detect antibodies to substance (reagin) derived from host tissues, now known to consist of the phospholipids cardiolipin and lecithin; they originated with Wassermann's test and are now represented by the VDRL and RPR (rapid plasma reagin) tests. Treponemal antigen tests detect specific antitreponemal antibodies; they originated with the TPI (*T. pallidum* immobilization) test and are represented by the FTA-ABS (fluorescent treponemal antibody absorption) test, the MHA-TP (microhemagglutination assay—*T. pallidum*), and assays using ELISA (enzyme-linked immunosorbent assay) methods. The term "serologic tests for syphilis" is occasionally used with reference only to nontreponemal antigen tests.

Serum bactericidal activity t., determination, by serial dilution, of the titer of serum that will in combination with the antibiotic in serum, kill 99.9 percent of the starting inoculum mixed with the serum sample; used to monitor antibiotic therapy in endocarditis, osteomyelitis, and other serious bacterial infections.

Serum neutralization t., a test of the antimicrobial activity of a serum done by inoculating a mixture of the serum and the virus or other microorganism being tested into a susceptible animal; also called protection t.

Shadow t. (retinoscopy)., an objective method of investigating, diagnosing and evaluating refractive errors of the eye, by projection of a beam of light into the eye and observation of movement of the illuminated area on the retina surface and of the refraction by the eye of the emergent rays.

Shear's t., (for vitamin D), to the oil add an equal volume of acid aniline (1 part concentrated HCl and 15 parts aniline). Mix and boil. A green color changing to red indicated vitamin D.

Sheep cell agglutination t., (SCAT), any agglutination test using sheep red blood cells, e.g., the Rose-Waaler test.

Short increment sensitivity index (SISI) t., tones of 1 to 5 decibel increments in intensity and lasting 0.5 seconds are superimposed on a continuous (carrier) tone of the same frequency at random intervals, the carrier tone being 20 decibels above speech reception threshold; only patients with cochlear damage can detect these increments.

Sia t., (for macroglobulinemia), a simple screening test performed by adding a drop if serum to 10 to 100 ml of cold distilled water; a positive reaction is indicated by the formation of a heaving cloud of precipitate at the bottom of the container. It is not diagnostic, because it may be positive in other conditions, as in rheumatoid arthritis.

Sicard-Cantelouble t., place 4 ml of spinal fluid in a specially graduated tube, add 12 drops of a 33 percent trichloracetic acid, mix, and read the amount of protein precipitated after twenty-four hours sedimentation.

Sickling t., a method to demonstrate hemoglobin S and the sickling phenomenon in erythrocytes, particularly in the heterozygous state, performed by reducing the enviromental oxygen to which the red cells are exposed. This may be done by simply sealing a drop of blood under a cover slip or, to hasten the morphologic change, by adding 2 percent sodium metabisulfite or sodium dithionite to the preparation.

Siebold-Bradbury t., (for salicylic acid in urine), alkaline with potassium carbonate, add a solution of lead nitrate in excess, filter, and a dilute solution of ferric chloride; a violet color will be produced.

Sign t., a nonparametric statistical test of the null hypothesis that a sample is drawn from, a population with median 0 based on the number of observations having positive signs (which under the null hypothesis has a binomial distribution with $p = 0.5$).

Signed rank t., a nonparametric statistical test of the null hypothesis that a sample is drawn from a population with median 0 (or that the median difference between matched pairs in two populations is 0) versus the alternative hypothesis that the median is nonzero based on the signed rank statistic calculated as the sum of the ranks of the positive sample observations (or positive differences between matched pairs) when all of the observations (differences) are arranged in order by absolute value. Also called Wilcoxon's signed rank t.

Silver t., (for dextrose in the urine), boil the urine with silver nitrate solution and an excess of ammonia, metallic silver will be deposited. Tartaric acid and aldehyde also produce this reaction.

Simonelli's t., (for renal inadequacy), iodine is administered and the urine and saliva tested for iodine; if iodine does not appear in the urine at the same time as in the saliva, the kidneys are diseased.

Sims' t., a postcoital test for the ability of the spermatozoa to penetrate the cervical mucus.

Skatole t., see specific tests, including Herter's t. (2), Kondo's t., nitroso-indole-nitrate t.

Skin t., any test in which an antigen is applied to the skin in order to observe the response of the patient, described according to method of applications as patch tests, scratch tests and intradermal tests. Skin tests are used to determine immunity to infectious diseases (e.g., tuberculin test), to identify allergens producing allergic reactions, and to assess ability to mount a cellular immune response (using a battery of antigens that give positive tests in most normal individuals).

Skin window t., a technique used to study the inflammatory process; an area of skin is abraded until capillary bleeding occurs and a cover slip or chamber containing balanced salt solution is applied. This permits direct observation of inflammatory cells migrating into the site. Polymorphonuclear leukocytes predominate at about 4 days.

Smear t., a method of staining smears of various body secretions, from the respiratory, digestive or genitourinary tract, for the examination of exfoliated cells, to detect the presence of a malignant process.

Smith's t., (for bile pigments), overlay the suspected liquid with tincture of iodine diluted 1:10; a green ring or plane appears at the junction of the two liquids in the tube.

Snellen's t., 1. (for pretended blindness in one eye), the patient is requested to look at alternate red and green letters; the admittedly sound eye is covered with a red glass and if the green letters are read, evidence of fraud is present. 2. Determination of visual acuity by means of Snellen's test types.

Snider's match t., (a screening test for pulmonary ventilation), an ordinary book match which is burned nearly half-way is held 6 inches from the mouth of the patient, who attempts to extinguish it by exhaling, after taking as deep a breath as possible, and without bringing the lips together.

Sniff t., when a patient sniffs, the paralyzed half of the diaphragm is seen to rise and the intact half to descend, as observed by fluoroscopy.

Soldaini's t., (for glucose in the urine), dissolve 15 gm of copper carbonate and 416 gm of potassium bicarbonate in 1400 ml of water for a reagent; 2. parts of urine are boiled with 1 part of the reagent. A yellow precipitate of cupric oxide shows the presence of dextrose.

Solera's t., (for thiocyanates), saturate filter paper with 0.5 percent starch paste containing 1 percent of iodic acid; dry and preserve as test paper. A piece of this paper moistened with saliva will turn blue if thiocyanate is present.

Solubility t., see bile solubility t.

Sonnenschein's t., (for strychnine), the suspected substance is dissolved in a drop of sulfuric acid, some cerosoceric oxide is added, and stirred with a glass rod; a deep-blue color is formed, changing to violet, and finally to cherry red in the presene of strychnine.

Soy bean t., see urease t.

Spavin t., a test for spavin in horses made by holding up the limb with the hock bent sharply; the horse is then started suddenly, and in cases of spavin the first steps are very lame. Also called hock t.

Specific gravity t., see specific tests, including Fishberg's concentration t., urine concentration t., Volhard's t. (2) See also specific gravity, methods for, under method.

Sphenopalatine t., the sphenopalatine ganglion is anesthetized with novocain in order to determine whether the efferent current which is motivating a symptom is routed through either sphenopalatine ganglion, and if so, whether the left one or the right one.

Spiegler's t., (for albumin), acidulate with acetic acid and filter; prepare a reagent with 8 gm of mercuric chloride, 10 gm of sodium chloride, and 4 gm of tartaric acid in 200 ml of water and 20 ml of glycerin; overlay the reagent with filtrate. If albumin is present, a white ring appears at the junction of the liquids.

Spiro's t., 1. A test for the determination of ammonia and urea, embracing a combination of Folin's method for urea and the Sjöqvist method for urea. 2. (for hippuric acid), warm the unknown with acetic anhydride, anhydrous sodium acetate, and benzaldehyde. Cool, and crystals of phenylaminocinnamic acid-lactimide form.

Split-renal function t., see Howard's t.

Sponge t., a test performed by passing a hot sponge up and down the spine; if any lesion of the spine is present, pain is felt as the sponge passes over its locality.

Stanford-Billet t., a modification of Binet's test, translated, adapted, and standardized on children in the United States.

Starch t., see iodine t. (1).

Station t., a test for disturbance of coordination, made by placing the patient in an erect posture, with the heels and toes of the two feet together; if the swaying of the body is beyond normal, coordination may be defective.

Staub-Traugott t., a second of dextrose by mouth to a normal person one hour after a first dose does not elevate the blood sugar level.

Steapsin t., see ethyl butyrate t.

Stein's t., inability to stand on one foot with the eyes shut; seen in disease of the labyrinth.

Steinle-Kahlenberg t., heat a chloroform solution of a sterol with antimony pentachloride; the purple color changes to cobalt blue in the light.

Stenger's t., a test for detecting simulated unilateral hearing loss—a signal is presented at an intensity less than the admitted threshold to the affected ear and a less intense signal of the same frequency is presented simultaneously to the unaffected ear. If the subject is feigning a loss of hearing, the subject will not be able to detect the signal in the unaffected ear.

Stock's t., (for acetone in urine), the distillate of the urine is used; 50 to 100 ml of urine is made acid by the addition of either acetic, hydrochloric, or sulfuric acid. The first 10 ml distillate will contain all the possible acetone. About 1 inch of the distillate is placed in a test tube; a drop or two of a 10 percent solution of hydroxylamine hydrochloride is added, and sufficient sodium hydroxide or carbonate solution to render the solution alkaline to liberate hydroxylamine; the mixture is shaken and a couple of drops of pyridine is added; if acetone is present, the ether will turn a distinctive green blue.

Stokvis' t., (for bile pigment), with 25 ml of urine mix 8 ml of a 1:5 zinc acetate solution; wash the precipitate in water on a filter, and dissolve in ammonia water. Filter again, and in a short time the filtrate shows a bluish green tint.

Stoll's t., a technique for the quantitative estimation of the worm burden of an individual based on collection of a 24-hour stool specimen and counting the number of ova present in an aliquot

Storck's t., (for human milk), catalase present in human milk decompose hydrogen dioxide.

Strange's t., see Henderson's t.,

Strassburg's t., (for bile acids in albumin-free urine), add cane sugar to the urine; dip filter paper into it and dry; a drop of sulfuric acid on the paper will cause a red or violet spot if bile acids are present.

Straus' biological t., (for glanders), when material containing virulent glanders bacilli is inoculated in the peritoneal cavity of male guinea pigs, scrotal lesions develop.

Stress t's, exercise t's.

Struve's t., (for blood in the urine), alkalinize the urine and add tannic and acetic acids until the reaction becomes acid and a dark precipitate is formed. When this is dried, crystals of hemin may be obtained from it by adding ammonium chloride and glacial acetic acid.

Strychnine t., see specific tests, including Alien's t. (3), Brieger's t. (2), Sonnenschein's t., Wemell's t.

Student's t t., see t-t.

Stypven time t., a test similar to the Quick one-stage prothrombin time test, but performed with Russell's viper venom (Stypven) as the thromboplastic agent; useful in defining deficiencies of blood coagulation factor X.

Sucrose lysis t., (for paroxysmal nocturnal hemoglobinuria), the patient's whole blood is mixed with isotonic sucrose solution, which promotes binding of complement to red cells. Incubated, and examined for hemolysis; greater than 10 percent hemolysis is indicative of PNH.

Sugar t., see tests listed under dextrose t., levulose t. and maltose t.

Sulfur t., (for protein), the suspected liquid is heated with an excess of sodium hydroxide and a small quantity of acetate of lead; if proteins are present, a black precipitate of lead sulfide is formed.

Sulkowitch's t., (for calcium in urine), the precipitation of calcium in urine as an oxalate with use of a reagent consisting of 2.5 gm of oxalic acid, 2.5 gm of ammonium oxalate, and 5 ml of glacial acetic acid dissolved in 150 ml of distilled water.

Sullivan's t., (for cysteine), to 1 or 2 ml of the known solution, add 1 to 2 drops of a 0.5 percent solution of 1,2-naphthoquinone 4-sodium sulfonate and then 5 ml of a 20 percent sodium thiosulfate made up in 0.25 normal sodium hydroxide. A brilliant red color indicates a free SH group cysteine rather than cystine.

Susceptibility t., (for testing the susceptibility of pathogenic bacteria to antibiotics), see dilution t. and disk diffusion t.

Syphilis t., see serologic t. for syphilis.

Szabo's t., (for HCl in the stomach contents), add to the suspected liquid a reagent containing equal parts of a 0.5 percent solution of sodioferric tartrate and ammonium thiocyanate; if HCl is present, the reagent is changed from a pale yellow to a brownish red.

T-t., a statistical hypothesis test based on the t-distribution (qv) used to test for a difference between the means of two groups. Also Called also student's t-t.

Tannic acid t., (for nucleoalbumin), see Ott's t.

Tanret's t., (for albumin), Tanret's reagent gives a white precipitate with albumin.

Tardieu's t., (for infanticide), presence of air bubbles in gastric mucosa after establishment of fetal respiration.

Taurine t., see Long's t.

Taylor's t., a modification of Schönbein's test for blood, the blue precipitate forming a deep sapphire blue solution when taken up by alcohol or ether.

Teichmann's t., (for blood), the suspected liquid is put under a coverglass with a crystal of sodium chloride and a little glacial acetic acid; heat carefully without boiling and then cool. If blood is present, rhombic crystals of hemin will appear.

Tensilon t., (for myasthenia gravis), after administration of Tensilon (edrophonium chloride), the patient's eye signs (ptosis and extraocular muscle abnormalities) markedly decrease.

Terman t., the Stanford's modification of the Binet's test.

Thalleioquin t., (for quinine), a neutralized solution of the suspected liquid is treated with chlorine, or bomine water, and then with an excess of ammonia; a green substance, thalleioquin, will be formed.

Thematic apperception t., (TAT), a projective test in which the subject tells a story based on each of a series of standard ambiguous pictures, so that his responses reflect a projection of some aspect of his personality and current psychological preoccupations and conflicts.

Thermoagglutination t., a test to detect antigenic variants, in which slightly rough strains may be detected by their agglutination upon boiling saline for two hours.

Thiamine t., see thiochrome t.

Thiochrome t., (for thiamine), oxidize the thiamine to thiochrome and then recognize the latter by its blue-violet fluorescence in ultraviolet radiation.

Thiocyanate t., see ferric chloride t. (1), Solera's t.

Thomas' t., with the patient supine, when one leg is flexed so that the knee touches the chest and the lumbar spine is flattened, the angle taken by the other hip is the degree of flexion deformity.

Thompson's t., (for gonorrhea), see two-glass t.

Thormählen's t., (for melanin in urine), treat urine with a solution of sodium nitroprusside, potassium hydroxide, and acetic acid; if melanin is present, a deep-blue color will form.

Three-glass t., on arising in the morning the patient urinates successively into three glass receptacles labeled I, II and III. In acute anterior urethritis the urine in I will be turbid from pus, while II and III will be clear; but in posterior urethritis the urine in all three glasses will be turbid. Blood in I only comes from the anterior urethra, but if it comes from the posterior urethra all three will contain blood. Shreds in glass III point to chronic prostatitis.

Thromboplastin generation t., a sensitive test for delineation of defects in formation of intrinsic thromboplastin (prothrombinase, intrinsic prothrombin-converting principle) and hence deficiencies of the factors involved. Patient plasma, serum, calcium chloride, and autologous platelets or platelet lipid substitute are incubated concurrently, and, at appropriate intervals, the clotting times of normal citrated plasma substrate, to which aliquots of the incubation mixture are added in sequential fashion, are determined.

Thudichum's t., (for creatinine), add to the suspected substance a dilute solution of ferric chloride; a dark-red color indicates the presence of creatinine.

Thumb-nail t., (for fractured patella), the examiner's thumbnail is passed over the subcutaneous surface of the patella; a fracture will be felt as a sharp crevice.

Thymol turbidity t., a flocculation test formerly used as a test of liver function; a positive result (formation of a precipitate when a supersaturated thymol solution is added to serum) reflects serum protein abnormalities, chiefly elevated levels of gamma or beta globulins.

Thyroid function t., see specific tests, including acetoni-strite t., Kottmann's t., Loewi's t., quadriceps t., and thyroid activity, method for, under method.

Thyroid suppression t., (for hyperthyroidism), after administration of liothyronine for several days, radioactive iodine uptake is decreased in normal persons but not in those with hyperthyroidism.

Tidy's t., (for albumin in urine), 1. Add equal volumes of phenol and glacial acetic acids; albumin will form a white precipitate. 2. Add 15 drops of alcohol and 15 drops of phenol; albumin will form a white precipitate.

Tine t., tine tuberculin t., (Rosenthal), four tines or prongs 2 mm long, attached to a plastic handle and coated with dip-dried old tuberculin (OT) are pressed into the skin of the volar surface of the forearm, where they deposit a dose of the tuberculin in the outer layer. The skin is checked 49 to 72 hours later for the presence of palpable induration; if the induration around one or more of the puncture wounds is 2 mm or more in diameter, the test is considered positive.

Tizzoni's t., (for iron in tissues), treat a section of tissue with 2 percent solution of potassium ferrocyanide. and then with a 0.5 percent solution of HCl the tissue will be stained a blue color if iron is present.

TNT t., see Webster's t.

Toad t., 1 See male toad t. 2 See Xenopus t.

Tobey-Ayer t., (in the diagnosis of lateral sinus thrombosis), after spinal puncture a manometer is attached to the puncture needle: compression on both jugular veins causes the fluid to rise in the manometer; pressure on one jugular vein alone, causes a rise in spinal fluid pressure if the lateral sinus is normal but little or no rise if there is thrombosis of the sinus on the same side as compression of the vein. The significance of the test is greater on the right side than on the left.

Tolerance t., 1. An exercise test to determine the efficiency of the circulation. 2. A test to determine the body's ability to metabolize a substance or to endure administration of a drug.

Tollens, Neuberg, and Schwket t., (for glycuronic acid), extract the glycuronic acid from acidified urine with ether, add water, evaporate the ether, and make orcinol test.

Tone decay t., an audiometer test in which the patient is asked to raise his hand as long as he hears a continuous tone at his threshold level and to lower it when it becomes inaudible; whenever he lowers it before 60 seconds, the intensity is raised by 5 decibels and the amount of tone decay from the initial threshold level in decibels is determined.

Tongue t., a slight blow upon the tongue produces a contraction with the appearance of deep depressions seen in tetany.

Topfer's t., quantitative tests for hydrochloric acid in gastric contents. 1. (for total acidity) 1 percent solution of phenolphthalein is used as the indicator 2. (for free HCl), 0.5 percent alcoholic solution of p-dimethylaminoazobenzene is used as the indicator. 3. (for combined HCl), 1 percent aqueous solution of sodium alizarin sulfonate is used as the indicator.

Torquay's t., (for bile), a small amount of the suspected liquid is added to a test tube containing an aqueous solution of methyl violet, 1:2000. Bile will change the blue color to red.

Tourniquet t., 1. (for capillary fragility), after application of pressure midway between diastolic and systolic for 5 minutes by a manometer cuff, the petechiae are counted in a previously marked area, 2.5 cm in diameter, on the inner aspect of the forearm, about 4 cm below the crease of the elbow. A number between 10 and 20 is marginal, above 20, abnormal. Also called Hess' capillary t. 2. (for collateral circulation), after hyperemia of the limb has been artificially produced by application of the tourniquet, the tourniquet is removed and the extent of collateral circulation is determined by compressing the main artery; also called Matas' t. 3. (for collateral circulation in patients with varicose veins) a bandage is applied to the upper part of the leg below the knee and the patient walks around with it on varicose veins of the leg will become evacuated from continuous compression if there is sufficient collateral circulation in the deep veins. Also called Perthes' t.

Toxigenicity t., (*in vitro*), (for detection of toxigenic strains of *Corynebacterium diphtheriae*), a primary culture is streaked onto a plate of tellurite agar containing a strip of filter paper perfused with diphtheria antitoxin. The exotoxin produced by the bacteria forms a band of precipitation with antitoxin diffusing from the filter paper. Called also Elek t.

TPI t., see *Treponema pallidum* immobilization t.

Trapeze t., when the patient hangs from a trapeze, a spinal deformity will disappear if the deformity is postural but will remain if it is structural.

Trendelenburg's t., 1. Raise the leg above the level of the heart until the veins are empty, then lower it quickly. If the veins become distended at once, varicosity and incompetence of the valves are indicated. 2. the patient, standing erect, stripped, with back to the examiner, is told to lift one leg and then the other: when weight is supported by the affected limb, the pelvis on the sound side falls instead of rising; seen, in disturbances of the gluteus-medius mechanism, as in deformity of the femoral neck, dislocated hip joint, and weakness or paralysis of the gluteus-medius muscle.

Treponema pallidum **complement fixation t.,** nontreponemal antigen serologic tests for syphilis using complement fixation rather than flocculation as the indicator reaction. Once widely used to confirm positive results of flocculation procedures, they have now been replaced by treponemal antigen tests.

Treponema pallidum **immobilization (TPI) t.,** the first treponemal antigen serologic test for syphilis, introduced in 1949, now little used; live *T. pallidum* is mixed with patient serum and complement and examined microscopically to determine the proportion of treponemes that are immobilized by specific antibodies in the serum.

Tretop's t., to fresh urine in a test tube, a few drops of 40 percent formalin are added; albumin in the urine is coagulated.

Triboulet's t., (for tuberculous ulceration of the intestines), lump of feces as large as a walnut is dissolved in 20 ml of distilled water and filtered; 3 ml of the filtrate is diluted with 12 ml of distilled water; 20 minims of Triboulet's reagent (sublimate 3.5, acetic acid 1, distilled water 100) are added. As a control, the same solution is prepared without Triboulet's reagent. The test tubes containing the two solutions are well shaken, and are compared after five and twenty-four hours. A positive reaction is indicated by a cloudy grey or brown deposit.

Trichophytin t., (for trichophyton infection), when filtrates of the fungus are injected into persons who have been infected with the disease, a reaction is produced somewhat resembling the tuberculin reaction.

Tricresol peroxidase t., (for raw milk), see Kastle's t.

Triketohydrindene hydrate t., to 25 ml of water, add 10 mg of aminoacetic acid. To 1 ml of this solution, add a solution of 50 mg of sodium acid in 2 ml of water, then add 0.2 ml of a solution of 5 mg of triketohydrindene hydrate (Ninhydrin) in 1 ml of water. Add the suspected matter and boil for 1-2 minutes. A violet color indicates a tree carboxyl and alpha-amino group in proteins, peptones, peptides, or amino acids.

Trommer's t., (for dextrose in the urine), to 2 parts of urine, add 1 part of potassium or sodium hydroxide, then add a very dilute solution of copper sulfate drop by drop, and boil the whole. Sugar, if present, causes precipitation of an orange-red deposit.

Trousseau's t., (for bile in urine), tincture of iodine diluted with 10 parts of alcohol is added to urine in a test tube; a green ring is formed where the liquids touch if bilirubin is present.

Tsuchiya's t., (for albumin), a modified test in which Tsuchiya's reagent is used instead of Esbach's reagent.

Tuberculin t., any of a large number of skin tests for tuberculosis using a variety of different types of tuberculin and methods of application. The most reliable procedure, now standard, is intradermal injection (the Mantoux's test) of PPD (purified protein derivative); a positive result consists of a palpable and visible area of erythema and induration greater than 10 mm in diameter developing around the site of injection 48 to 72 hours after the injection. Intermediate strength tuberculin (5 TU) is generally used to test adults; a positive result is virtually diagnostic of a previous or current infection with *Mycobacterium tuberculosis*. Persons with a negative test are retested with second strength tuberculin (250 TU); in this test, a positive reaction is frequently due to atypical mycobacteria infection and is thus nonspecific; a negative result indicates either absence of tuberculosis or the presence of cutaneous anergy due to overwhelming tuberculosis infection or to an associated immunosuppressive illness, e.g., Hodgkin's disease or sarcoidosis.

Tuberculin t., Sterneedle t., the needle points of the Sterneedle are dipped into 1 to 2 drops of tuberculin PPD, and then placed on the forearm, where the six needle points are caused to penetrate the skin (by means of a spring device in the handle), through the PPD solution, to a depth of 1 mm, thus depositing tuberculin in the outer layer of the skin. Palpable, coalescing induration (edema) extending more than

5 mm around the puncture wounds in three to seven days indicates a positive reaction. In England, it is known as the Heaf's test.

Tuberculosis t., see specific tests, including Craig's t., Mantoux's t, mirror t., niacin t. (1), (2), Romer's t., tine t., Triboulet's t., tuberculin t., tuberculin t., Sterneedle t., urorosein t., Vollmer's t.

Tuffier's t., in aneurysm, when the main artery and vein of a limb are compressed, swelling of the veins of the hand or foot will occur only if the collateral circulation is free.

Two-glass t., (for urethritis), the patient collects his urine on rising, the first part in one glass and the second part in a separate glass. If he has anterior urethritis, the first portion will be turbid and the second portion clear; if he has both anterior and posterior urethritis, both portions will be turbid.

Two-stage prothrombin t., a method of quantitating prothrombin after tissue thromboplastin and excess Factor V have converted it to thrombin, by determining the clotting time of a standard fibrinogen solution to which the previously generated thrombin has been added.

Two-tailed t., a hypothesis test (qv) in which the critical region comprises both tails of the distribution of the test statistic and the null hypothesis is tested against a two-sided alternative that includes deviation from the null hypothesis in both directions.

Typhoid fever t., see specific tests, including Ehrlich's t. (1), miostagmin t., Moretti's t., Petzetaki's t., urorosein t.

Tyrosine t., see specific tests, including Hoffmann's t., Morner's t. (1), Piria's t., Scherer's t. (3), Udranszky's t. (2), Wurster's t. (2).

Tyson's t., (for bile acids in urine), 180 to 240 ml of urine are evaporated to dryness on the water bath. The residue is extracted with absolute alcohol, and to the extract 12 to 14 volumes of ether are added. The bile acids are precipitated, then are filtered off, dissolved in water, and the aqueous solution decolorized with animal charcoal.

Tzanck's t., examination of tissue from the floor of a lesion, in vesicular or bullous diseases, to discover the type of cell present as a means of diagnosing the disease. Multinucleated giant cells are pathognomonic of varicella, herpes simplex, herpes zoster, or pemphigus.

Udránszky's t., 1. (for bile acids), take 1 ml of a solution of the suspected substance, add a drop of 0.1 percent solution of furfurol in water, underlay with strong sulfuric acid, and cool; if bile is present, a bluish-red color is formed. 2. (for tyrosine), take 1 ml of the suspected substance in solution, add a drop of 0.5 percent aqueous solution of furfurol, and underlay with 1 ml of concentrated sulfuric acid; a pink color shows the presence of tyrosine.

Uffelmann's t., (for hydrochloric acid and lactic acid in the gastric contents), to a quantity of material taken from the stomach, add a few drops of a reagent containing 3 drops of a solution of ferric chloride, 3 drops of a concentrated solution of phenol, and 20 ml of water; hydrochloric acid, if present, decolorizes this solution, while lactic acid turns it yellow.

Ulrich's t., (for albumin), the reagent consists of saturated solution of common salt 98 ml, glacial acetic acid, 2 ml. It must be perfectly clear. Boil a few milliliters of this fluid in a test tube, and immediately overlay with the urine. Albumin and globulin give a white ring at the zone of contact.

Ultzmann's t., (for bile pigments), to 10 ml of the urine to be tested, add 3 or 4 ml of a 1.3 solution of potassium hydroxide and an excess of HCl; bile pigments will cause an emerald-green coloration.

Umber's t., (for scarlet fever), to a small quantity of urine, add 2 drops of a solution made with 30 ml concentrated hydrochloric acid, 2 gm of paradimethylaminobenzaldehyde and 70 ml of water; a red reaction indicates scarlet fever.

Unheated serum reagin (USR) t., a modification of the VDRL test using unheated serum, used primarily for screening.

Uracil t., see Wheeler-Johnson t.

Urea t., see specific tests, including Benedict's t. (2), biuret t. (2), diacetyl t., Marshall's t., Schiff's t. (4), Schroeder's t., Spiro's t. (1), urease t., Van Slyke's t. (2). See also urea, methods for, under method.

Urea clearance t., see blood-urea clearance t.

Urea concentration t., (for renal efficiency), a test based on the fact that urea is absorbed rapidly from the stomach into the blood, and is excreted unaltered by the kidneys: 15 gm of urea is given with 100 ml of fluid, and the urine which is collected at the end of two hours is tested for urea concentration. Also called MacLean-de Wesselow t., and Jones-Cantarow t.

Urease t., 1. A test for urea based on the conversion of urea into ammonium carbonate by the urease of soybean: see Marshall's method and urease, methods for, under method. 2. (for the production of urease by bacteria), a peptone agar medium containing urea concentrate and phenol red is prepared in slants. After inoculation of the surface and incubation, urease-positive cultures produce an alkaline reaction (red color) in the medium *Proteus* cultures show an early urease-positive reaction; other genera may have a delayed response.

Urecholine supersensitivity t., (for neurogenic bladder), administer 2.5 mg of Urecholine (bethanechol) subcutaneously; the bladder is neurogenic if it exhibits a rise in intravesical pressure more than 15 cm greater than that of a control.

Uric acid t., see specific tests, including; Porter's t. (1), Salkowski-Ludwig t., Schiff's t. (5), von Jaksch's t. (4), Weidel's t. (1). See also uric acid, methods for, under method.

Urine concentration t., under a controlled diet the specific gravity of the urine should reach 1.18 or more at certain times.

Urobilin t., see specific tests, including Hitdebrandt's t., Schlesinger's t., See also urobilinogen, methods for, under method.

Urochromogen t., see Weiss' t.

Urorosein t., urorrhodin t., add to the urine half as much concentrated hydrochloric acid and a few drops of a 1 percent solution of potassium nitrate; a red color indicates urorosein (urorrhodin); seen in typhoid fever, nephritis, pulmonary tuberculosis, and other diseases.

USR t., unheated serum reagin t.

Valenta's t., (for foreign fats in butter), the butter is heated with an equal amount of glacial acetic acid and then cooled. If opacity begins to show at 96°F, there is adulteration; if opacity is not observed until about 62°F, the butter is pure.

Valsalva's t., (for pneumothorax), after a deep inspiration, the mouth and nose are held tightly closed, and a strong attempt at expiration is made.

van den Bergh's t., a test for bilirubin in which diazotized serum or plasma is compared with a standard solution of diazotized bilirubin.

van den Velden's t., see Maly's t.

Van Slyke's t., 1. (for amino-nitrogen) nitrous acid acting on amino-nitrogen sets free nitrogen gas, which is collected and its volume determined. 2. (for urea) treat the sample with urease, pass the ammonia so formed into fiftieth normal acid, and titrate the excess of acid.

Van Slyke-Cullen t., see under method.

Vaughan-Novy t., (for tyrotoxicon), adding 2 or 3 drops each of sulfuric and carbolic acids and a few drops of an aqueous solution of the suspected substance to tyrotoxicon gives a yellow or orange red color.

VDRL (Venereal Disease Research Laboratory) t., the standard nontreponemal antigen serologic test for syphilis, a slide flocculation test using heat-inactivated serum and VDRL antigen, a standardized mixture of cardiolipin, lecithin, and cholesterol. Positive tests are seen in about 70 percent of cases in primary syphilis, 100 percent in secondary syphilis, and 70 percent in tertiary syphilis. There is a 20 to 40 percent false positive rate; see biologic false-positive under false-positive t.

Ventilation t., measurement of the quantity of air expired by a person during a period of exercise.

Visscher-Bowman t., (for pregnancy), a chemical test for pregnancy, depending on the presence of anterior pituitary hormones in the urine.

Vitali's t., 1. (for alkaloids) evaporate with fuming nitric acid and add a drop of potassium hydroxide; color reactions will occur. For atropine the color is violet, turning to red. 2. (for alkaloids) add sulfuric acid, potassium chlorate, and an alkaline sulfide; various color reactions will follow. 3. (for bile pigments) add a few drops of potassium nitrate in solution and dilute sulfuric acid. The color reactions are green, followed by blue or red and yellow. 4. (for bile pigments) add quinine bisulfate in solution and follow with ammonia water, sulfuric acid, a crystal of sugar, and alcohol; a violet color results. 5. (for thymol) distill, and pass the vapor through a mixture of chloroform and potassium hydroxide solution; a red color results. 6. (for pus in the urine) the urine is acidified with acetic acid and filtered. On the filter paper thus obtained a small quantity of guaiacum is B dropped. The paper will turn dark blue if pus is present.

Vitamin t., see specific tests, Gothlin's t., Harris-Ray t., Rosenheim-Drummond's t., Rotter's t., Schopfer's t., Shear's t., thiochrome t.

Voelcker-Joseph t., see indigo carmine t.

Vogel-Lee t., (for mercury), add 3 percent of hydrochloric acid and concentrate the urine to one fifth its original volume. Add a piece of clean copper wire. A silvery film indicates mercury. To confirm, place the wire in a tube with a plug of gold foil and distill the mercury over onto the gold. Sublime a crystal of iodine onto the mercury and form the red iodide of mercury.

Voges-Proskauer t., (for differentiation of Enterobacteriaceae), a test for the production of acetylmethylcarbinol from glucose in bacterial cultures. An appropriate culture is treated with a solution of potassium hydroxide and creatinine. Development of a red color indicates a positive reaction. *Enterobacter, Klebsiella,* and *Serratia* are V-P positive; *Erwinia, Pectobacterium,* and *Yersinia* are variable; *Escherichia* and other genera of Enterobacteriaceae are V-P negative.

Vollmer's t., (obs), a tuberculin patch test.

von Aldor's t., (for proteoses), precipitate the urine with phosphotungstic acid, wash the precipitate with alcohol, bring into solution with potassium hydroxide, and apply the biuret test.

von Jaksch's t., 1. (for free HCl in gastric juice) a test paper prepared with benzopurpurine B takes on a fine violet color if HCl is present. If present in considerable amount, it becomes dark blue. 2. (for dextrose in urine) add to the urine a mixture of 3 parts of sodium acetate and 2 parts of phenylhydrazine hydrochloride, warm it, and put the test tube in hot water for half an hour. On cooling, yellow needles of phenylglucosazone are seen as a precipitate. 3. (for melanin) add to the suspected liquid a few drops of a solution of ferric chloride. If melanin is present, a grey appearance is produced. After precipitation add more ferric chloride, and the precipitate will be redissolved. 4. (for uric acid) heat the powder slowly on a glass dish with a few drops of bromine water or chlorine water; the substance becomes red. After cooling, add ammonia, and it becomes purplish red.

von Maschke's t., (for creatinine), to the suspected solution, add a few drops of Fehling's solution, after mixing with a cold solution of sodium carbonate; an amorphous, flocculent precipitate proves the presence of creatinine.

von Pirquet's t. see Pirquet's t.

von Recklinghausen's t., (of heart function), a test based on the proposition that the product of the frequency of the pulse and the amplitude of the blood pressure is equal to the amount of blood expelled by the heart in a second, divided by the distensibility of the circulatory system.

von Zeynek and Mencki t., (for blood), precipitate the urine with acetone, extract the precipitate with acidified acetone, and examine the colored extract under the microscope for small hemin crystals.

Waaler-Rose t., see Rose-Waaler t.

Wada's t., (for cerebral dominance of language function), amobarbital is injected into an internal carotid artery to produce transient hemiparesis of the contralateral limbs. Injection into the artery of the hemisphere dominant for language produces a transient aphasia, into that of the nondominant hemisphere does not interfere with language function.

Wagner's t., (for occult blood), see benzidine t.

Walter's bromide t., a test based on the fact that in normal persons the ratio of the amount of bromide in the blood and cerebrospinal fluid is constant; in persons with mental disorder, the ratio may vary.

Wang's t., (quantitative test for indican), the indican is converted into indigosulfuric acid and titrated by means of a potassium permanganate solution.

Warren's t., see Trommer's t.

Wassermann's t., the original (1906) nontreponemal antigen serologic test for syphilis.

Water-gurgle t., (for structure of the esophagus), the swallowing of water causes a peculiar gurgle heard on auscultation.

Water provocative t., see drinking t.

Watson-Schwartz t., a simple qualitative procedure, depending upon the chloroform and butanol-insolubility of porphobilinogen aldehyde, for differentiating porphobilinogen from urobilinogen and other Ehrlich's reactors; it is of value in the diagnosis of acute porphyria.

Weber's t., 1. (for differentiating between hearing impairment of conductive or sensorineural origin), the stem of a vibrating tuning fork is placed on the vertex or midline of the forehead; if the sound is heard best in the affected ear, the impairment is probably of the conductive type: if heard best in the normal ear, the impairment is probably of the sensorineural type (Friedrich Eugen Weber). 2. (for indican) boil 30 ml of suspected urine with an equal volume of hydrochloric acid containing a little nitric acid; cool it, and shake with ether; if indican is present, the ether will become red or violet and the froth will be blue (Ernest Heinrich Weber). 3. (for blood) mix the sample with 30 percent acetic acid and extract with ether; to the ethereal extract add an alcoholic solution of guaiac and hydrogen peroxide. A blue color indicates blood (Ernest Heinrich Weber).

Webster's t., (for TNT in urine), the urine is extracted with ether, then acidified with a mineral acid and again extracted with ether. In the latter extract, the presence of the azoxy-compound formed from TNT is shown by the development of a violet tint on the addition of alcoholic potash.

Weichbrodt's t., (for globulin), to 0.7 ml of spinal fluid, add 0.3 ml of a 1 percent solution of mercuric bichloride; a cloudiness or opalescence indicates globulin.

Weidel's t., 1. (for uric acid), the substance tested is treated with nitric acid, evaporated, and moistened with ammonia water; if uric acid is present, murexide will be formed, and a purple color is produced. Also called murexide t. 2. (for xanthine) warm with freshly prepared chlorine water containing a trace of nitric acid until gas ceases to be produced; contact with gaseous ammonia develops a pink or purple color. 3. (for xanthine bodies) dissolve in warm chlorine water, evaporate, and treat with ammonia water; a pink or purple color will form, changing to violet on the addition of sodium or potassium hydroxide solution.

Weil-Felix t., (for diagnosis of typhus and certain other rickettsial diseases), the blood serum of a patient with suspected rickettsial disease is tested against certain strains of *Proteus vulgaris* (OX-2, OX-19, OX-K). The agglutination reactions, based on antigens common to both organisms, determine the presence and type of rickettsial infection.

Weiss' permanganate t., see Weiss' t.

Weiss' t., (for urochromogen), to 2 ml of the urine, add 4 ml of distilled water and 3 drops of a 1:1000 solution of potassium permanganate; a canary yellow color indicates urochromogen.

Welland's t., see bar-reading t.

Wender's t., (for dextrose), make a reagent by dissolving 1 part of methylene blue in 300 parts of distilled water, alkalinize this with potassium hydroxide and heat with a suspected solution; dextrose, if present, will decolorize it.

Wenzell's t., (for strychnine), treat the suspected material with a solution of 1 part of potassium permanganate in 2000 parts of sulfuric acid; strychnine, even in very small proportion will cause color reactions.

Weppen's t., (for morphine), treat with sugar, bromine, and sulfuric acid; a red color shows the presence of morphine.

Wernicke's t., reaction in certain cases of hemianopia in which the stimulus of light thrown upon one side of the retina causes the iris to contract, while light thrown on the other side arouses no response.

Wetzel's t., (for carbon monoxide in blood), to the blood to be examined, add 4 volumes of water and treat with 3 volumes of a 1 percent tannin solution. If CO is present, the blood becomes carmine red; normal blood slowly assumes a greyish hue.

Weyl's t., 1. (for creatinine) to the suspected solution, add a little of a dilute solution of sodium nitroprusside, and then carefully put in a few drops of a weak solution of sodium hydroxide: a ruby-red color results, changing to blue on warming with acetic acid. 2. (for nitric acid in the urine) distill 200 ml of urine with 0.2 part of sulfuric or hydrochloric acid, receiving the distillate in a potassium hydroxide solution. If metaphenyl-diamine is added, a yellow color will form; if there is added pyrogailic acid in aqueous solution with a little sulfuric acid, the color will be brown; but sulfanilic acid in solution, followed in ten minutes by naphthylamine hydrochlorate, produces a red tint.

Wheeler-Johnson t., (for uracil and cytosine), to the unknown solution, add bromine water until the color is permanent, but avoid excess. Then add an excess of barium hydroxide. A purple color indicates one of these substances.

Whipple's t., see lipase t. (1), phenoltetrachlorophthalein t.

Whiteside's t., a test for the detection of subclinical mastitis in cows as indicated by an excessively high leukocyte count of the milk. Mix 2 ml of a normal solution of sodium hydroxide with 10 ml of milk; the development of a viscous mass is positive. A modified version consists in mixing 1 drop of milk with 5 drops of normal sodium hydroxide solution on a glass plate, and stirring for about 20 seconds with a glass rod. No changes in consistency—negative; threads, clumps, or flakes of coagulated material—positive; the development of a viscous mass with separation of a clear whey—strongly positive.

Widal's t., Widal's serum t., (for typhoid fever), a test for the presence of agglutinins to O and H antigens of *Salmonella typhi* and *Salmonella paratyphi* in the serum of patients with suspected *Salmonella* infection.

Wideroe's t., a test for the character of puncture fluids. A few drops of Millon's reagent is placed in a water glass, and 1 drop of the fluid to be tested is placed on the surface. A film of coagulated protein at once forms. If this film is coherent and can be lifted readily, the exudate is tuberculous; if less readily, it is inflammatory; if it breaks up so that it cannot be lifted at all, it is a transudate.

Widmark's t., a blood test for the diagnosis of alcoholic intoxication.

Wijs' t., an iodine number test which employs Wijs' iodine solution; iodine number—the amount of iodine in grams which 100 gm of the fat can take up; it indicates the amount of unsaturated fatty acids present in the fat.

Wilbrand's prism t., a small circle of white paper is placed upon a black surface, and the patient is seated before it with one eye bandaged. He is directed to look at the spot, and a strong prism is placed before the eye in such a way that the image of the spot is thrown upon the blind half of the retina. It is noticed if the eye at once moves to find the object again, and whether the movement is reversed when the prism is withdrawn. The presence of this reaction places the lesion in the cerebrum; the absence of the reaction locates it in the tract.

Wilcoxon's rank sum t., see rank sum t.

Wilkinson-Peter t., (for raw milk), benzidine and hydrogen peroxide give a blue color in raw milk, but not in heated milk.

Williamson's blood t., in a narrow test tube 4 ml of water and 2 ml of blood are placed; to this are added 1 ml of methylene blue (1:6000) and 4 ml of solution of potassium hydroxide. The tube is placed in a pot of boiling water. If the blood is from a diabetic patient, the blue soon disappears, but not otherwise.

Winckler's t., 1. (for alkaloids) a solution of mercuric chloride with an excess of potassium iodide is added; alkaloids will cause a white precipitate. 2. (for free HCl in the gastric juice) filter the juice into a porcelain cell with a few drops of the 5 percent alcoholic solution of alphanaphthol containing 1 percent or less of dextrose. Heat carefully, and a bluish-violet zone will appear, which rapidly grows darker. 3. (for iodine) sodium nitrate is mixed with a starch paste; iodine gives a blue color with it.

Winslow's t., test for respiration in doubtful death by observing a vessel of water placed at the bottom of the chest.

Wishart's t., (for acetonemia) a few drops of plasma are placed in a small test tube. Enough dry powdered ammonium sulfate is added to supersaturate, so that at the end of the test there will still be some of the solid sulfate in the bottom of the tube. A couple of drops of a fresh solution of sodium nitroprusside are next added and shaken, and finally 1 or 2 drops of ordinary ammonia water. On shaking, a purple color develops, a little more slowly than in the case of urine. The intensity of the color indicates the degree of acetonemia.

Witz's t., (for hydrochloric acid in the gastric juice), a 1:48 aqueous solution of methyl violet causes a violet color, changing to blue and then green.

Woldman's t., a test for gastrointestinal lesion based on the principle that free phenolphthalein may pass through a lesion in the gastrointestinal mucosa and appear in the urine.

Wolff-Junghans t., (for gastric cancer), quantitative estimation of the soluble albumin in the gastric extracts after giving a test meal; marked increase of dissolved albumin indicating malignant disease.

Woodbury's t., (for alcohol in the urine), to 2 ml of urine, 1 ml of sulfuric acid is added, and a crystal of potassium dichromate; a green color will soon form.

Worm-Müller t., (for dextrose in the urine), a test made by boiling in a test tube 0.33 ml of a 2.5 per cent solution of copper sulfate and 2.5 ml of a solution of potassium hydroxide. Boil each and mix, and a yellowish or red precipitate will be formed.

Wormley's t., (for alkaloids), 1. Made by treating with an alcoholic solution of picric acid; a yellow precipitate will be formed. 2. Made by treating with a solution of 1 part of iodine and 2 parts of potassium iodide in 60 parts of water; a colored precipitate will be formed.

Worsted t., see Holmgren's t.

Wurster's t., 1. (for hydrogen peroxide) test paper is saturated with the solutions tetramethylparaphenylenediamine; hydrogen peroxide turns it to a blue-violet color. 2. (for tyrosine) the suspected material is dissolved in boiling water and a little quinon; ruby-red color will form, changing slowly to brown.

X^2 **t.**, see chi-square t.

Xanthine t., see specific tests, including Hoppe Seyler's t. (2), Weidel's t. (2), (3).

Xanthoproteic t., see Mulder's t. (2).

Xenopus t., (for pregnancy), a female African toad (*Xenopus laevis*) is injected with 2 ml of urine, or 1 ml of an extract, into the dorsal lymph sac; a deposit of 5-6 or more eggs within four to twelve hours indicates pregnancy.

Xylidine t., see Schiff's t. (1).

D-xylose absorption t., D-xylose tolerance t., (for differential diagnosis in malabsorption syndromes), after the oral administration of 25 gm (sometimes 5 gm is used) of D-xylose dissolved in 250 ml of water, followed immediately by an additional 250 ml of water, to a fasting adult, the amount excreted in the urine during a five-hour period is determined. Since poor renal function may also result in low xylose absorption, blood levels are also determined at two hours. Normally, more than 4.0 gm of xylose should be excreted over the five-hour period; less than this amount suggests intestinal malabsorption. Blood values are normally more than 25 mg xylose per 100 ml of blood.

Young's t., (for cataract), on a disk with a varied number of pinholes in different portions, the patient's ability to recognize the number of holes is a test of the integrity of macular function.

Zaleski's t., (for carbon monoxide in blood) to 2 ml of blood, add an equal volume of water and 3 drops of a one-third saturated solution of copper sulfate: if carbon monoxide is present, a brick-red deposit is thrown down; otherwise, the precipitate is greenish brown.

Zappacosta's t., (for liver function), glycocyamine is injected intravenously; if in one quarter of an hour after the injection the substance is still present in the blood, liver function is impaired.

Zeisel's t., (for colchicine), dissolve in hydrochloric acid, boil with ferric chloride, and shake with chloroform; a brown or dark-red layer will form at the bottom.

Zinc fluorescence t., (for urobilin), see Schlesinger's t.

Zondek-Aschheim t., see Aschheim-Zondek t.

Zouchlos' t., (for albumin in the urine), 1. Precipitate the urine with a mixture of 1 part of acetic acid and 6 parts of a 10 percent solution of mercuric chloride. 2. Prepare reagent with 100 parts of a 10 percent solution of potassium thiocyanate and 20 parts of acetic acid; drop it slowly into the urine until the albumin appears as a white cloudiness 3. Add equal parts of succinic acid and potassium thiocyanate; albumin, if present, will be precipitated.

Zsigmondy's gold number t., see colloidal gold t.

Zwenger's t., 1. (for cholesterol), a crystal of cholesterol with 5 parts of sulfuric acid and 1 part water gives a red ring changing to violet. 2. See Liebermann's t.

6
Maneuvers

Maneuver: Any dexterous procedure.

Adson's m., see under tests.

Alien m., with the forearm flexed at a right angle, the arm is extended horizontally and rotated externally at the shoulder, the head being rotated to the contralateral shoulder; obliteration of the radial pulse suggest scalenus anticus syndrome.

Bracht's m., (for breech presentation), the breech is allowed to spontaneously deliver up to the umbilicus. The body and extended legs are held together with both hands maintaining the upward and anterior rotation to the fetal body. When the anterior rotation is nearly complete, the fetal body is held against the mother's symphysis. Maintenance of this position leads to spontaneous completion of delivery.

Brandt-Andrews m., a method of expressing the placenta from the uterus in the third stage of labor; the left hand grasps the umbilical cord while the right is placed on the maternal abdomen with the fingers over the anterior uterine surface. The right hand is gently pressed backward and slightly upward as the left applied gentle traction on the cord.

Chassard-Lapine m., the patient sits and bends forward as far as possible. The roentgen rays, directed from above, penetrate the spine and outline the sigmoid loops in a transverse projection.

Crede's m., see under method.

Engel-Lysholm m., a radiologic method of determining the size of the retrogastric organs or masses: the patient takes effervescent powders to fill his stomach with carbondioxide, and assumes a prone position; a lateral view of the abdomen with a horizontal beam, and a posteroanterior projection with a vertical beam are made.

Forward-bending m., a method of detecting retracton signs in neoplastic changes in the mammae; the patient bends forward front the waist with chin held up and arms extended toward the examiner. If retraction is present an asymmetry in the breast is seen.

Fowler m., a test for tight intrinsic muscles in ulnar deviation of the digits: in rheumatoid arthiritis a heavy, taut ulnar band is demonstrated when the digit is held in its normal axial relationship.

Halstead m., while the examiner exerts downward traction on the upper limb to be tested, the subject rotates his head toward the contralateral shoulder; obliteration of the radial pulse is suggestive of scalenus anticus syndrome.

Heiberg-Esmarch m., (obs), a pushing forward by the anesthetist of the patient's lower jaw in order to prevent the tongue from slipping backward.

Heimlich m., a method of dislodging food or other material from the throat of a choking victim: after wrapping the arms around the victim at the belt line and allowing his upper torso to hang forward, make a fist with one hand and grasp it with the other; with both hands placed against the victim's abdomen slightly above the navel and below the rib cage, forcefully press into the abdomen with a quick upward thrust. If the victim is sitting, stand behind him and perform the same procedure; if he is prone, turn him on his back, kneel astride the torso, place both hands at the location on the victim's abdomen as described above and press forcefully with a sharp upward thrust. The maneuver may be repeated several times if necessary.

Hoguet's m., in hernioplasty, conversion of the direct hernial sac to an indirect one by withdrawing the sac from beneath the deep epigastric vessels.

Hueter's m., downward and forward pressure on the patient's tongue by the left forefinger of the physician during introduction of a stomach tube.

Jendrassik's m., a procedure for emphasizing the patellar reflex: the patient hooks his hands together by the flexed fingers and pulls apart as hard as he can.

Kappeler's m., (obs), a drawing forward of the patient's lower jaw by the anesthetist.

Kocher m., operative mobilization of the duodenum for exposure of the retroduodenal, intrapancreatic and intraduodenal portion of the common bile duct.

Leopold's m.s, four maneuvers in palpating the abdomen for ascertaining the position and presentation of the fetus.

Lovset's m., extraction of the arms in breech birth by clockwise and counterclockwise rotation of the fetus, after it has been expelled up to the umbilicus.

McDonald m., measurement of the contour of the abdomen to calculate the duration of pregnancy.

Mauriceau m., a method of delivering the aftercoming head in cases of breech presentation.

Muller's m., an inspiratory effort with a closed glottis after expiration, used during fluoroscopic examination to cause a negative intrathoracic pressure with engorgement of intrathoracic vascular structures, which is helpful in recognizing esophageal varices, and distinguishing vascular from nonvascular structures.

Muller-Hillis m., procedures for ascertaining the relation between the size of the fetal head and the pelvis of the mother.

Munro Kerr m., a maneuver for ascertaining the proportion between the head of the fetus and the pelvis of the mother.

Pajot's m., for forceps traction along the axis of superior strait, one hand over the lock of the forceps pulls downward toward the floor, while the other hand applies horizontal traction.

Phalen's m., (for detection fo carpal tunnel syndrome), the size of the carpal tunnel is reduced by holding the affected hand with the wrist fully flexed or extended for 30 to 60 seconds, or by placing a sphygmomanometer cuff on the involved arm and inflating to a point between diastolic and systolic pressure for 30 to 60 seconds.

Pinard's m., a method of bringing down the foot in breech extraction.

Prague m., a method in breech presentation of engaging the head by bringing down the breech and making traction on the head with the finger, which is hooked over the nape of the neck.

Ritgen m., delivery of the fetal head by lifting the head upward and forward through the vulva, between pains, by pressing with the tips of the fingers upon the perineum behind the anus.

Saxtorph's m., see Pajot's m.

Scanzoni m., a method of forceps rotation of the fetal head in the posterior position of the occiput.

Schreiber's m., rubbing of the inner side of the upper part of the thigh while testing for patellar reflex.

Sellick m., the application of pressure to the cricoid cartilage in order to compress the esophagus and prevent passive regurgitation during endotracheal intubation.

Toynbee m., pinching the nostrils and swallowing; if the auditory tube is patent, the tympanic membrane will retract medially.

Valsalva's m., 1. Forcible exhalation effort against a closed glottis; the resultant increase in intrathoracic pressure interferes with venous return to the heart. 2. Forcible exhalation effort against occluded nostrils and a closed mouth; the increased pressure in the eustachian tube and middle ear causes the tympanic membrane to move outward.

van Hoorn's m., a maneuver like the Prague maneuver, with the addition of pressure on the fetal forehead from outside.

Wigand's m., external conversion of a transverse lie into cephalic presentation, accomplished by pushing fetal head down with one hand and its buttock up with the other.

7
Methods

Method: The manner of performing any act or operation; a proce-dure or technique.

Abbott's m., treatment of scoliosis by lateral pulling and counter pulling on the spinal column by means of wide bandages and pads until the deformity is overcorrected and then applying a plaster jacket to produce pressure, counter pressure, and fixation of the spine in its corrected position.

ABC (alum, blood, clay) m., a method of deodorizing and precipitating sludge by the addition of alum, charcoal (or some other material), and clay to the raw sewage.

Absorption m., the separate and selective removal of agglutinins from specific immune sera by the addition of homologous particulate antigen(s) (e.g., bacterial cells or red blood cells) to the immune sera, or by the passage of specific immune sera through columns containing antigen on an insoluble support (immunosorbent) with which the homologous antibody combines and is thereby removed from the serum.

Acid hematin m., (for hemoglobin), dilute the blood in tenth normal HCl and compare the color with a standard heme solution or glass standards.

Addis m., see under tests.

Alkali reserve, m's for, see Fridericia's m. Marriott's m. van Slyke and Cutlen's m. (1), and van Slyke and Fitz's m.

Allantoin, m's for, see Folin's m. (15), Plimmer and Skelton's m., Wiechowski and Handorsky's m.

Altmann-Gersh m., a method of preparing tissue for histologic study by freeze drying.

Amino acid nitrogen, m for, see nitrogen, amino acid m's for.

Ammonia nitrogen, m for, see nitrogen, ammonia, m's for.

Arnold and Gunning's m., (for total nitrogen), a modified form of the Kjeldahl process for urine.

Aronson's m., volatilizing formaldehyde gas from the solid polymer, trioxymethylene, by heat.

Askenstedt's m., (Parker's modification) (for indican), precipitate the urine with solid mercuric chloride; oxidize the indican to indigo with Obermeyer's reagent; shake out with chloroform and compare the blue color with a standard solution of indigo.

Austin and Van Slyke's m., (for chlorides in whole blood), lake the blood with distilled water, precipitate the proteins with picric acid, and then proceed as in McLean and van Slyke's method for chlorides in oxalated plasma.

Autenrieth and Funk's m., (for cholesterol), boil the blood or serum to saponify the fats; extract with chloroform and evaporate the chloroform; make a Liebermann-Burchard test on the residue and compare it with a standard solution of cholesterol.

Autoclave m., see Clark-Collip m. (2).

Baer's m., prevention of the reforming of adhesions by the injection of sterilized oil into an ankylosed joint.

Bang's m., 1. Estimation of the quantities of the sugar, albumin, urea, etc., in the blood by examination of a few drops only collected on blotting paper. 2. (for dextrose): to an excess of the boiling reagent (an alkaline solution of copper thiocyanate), add the urine and titrate the excess of copper thiocyanate with hydroxylamine sulfate. 3. (a micromethod for dextrose): boil the urine with an excess of the reagent ($KHCO_3$, 160 gm; K_2CO_3 100 gm; KCl 66 gm; $CuSO_4$-$5H_2O$. 4.4 gm; and water to 1 liter) and titrate excess of CuCl with a solution of iodine, using starch as an indicator.

Barger's m., a method for determining osmotic pressure from vapor pressure.

Barraquer's m., phacoerysis—removal of the lens in cataract by means of suction with an instrument known as erysiphake.

Bergonie's m., the application of general faradization for the reduction of corpulence.

Beta-hydroxybutyric acid, m's for, see Black's m. and van Slyke and Palmer's m.

Bethea's m., see under sign.

Bile pigments, m's for, see Meulengracht's m; Wallace and Diamonds m. and see under tests.

Bivine's m., treatment of strychnine poisoning by administration of chloral hydrate.

Black's m., (for beta-hydroxybutyric acid), evaporate the urine to a small volume, acidify, add plaster of Paris to form a coarse meal, extract the beta-hydroxybutyric acid with ether in a Soxhlet apparatus, evaporate to dryness, take up in water and determine the amount by a polariscope.

Bloor, Pelkan, and Allen's m., (for fatty acids and cholesterol), extract the lipoids by an alcohol-ether mixture, saponify, extract the cholesterol with chloroform and the soaps with hot alcohol. The cholesterol is then determined colorimetrically and the fatty acids nephelometrically.

Bock and Benedict's m., (for total nitrogen), it is similar to Folin and Farmer's method, except that the ammonia is distilled instead of aerated over into the acid.

Bogg's m., (for protein in milk), this is a modification of Esbach's method for protein in urine; the protein being precipitated with Bogg's reagent instead of with picric acid.

Brandt-Andrews m., see under maneuver.

Brehmer's m., treatment of pulmonary tuberculosis by the use of dietetic and physical measures.

Breslau's m., volatilizing formaldehyde from dilute (8 percent) solutions to prevent polymerization.

Brine flotation m., (for concentration of ova), suspend a portion of the stool in a saturated solution of sodium chloride; let it stand for a time and collect the ova from the surface.

Brunn's m., see Breslau's m.

Calcium m's for, see Clark-Collip m. (1), Corley and Denis'm; Kramer and Tisdall's m. (2), Lyman's m., McCrudden's m., and Shohl and Pedley's m., and see under tests.

Caliper m., a method for approximating fat content in the body by measuring the thickness of folds of the skin at stated areas of the body by means of specially designed calipers.

Callahan m., 1. A root canal filling method in which the root canal is first flooded with a chloroform-rosin solution and then gutta-percha is dissolved in the solution. 2. A method of tracing and opening up the root canal by destroying the pulp tissue by application of a 50 percent sulfuric acid solution.

Carbon dioxide, m., see Fridericia's m. and van Slyke and Cullen's m (1).

Carrel's m., 1. A method of end-to-end suture of blood vessels. 2. Treatment of wounds, based on thorough exposure of the wound, removal of all foreign material and devitalised tissue, meticulous cleaning, and repeated irrigation with a dilute sodium hypochlorite solution. The adjacent skin is protected with petrolatum gauze. 3. A method of determining when to make secondary closure of wounds. A loop of material is taken from the wound, spread on a slide, stained, and the number of bacteria counted.

Castaneda's m., (for rickettsiae in smears), (1) A thin smear is made in a phosphate buffer (pH 7.6) and air-dried, (2) Stained with methylene blue solution for 3 minutes, (3) Counterstained with safranine solution, and (4) Washed, blotted, and dried. Rickettsiae appear pale blue; cell nuclei and protoplasm are red.

Cathelin's m., introduction of anesthetics into the epidural space through the sacrococcygeal ligament.

Chandler s m., (for fibrinogen), precipitate the fibrinogen with calcium chloride, centrifugalize, and determine the nitrogen in the clot.

Chick-Martin m., a method for testing the bactericidial value of disinfectants for water supplies in the presence of organic matter. The procedure originally incorporated 3 percent human feces. In the revised method, serial dilutions of disinfectant are incubated with a specified quantity of yeast and *Salmonella typhi* for a period of 30 minutes. The effectiveness is expressed by the ratio: effective concentration of phenol divided by effective concentration of test disinfectant (Chick-Martin coefficient).

Chlorides. m's for, see Austin and van Slyke's m., Dehn and Clark's m., McLean and van Slyke's m., Mohr's m., Volhard and Arnold's m., Volhard and Harvey's m., and Whitehorn's m.

Chloropercha m., a method of filling a root canal with gutta-percha dissolved in a chloroform-rosin solution; see Callahan's m. (def. 1) and Johnson's m.

Cholesterol, m's for, see Autenrieth and Funk's m., Bloor, Pelkan, and Alien's m., and Myers and Warden's m. and see under tests.

Ciaccio's m., treatment of tissue for the purpose of rendering visible the intracellular lipoids; they are fixed with acid chromate solution and stained with Sudan III.

Clark-Collip m., 1. (for calcium in serum), dilute the serum and add ammonium oxalate; wash the precipitate, dissolve with sulfuric acid, and titrate with potassium permanganate. 2. (for urea in blood), to 5 ml of blood filtrate add 1 ml of NH_4Cl and heat in autoclave at 150°C for ten minutes. Make alkaline, distil into acid, and titrate, using methyl red as indicator.

Clausen's m., 1. (for lactic acid in blood), remove the glucose by adding copper sulfate and calcium hydroxide, filter, and proceed with filtrate as in Clausen's method for lactic acid in urine. 2. (for lactic acid in urine), extract the lactic acid from the urine with ether, convert it into acetaldehyde by treatment with sulfuric acid, add sodium bisulfite, and titrate with standard iodine solution.

Closed-plaster m., treatment of wounds, compound fractures, and osteomyelitis by enclosing the limb in an immobilizing plaster cast as in (a) Orr treatment—treatment of compound fractures and osteomyelitis by debridement of wound, alignment of the wound, alignment of fracture, drainage with petrolatum gauze, and immobilization of limb in a plaster cast which is left on until the wound discharge is softened the plaster, and (b) Trueta treatment—immediate treatment of fractures as follows: (1) adopt surgical treatment as soon as possible; (2) thoroughly wash wound and entire limb with water, soap, and a nail brush, shave hair, paint surrounding skin with weak alcoholic solution of iodine, avoiding the wound; (3) debride wound; (4) open neighboring cellular spaces and remove hematomas; (5) remove completely denuded or displaced bone fragments and all foreign matters; (6) reduce fracture; (7) dress wound with sterile gauze and immobilize with plaster, including two adjacent joints if possible; (8) give injection of tetanus antitoxin.

Converse m., reconstruction of the ear lobe by raising a flap of skin below the auricle with a superior base about one third larger than the proposed lobe; a full-thickness skin graft covers the defect at the site of the flap except for the last third of the medial aspect of the pedicle.

Corley and Denis'm., (for calcium in tissues), if there is only a small amount of organic material, it may be removed by washing, aided by nitric acid. With more organic material, add 5 volumes of tenth normal sodium hydroxide and heat in autoclave at 180°C for two hours. Precipitate as oxalate, dissolve in sulfuric acid, and titrate with potassium permanganate.

Corning's m., anesthesia produced by injection of a local anesthetic into the subarachnoid space around the spinal cord.

Corri's m., (for lactic acid in tissues), precipitate the protein with $HgCl_2$, remove the mercury from the filtrate with H_2S, and determine lactic acid by Clausen's method.

Couette m., a method for measuring viscosity by calculating the rate of movement of an inner cylinder separatd from an outer cylinder by a thin layer of the fluid whose viscosity is being tested.

Coutard's m., a method of X-ray irradiation by protracted and fractionated dosage.

Creatine, m's for, see Folin's m. (7, 8), Folin, Benedict, and Myers' m. Folin and Wu's m. (2), and Meyer's m.

Creatinine, m's for, see Folin's m. (9), Folin and Wu's m. (1,2). and Shaffer's m. and see under tests.

Credé's m., 1. Method of expressing the placenta by forcing the uterus down into the pelvis and at the same time squeezing the uterus from all sides so that its contents are expelled. 2. a similar method for expressing urine from the bladder, especially in paralytic bladder. 3. the placing of a drop of 2 percent solution of silver nitrate in each eye of a newborn child for the prevention of ophthalmia neonatorum.

Cronin m., an operation to correct a flat nasal tip with short columella by using bilateral flaps of skin elevated in the floor of the nostrils.

Crystallizing oxyhemoglobin, m. for, see Reichert's m.

Cuignet's m., method of doing retinoscopy—see Shadow's test.

Cup plate m., see ring test (def. 1), under tests.

Dakin-Carrel m., Carrel's treatment—treatment of wounds, based on through exposure of the wound, removal of all foreign materials and devitalized tissue, meticulous cleansing, and repeated irrigation with a dilute hypochlorite solution. The adjacent skin is protected with a petrolatum gauze.

Dehn and Clark's m., (for chlorides), oxidize any interfering organic matter with sodium peroxide and then proceed with Volhard and Arnold's method.

Denis' m., (for magnesium in serum), remove the calcium by the Clark-Collip method, precipitate as magnesium ammonium phosphate, dissolve the precipitate in tenth normal HCl, reduce it with aminonaphthol-sulfonic acid and compare the blue color with a standard solution of ammonium magnesium phosphate in 0.1 percent HCl.

Denis and Leche's m., (for total sulfate), add acid and autoclave the decompose protein, then precipitate with barium chloride, dry and weigh.

Denman's m., a mechanism of spontaneous version in shoulder presentations in which the head rotates behind and as the breech descends the shoulder ascends in the pelvis, the breech finally coming down and emerging.

Dextrose, m's for, see glucose (dextrose), m's for.

Dickinson m., a method of controlling postpartum hemorrhage: the entire uterus is grasped through the abdominal wall, lifted out of the pelvis, and compressed against the spinal column.

Direct m., in ophthalmosoopy, that in which the ophthalmoscope is held close to the eye examined and an erect virtual image is obtaied of the fundus.

Direct aeration m., (for urea in blood), see Myers' m.

Direct centrifugal flotation m., see Lane m.

Disk diffusion m., see disk diffusion test, under tests.

Domagk's m., (for demonstration of reticuloendothelial cells), a culture of gram-positive staphylococci in physiologic salt solution is injected into the femoral vein of a rat which is then killed in fifteen to thirty minutes. In formalin-fixed sections stained by cresyl violet or by Gram's stain followed by alum-carmine, Kupffer's cells and other cells of the reticuloendothelial system stand out strikingly.

Douglas' m., a mechanism of spontaneous evolution of the fetus in the back anterior position with prolapse of the arm: the head, arrested above inlet, rotates to the pubis; the neck is applied to the pelvis brim; the chest; abdomen, and breech roll alongside the shoulder; the legs drop out, followed by the other arm and the head.

Duke's m., the period of duration of bleeding that follows controlled, standerdized puncture of the earlobe (Duke method) or forearm (Ivy method); a relatively inconsistent measure of capillary and platelet function.

Eggleston's m., a method of administering digitalis leaf.

Eicken's m., examination of the hypopharynx, with the cricoid cartilage drawn forward.

Ellinger's m., (for indican), precipitate the urine with basic lead acetate and filter. To the filtrate add Obermayer's reagent. Shake out the indigo with chloroform, evaporate off the chloroform, and titrate the residue with potassium permanganate.

Epstein's m., (for dextrose), a modification of the Lewis and Benedict method, making it possible to make the test with very little blood.

Fahraeus m., the original (1918) method for determination of the erythrocyte sedimentation rate (ESR); no longer used.

Fatty acids, m. for, see Bloor, Pelkan, and Alien's m.

Faust's m., a method of diagnosing helminth and protozoan infections by centrifugation of washed feces wtih zinc sulfate of a specific gravity of 1.180, after which eggs and protozoan cysts may be removed from the supernatant layer.

Fibrinogen, m. for, see Chandler's m.

Fichera's m., treatment of cancer by hypodermic injection of autolysed human fetal tissue.

Fick m., a restatement of the law of conservation of mass used in making indirect measurement, e.g., of cardiac output: the amount of blood traversing the pulmonary capillaries per unit of time is a measure of cardiac output and, because gas diffusion across the pulmonary alveolar walls depend on pulmonary blood flow, the cardiac output (liters per min.) equals O_2 absorption (cc per minute) divided by the arterial O_2 minus the mixed venous) O_2 (cc per liter).

Fishberg's m., one for determining specific gravity of the urine, which serves as a concentration test of renal function.

Fiske's m., (for total fixed base), remove phosphates with ferric chloride, convert fixed bases into sulfates by heating in H_2SO_4, ignite, take up in water, precipitate sulfates as benzidine sulfate, and titrate with alkali.

Fiske-Subbarow m., 1. (for acid-soluble phosphorus in blood), destroy organic matter by heating with sulfuric and nitric acids, precipitate the phosphates as magnesium ammonium phosphate, and reduce the precipitate with para-amino-naphthol-sulfonic acid. Compare the blue color with a standard phosphate solution. 2. (for inorganic phosphates), the phosphates are precipitated as ammonium phosphomolybdate. This is then reduced by para-amino-naphthol-sulfonic acid and the blue color compared colorimetrically with a standard solution.

Fitz Gerald m., treatment of disorder by mechanical stimulation of a body area located in the same longitudinal zone as the disorder.

Fixed base, m. for. see Fiske's m.

Flash m., the process of heating milk to destroy microorganisms that would cause spoilage. The milk is held at 62°C for 30 minutes or heated rapidly to 80°C and held for15 to 30 seconds and then chilled. The procedure kills most pathogenic bacteria while retaining the flavor of the liquid.

Flotation m., any method for separating cysts and ova from the heavier component of the stool and which depends upon the use of a solution intermediate in density between the parasitic material (which floats) and the bulk of the feces (which remains as sediment after centrifugation).

Folin's m., 1. (for acetone), aerate the acetone from the urine over into an alkaline hypo-iodite solution of known strength. The acetone is thus changed to iodoform and the excess of iodine is titrated with a standard thiosulfate solution, using starch as an indicator. 2. (for acetone), micromethod: aerate the acetone over into a solution of sodium bisulfite and then determine the amount of nephelometric comparison with a standard acetone solution using Scott and Wilson's reagent. 3. (for amino acids in blood), make 10 ml of protein-free blood filtrate slightly alkaline to phenolphthalein. Add 2 ml of beta-naphthaquinone solution and place in the dark. The next day add 2 ml of acetic acid-acetate solution and 2 ml of 4 percent thiosulfate solution. Dilute to A 25 ml and compare the blue color with a standard aminoacid solution similarly treated. 4. (for amino acid nitrogen in blood), treat the urine with permutit to remove the ammonia and then with beta-naphtha-quinone sulfonic acid. The red color is compared with a standard amino acid solution. 5. (for ammonia nitrogen), sodium carbonate is added to the urine to free the ammonia, which is aerated into standard acid and titrated. 6. (for blood sugar), to 2 ml of neutral protein-free blood filtrate, add 2 ml of the folin copper solution and heat in boiling water bath ten minutes. Cool and add 2 ml of acid molybdate reagent. Dilute to 25 ml mark and compare the blue color with a standard glucose solution similarly treated. 7. (for creatine), precipitate the proteins of the blood with picric acid and filter. To the filtrate add sodium hydroxide and compare color with a standard solution of creatine. 8. (for creatine in urine); change creatine into creatinine by heating at 90° C for three hours in the presence of third normal HCl. Determine creatinine by picric acid and alkali and deduct the preformed creatinine. 9. (for creatinine in urine), to the urine add picric acid and sodium hydroxide and compare the red color with a half normal solution of potassium bichromate. 10. (for ethereal sulfates), remove the inorganic sulfates with barium chloride and then the conjugated sulfates after hydrolyzing with boiling dilute hydrochloric acid. 11. (for inorganic sulfates), acidify the urine with hydrochloric acid, precipitate with barium chloride, filter, dry, ignite and weigh. 12. (for protein in urine), add acetic acid and heat, wash, dry, and weigh the precipitate. 13. (for total acidity), add potassium oxalate to the urine to precipitate the calcium which should otherwise precipitate at the neutral point, and titrate with tenth normal sodium hydroxide, using phenolphthalein as an indicator. 14. (for total sulfates), boil the urine for thirty minutes with dilute hydrochloric acid, precipitate with barium choride, filter, dry, ignite, and weigh. 15. (for urea and atlantoin), decompose the urea by heating with magnesium chloride and hydrochloric acid. Distil off the ammonia, and titrate.

Folin, Benedict, and Myers's m., (for creatine in urine), to 20 ml of urine add 20 ml of normal HCl and autoclave at 120°C for one-half hour. Neutralize, add picric acid and alkali, and compare the color with a standard solution of potassium bichromate.

Folin and Wu's m., 1. (for creatinine), the color produced by the unknown (protein-free blood filtrate or urine) in an alkaline solution of picric acid is compared in a colorimeter with the color produced by a known solution of creatinine or with a standard solution of potassium bichromate. 2. (for creatine plus creatinine), the creatine of a protein-free blood filtrate is changed to creatinine by heating with dilute HCl in an autoclave, and the creatinine thus produced together with the preformed is determined colorimetrically after adding an alkaline picrate solution. 3. (for glucose), the protein-free blood filtrate is boiled with a dilute alkaline copper tartrate solution, the cuprous oxide is dissolved by adding a phosphomolybdic-phosphoric acid solution, and the blue color produced is compared with the color from sugar solutions of known strength. 4. (nonprotein nitrogen), the total nonprotein nitrogen in the protein-free blood filtrate is determined by setting free the nitrogen as ammonia by the Kjeldahl process, nesslerizing this ammonia, and comparing with a standard, 5. (for protein-free blood filtrate), lake the blood with distilled water, add sodium tungstate and sulfuric acid, and filter. 6. (for urea), change the urea to ammonia by means of urease, and nesslerize. 7 (for uric acid), uric acid is precipitated from the protein-free blood filtrate or from urine by silver lactate, treated with phosphotungstic acid, and the blue color compared with the color produced by known amounts of uric acid.

M's for (volatilizing) formaldehyde gas, see Aronson's m., Breslau's m. Schlossmann's m., and Trillat's m.

Formol titration, m's of, see Malfatti's m., and Sorensen's m.

Freiburg m., twilight sleep—a condition of analgesia and amnesia, produced by hypodermic administration of morphine and scopalmine. In this state the patient, although responding to pain, does not retain it in her memory. Formerly widely used in obstetrics.

Frey and Gigon's m., (for amino acid nitrogen), a modified form of Sorensen's method in that the ammonia is aspirated off after adding the barium hydroxide.

Fridericia's m., (for alveolar carbon dioxide tension), the carbon dioxide is absorbed into a solution of potassium hydroxide and the decrease in volume read in percentage in a special apparatus.

Fulleborn's m., (for ova in stools), grind 1 gm of stool and mix with 20 ml of a saturated solution of sodium chloride. Allow to stand one hour or more, then float cover glasses on the surface and transfer them, without draining, to slides.

Gasometric m., (for urea), see Stehle's m.

Gerota's m., injection of the lymphatics with a dye; such as prussian blue, which is soluble in chloroform or ether, but not in water.

Girard's m., treatment of sea sickness by hypodermic or oral administration of atropine sulfate and strychnine sulfate.

Givens' m., (for peptic activity), varying amounts of diluted gastric juice are added to a series of tubes containing pea globulin, the mixtures are incubated, and the amount of digestion noted.

Glucose (dextrose), m's for, see Bang's m., Epstein's m,. Folin's m. (6), Folin and Wu's m. (3). Hagedorn and Jensen's m., Lewis and Benedict's m., Peter's Power and Wilder's m., Stammer's and Summer's m. See also dextrose test, under tests.

Gold number m., see colloidal gold test.

Gram's m., an empirical staining procedure devised by gram in which microorganisms are stained with crystal violet, treated with 1:15 dilution of Lugol's iodine, decolorized with ethanol or ethanol-acetone and counterstained with a contrasting dye, usually safranin. Those microorganisms that retain the crystal violet stain are said to be gram-positive, and those that lose the crystal violet stain by decolorization but stain with the counterstain are said to be gram negative.

Greenwald's m., (for non-protein nitrogen), the proteins are precipitated by trichloracetic acid, the filtrate is decomposed by sulfuric acid as in the Kjeldahl method, the ammonia is distilled off and the amount titrated with tenth normal sodium hydroxide.

Greenwald and Lewman's m., (for titratable alkali of blood), the protein of the blood is precipitated with an excess of picric acid. Both the free and the total picric acid in the filtrate are then determined. The difference represents the picric acid which is combined with the bases of the blood.

Griffith's m., (for hippuric acid), extract the hippuric acid with ether. Distil off the ether and destroy urea in the residue with sodium hypobromite solution. Determine the nitrogen in the residue by the Kjeldahl method.

Gross's m., (for tryptic activity), add increasing amounts of a trypsin solution to a series of tubes of pure. Fat-free casein which have been heated to 40°C. Incubate at 40°C for fifteen minutes. Test by adding a few drops of acetic acid (dilute) to each tube. A precipitate on acidification indicates that digestion is incomplete or lacking: no precipitate indicates digestion.

Guanidine, m's for, see Pfiffner and Myers' m. and Weber's m.

Guinard's m., application of calcium carbide to ulcerating tumors.

Hagedorn and Jensen's m., (for sugar in blood), precipitate the protein with zinc hydroxide. Heat the filtrate with potassium ferricyanide solution and determine the amount of ferricyanide reduced by adding an iodide solution and titrating the iodine set free with sodium thiosulfate.

Hall's m., for total purine nitrogen), remove phosphates by means of magnesia mixture and precipitate the purine bodies in a specially graduated tube by means of silver nitrate and ammonium hydroxide. After twenty-four hours read the volume of the purine precipitate.

Hamilton's m., (in postpartum hemorrhage), compress the uterus between a fist in the vagina and a hand pressing down the abdominal wall.

Hammer-Schlag's m., (for specific gravity of blood), prepare a mixture of benzene and chloroform of about 1.050 specific gravity. Into this let fall a drop of blood and add benzene or chloroform until the drop neither rises nor sinks. Then take the specific gravity of the mixture.

Heintz's m., (for uric acid), precipitate the urine by adding hydrochloric acid, filter off the crystals, wash, dry, and weigh.

Hemoglobin, m's for, see acid hematin m., Dare's m., and Sahli's m: and see under tests..

Henriques and Sorensen's m., (for aminoacid nitrogen by solution of formaldehyde titration), see Sorensen's m.

Herter and Foster's m., (for indole in feces, modified by Bergeim), make the feces alkaline and distil. Make the distillate acid and distil again. To the second distillate add beta-naphtha-quinone sodium monosulfonate and alkali. Extract the blue color with chloroform and compare it with a standard solution of indole containing 0.1 mg of indole per milliliter.

Heublein m., ionizing irradiation of the whole body with low-dose increments protracted for ten to twenty hours per day over several days.

Hippuric acid m., see Griffith's m.and Roafs m., and see under tests.

Hirschberg s m., measurement of the deviation of a strabismic eye by observing the reflection of a candle from the cornea.

Holding m., see flash method.

Howard's m., (of artificial respiration), the patient is placed on his back, hands under his head, with a cushion so placed that his head is lower than his abdomen. Manual rhythmical pressure is then applied upward and inward against the lower lateral parts of the chest.

Howell's m., (for clotting time of blood), place 5 ml of blood in a 21 mm. test tube with suitable precautions. Tilt the tube every two minutes and note time of clotting.

Hunter and Given's m., (for uric acid and purine bases), precipitate and decompose precipitate as in the Krueger-Schmidt method. Determine the uric acid in an aliquot part and in the remainder destroy the uric acid by oxidation and determine the purine bases as in the Krueger-Schmidt method.

Hydrogen ion concentration, m. for, see Levy, Rowntree and Harriott's m., indican m's for, see Askenstedt's m. and Ellinger's m. and see under tests.

Indole, m's for, see Herter and Foster m. and see under tests.

Inorganic phosphates, m. for, see phosphates, inorganic, m. for.

Inorganic sulfates, m's for, see sulfates, inorganic, m's for.

Iodine, m's for, see specific methods, including Kendall's m., Leipert's m.

Iron m's for, see Walker's m., Walter's m., and see under tests.

Ivy's m., see Duke method.

Japanese m., a method for fixing paraffin sections to glass slides with the use of Mayer's albumin.

Johnson m., a modification of the Callahan method (def. 1) in which the canal is initially flooded with alcohol, allowing diffusion of the chloroform component of the chloroform-rosin solution: alcohol deep in the dentin facilitates rosin dissolved in the chloroform to be diffused into the dentin.

Kaiserling's m., a procedure for preserving the natural colors in museum preparations, employing formaldehyde and potassium acetate.

Karr's m., (for urea in blood), change the urea to ammonium carbonate by means of urease, nesslerize directly and compare the color with that of a standard urea solution similarly treated.

Kendall's m., for iodine in thyroid tissue), oxidize the organic matter by fusion in KNO_3 and strong KOH. Acidify, oxidize with bromine, add an excess of KI, and titrate the liberated iodine with sodium thiosulfate.

Kety-Schmidt m., a method of measuring perfusion flow of blood through brain tissue.

Kirstein's m., inspection of the larynx without a laryngoscope by having the patient incline his head far back and depressing the tongue.

Kjeldahl's m. (1883), a method of determining the amount of nitrogen in an organic compound. It consists in heating the material to be analyzed with strong sulfuric acid. The nitrogen is thereby converted to ammonia, which is distilled off and caught in tenth normal solution of sulfuric acid. By titration the amount of ammonia is determined, and from this the amount of nitrogen is estimated.

Kluver-Barrera m., a histologic staining method in which myelin sheaths are stained blue-green and the cells purple.

Koch and McMeekin's m. (for total nitrogen), destroy organic matter with sulfuric acid and hydrogen peroxide, and nesslerize the resulting solution directly.

Korotkoffs m., the auscultatory method of determining blood pressure.

Kramer and Gittleman's m. (for sodium in serum), dry and ash the serum. Take it up in 0.1 percent HCl and make slightly alkaline with KOH. Precipitate with the pyroantimonate reagent and alcohol, dissolve precipitate in strong HCl add potassium iodide, and titrate with sodium thiosulfate.

Kramer and Tisdall's m., 1. (for potassium in serum), precipitate with sodium cobaltinitrite reagent, treat precipitate with acid permanganate solution, then with sodium oxalate, and titrate with standard permanganate. 2. (for calcium in serum), precipitate the calcium as oxalate. Wash, dissolve, and titrate with potassium permanganate.

Kristeller's m., a method of expelling the fetus in labor. The fetal head should be in the vulva and the abdomen must be sufficiently relaxed so that the assistant may grasp the fundus. The grip on the fundus is made by the fingers of the two hands parallel behind and the thumb in front, the line of force being in the direction of the axis of the inlet. The expression should be done in one or two sustained efforts.

Krogh's m., (for urea), the urea is oxidized by sodium hypobromite to carbon dioxide and nitrogen in an alkaline solution which absorbs the carbon dioxide. The remaining nitrogen is then measured.

Krueger and Schmidt's m., (for uric acid and purine bases), precipitate the uric acid with copper sulfate, decompose the precipitate with sodium sulfite, acidify, concentrate and let uric acid crystals separate. Determine the nitrogen in them by the Kjeldahl method. Reprecipitate the purine bases with copper sulfate, filter, wash, and determine the nitrogen in the precipitate by the Kjeldahl method.

Kwilecki's m., (for albumin), 10 drops of a 10 percent solution of ferric chloride are added to the urine before proceeding with the regular method of Esbach.

Laborde's m., the making of rhythmic traction movements on the tongue in order to stimulate the respiratory center in asphyxiation.

Lactalbumin, m. for, remove casein from the milk with magnesium sulfate. Add Alman's reagent to the filtrate, determine the nitrogen in the precipitate with the Kjeldahl method, and multiply the result by 6.37.

Lactic acid, m's for, see specific methods, including Clausen's m. (1), (2), Corri's m., von Furth and Charnass' m. See also lactic acid test, under tests.

Lamaze m., psychoprophylactic method of preparing for delivery, involving education the prospective mother in the physiology of pregnancy and parturition and in techniques (e.g., breathing exercises and bearing down) to ease delivery.

Lane m., a method of diagnosing hookworm infection by centrifugation of 1 ml of washed feces mixed with brine, the tube being covered with a cover slip on which the eggs can be counted. Called also direct centrifugal flotation method, or DCF.

Lateral condensation m., a method of filling a root canal in which the main portion of the canal is filled with a primary gutta-percha cone or silver point and sealer cement or paste and the remaining space is packed with auxiliary gutta-percha cones. Spreader sites and pluggers are used to force gutta-percha into the canal laterally and sometimes vertically. Called also multiple cone m.

Leboyer m., a method of delivery of the infant based upon the theory that the violence associated with birth causes emotional trauma to the infant and that this trauma will affect the child's personality throughout his life. The concepts of this method emphasize that the delivery should be gentle and controlled, without unnecessary intervention; the infant should be handled gently, with the head, neck, and sacrum supported; the infant should not be overstimulated and should be allowed to breathe spontaneously, without painful stimuli, such as spanking. Called also Leboyer technique.

Leipert's m., (for iodine in blood), destroy organic matter with chromic-sulfuric acid. Reduce iodic acid to free iodine with arsenous acid, distil off the iodine, and titrate.

Levy, Rowntree, and Marriotfs m., (for hydrogen ion concentration of blood, kdialyze the blood through a collodion tube against neutral physiologic salt solution; then match the color produced by phenolsulfonphthalein in the dialysate and in solution of known hydrogen ion concentration.

Lewis and Benedict's m., (for dextrose)! the proteins of the blood are precipitated by means of picric acid, sodium carbonate is added, and the color of the picramic acid solution is compared with that of a standard glucose solution.

Lewisohns m.(obs.), a method of indirect transfusion by adding sodium citrate to the blood.

Lime m., a method of generating or volatilizing formaldehyde gas. Forty percent formaldehyde, containing 10 percent of sulfuric acid, is poured over quicklime in a suitable container; 1-1/2 to 2 pounds of lime should be used for each pint of the solution.

Lovset's m., see under maneuver.

Lyman's m., (for calcium), precipitate the calcium from the protein-free blood filtrate or from urine as calcium oxalate, redissolve in dilute acid and reprecipitate as calcium ricinate, and determine the amount nephelometrically.

McCrudden's m., (for calcium and magnesium), make 200 ml of urine faintly acid to litmus, add 10 ml of concentrated hydrochloric acid, precipitate with oxalic acid, filter, ignite, and weigh as calcium oxide, or filter and titrate the precipitate with potassium permanganate. This gives the calcium. For the magnesium, add to the filtrate from the calcium, nitric acid, evaporate to dryness, and heat until the residue fuses. Take up in water, add sodium acid phosphate and ammonia, filter, wash, ignite, and weigh as the pyrophosphate.

McLean and Van Slyke's m., (for chlorides), precipitate the chlorides from oxalated plasma with an excess of silver nitrate and titrate the excess with potassium iodide and starch.

Magnesium, m's for, see Denis' m and McCrudden's m.

Malfatti's m., (for ammonia nitrogen by solution of formaldehyde titration), add potassium oxalate to the urine and make neutral to phenolphthalein with tenth normal sodium hydroxide; add the neutral solution of formaldehyde and titrate again.

Marriott's m., (for alkali reserve), the patient rebreathes the air in a bag until its carbon dioxide tension is virtually that of venous blood. This air is then bubbled through a standard bicarbonate solution until the solution is saturated and the color produced is compared with standard color tubes.

Marshall's m., (for urea), the urea is changed into ammonium carbonate by the enzyme urease and the ammonia titrated with tenth normal hydrochloric acid, using methyl orange, as indicator.

Meltzer's m., insufflation, through an endotracheal tube, of air containing an anesthetic vapor; employed in thoracic surgery.

Messinger and Huppert's m., (for acetone), the same as the method of Folin and Hart except that the acetone is distilled instead of aspirated.

Mett's m., (for peptic activity), see Nirenstein and Schiffs m.

Meulengracht s m., (for bile pigment in serum), the serum is diluted until the yellow color corresponds to that of a standard potassium bichromate solution.

Meyer's m., (for creatine), a modification of Folin and Benedict's method in that the creatine is changed into creatinine after adding hydrochloric acid by digesting in an autoclave.

Moerner-Sjoqvist m., see Sjoqvist's m.

Mohr's m., (for chlorides), oxidize interfering organic matter by igniting with potassium nitrate. To the solution of the ash add potassium chromate and titrate with standard silver nitrate until the red silver chromate appears.

Monias and Shapiro's m., convert the indican into indigolignon and compare with a standard.

Multiple cone m., see lateral condensation m.

Murphy m., 1. Suture of an artery by invaginating the ends over a cylinder in two pieces which can then be removed. 2. Continuous proctoclysist—the continuous administration per rectum of saline solution, drop by drop, from an elevated reservoir. Called also murphy drip.

Myers' m., (for urea in blood), change the urea to ammonium carbonate by the action of urease, aerate off the ammonia into an acid solution and nesslerize; called also direct aeration m.

Myers and Wardell's m., (for cholesterol), dry the blood on plaster of Paris and extract the cholesterol with chloroform. Add acetic anhydride and sulfuric acid and compare the color with that of a standard solution of cholesterol similarly treated.

Neumann's m., local anesthesia for surgery on the ear by the subperiosteal injection of a solution of cocaine and epinephrine.

Nikiforoff's m., a method of fixing blood films by placing them for from five to fifteen minutes in absolute alcohol, pure ether, or equal parts of alcohol and ether.

Nimeh's m., a method of determining the size of liver and spleen, based on measurements made on flat films of the hepatic and splenic regions taken separately without any preparation or after retroperitoneal insufflation of carbon dioxide gas. The ventricle diameter is the index of the size of the liver, the broad diameter that of the spleen.

Nirenstein and Schiffs m., (for peptic activity), Mett's tubes are placed in the solution to be tested and incubated for twenty-four hours. The length of the column digested at each end is then determined.

Nitrogen, amino acid, m's for, see Folin's m. (4), Frey and Giron's m., Sorensen's m., van Slyke's m., and van Slyke and Meyer's m.

Nitrogen, ammonia, m's for, see Folin's m. (5), Malfatti's m. and see under tests.

Nitrogen, nonprotein, m's for, see Folin and Denis' m. (4), Folin and Wu's m. (4), and Greenwald's m.

Nitrogen, purine, m. for, see Hall's m.

Nitrogen, total, m's for, see Arnold and Gunning's m, Bock and Benedict's m., Koch and McMeekin's m., Taylor and Hulton's m.

Oberst's m., local anesthesia produced by injecting saline solution or distilled water into the subcutaneous connective tissue.

Ogata's m., a method of stimulating respiration by stroking the chest.

Ogino-Knaus m., the rhythm method of birth control.

Optical density m., the measuring of growth rates of cells by taking the optical density or turbidity of a dense population and comparing this with optical densities of known dilutions of the sample.

Orr m., see closed plaster method.

Orsi-Grocco m., palpatory percussion of the heart.

Osborne and Folin's m., (for total sulfur in urine), destroy the organic matter in the concentrated urine and oxidize the sulfur by fusing with sodium peroxide. Precipitate with barium chloride, wash, dry, ignite, and weigh.

Ova concentration, m. for, see brine flotation m.

Oxalic acid, m. for, see Salkowski, Autenrieth and Barth's m.

Panoptic m., a solution containing azure ll-eosin, azurell, glycerin, and methanol; used for staining protozoan parasites such as *Plasmodium* and *Trypanosoma Chlamydia* for differential staining of blood smears, and for viral inclusion bodies, stained elements appear pink to purple to blue.

Pap's silver m., a method for demonstrating reticulum.

Parker's m., (for indican), see Askenstedt's m.

Peptic activity, m's for, see specific methods, including Givens' m., Nirenstein and Schiff's m.

Peter's m., (for dextrose), boil the unknown in an excess of the reagent, filter off the reduced copper, and titrate the filtrate with potassium iodide and standard thiosulfate solution.

Pfiffner and Myers' m., (for guanidine in blood), a colorimetric method by the use of an alkaline nitroprusside-ferricyanide reagent.

Phenol, m's for, see Tisdall's m. See also phenol test under tests.

Phosphates, inorganic, m's for, see Fiske and Subbarow'g m. (2).

Phosphorus, m. for, see uranium acetate m.

Phosphorus, acid-soluble, m. for, see Fiske and Subbarow's m. (1).

Plimmer and Skelton's m., (for allantoin), determine the urea and allantoin by Folin's method (15), and the urea alone by Marshall's urease method. The difference is allantoin.

Point source m., a method of intracavitary irradiation of the bladder wall utilizing a small point source of radiation at the center of a Foleys catheter bag inflated with a radiopaque solution containing methylene blue or indigo carmine.

Potassium, m. for, see Kramer and Tisdall's m. (1).

Power and Wilder's m., (for glucose in urine), remove interfering substances with mercuric sulfate. To the filtrate add alkaline ferricyanide; heat for ten minutes, cool, and add Kl and an acid zinc sulfate solution. Titrate the liberated iodine with standard thiosulfate solution

Price-Jones m., a frequency distribution curve of erythrocyte diameters in peripheral blood smear, estimated visually with the aid of an optical micrometer.

Protein in milk, m. for, see Bogg's m.

Protein-free blood filtrate, m's for, see Folin's m. (6), and Folin and Wu's m. (5).

Purdy's m., the use of the centrifuge for the determination of the quantity of albumin, chlorides, sulfates. etc.

Purine bodies, m's for, see Hunter and Given's m; Krueger and Schmidt's m., Salkowski's m. Satkowski and Arnstein's m., and Welker's m. and see under tests.

Purine, nitrogen, m. for, see Hall's m.

Radioactive balloon m., a method of intracavitary irradiation of the bladder wall utilizing a Foley catheter bag filled with a radioactive solution.

Raiziss and Dubin's m., (for ethereal and inorganic sulfates), oxidize the urine by Benedict's method, precipitate the sulfate with benzidine hydrochloride, as in the method of Rosenheim and Drummond, and titrate with tenth normal potassium permanganate.

Rehfuss' m., see under tests.

Retrofilling m., a method of filling root canal of a tooth from the apex of a root which has been surgically exposed; zinc free silver alloy is the most commonly used filling material.

Rhythm m., a method of preventing conception by restricting coitus to the so-called safe period, avoiding the days just before and after the expected time of ovulation.

Rideal-Walker m., a method for testing the bactericidal activity of a disinfectant as compared with that of phenol. Cultures of *Salmonella typhi* are incubated with serial dilutions of the test compound, with dilutions of phenol as standards. Samples are removed at intervals, transferred to sterile broth, and the resulting cultures incubated and examined for bacterial growth. Activity is expressed as the ratio of effective concentration of test compound divided by that of phenol (phenol coefficient).

Ritchie's formolether m., a method whereby feces, fixed in a formol-saline solution, are subjected to extraction with ether to remove fatty materials, and the washed sediment examined for protozoan cysts and helminth ova.

Ritgen's m., see under maneuver.

Roaf's m., (for the preparation of hippuric acid), add 125 gm of ammonium sulfate and 7.5 gm of concentrated sulfuric acid to 500 ml of urine of a horse. Hippuric acid will crystallize out.

Romanovsky's (Romanowsky's) m., the prototype of the many eosin-methylene blue stains for blood smears and malarial parasites, including Giemsa stain, Leishman's stain, and Wright stain.

Rosenheim and Drummond's m., (for ethereal and inorganic sulfates), precipitate the sulfates with benzidine hydrochloride and titrate the acid in the benzidine sulfate with tenth normal potassium hydroxide.

Ruhemann's uricometer m., (for uric acid), urine is added in a specially graduated tube to a mixture of carbon bisulfide and iodine solution until the carbon bisulfide is decolorized.

Sahli's m., (for estimation of hemoglobin), convert the hemoglobin into acid hematin by, adding HCl and compare the color with a standard color scale.

Salkowski's m., (for purine bodies and uric acid), precipitate as silver magnesium salts, decompose the precipitate with hydrogen sulfide, precipitate uric acid by means of sulfuric acid, and the purine bodies as silver salts.

Salkowski and Arnstein's m., (for purines), precipitate the urine with magnesia mixture and to the filtrate add 3 percent ammoniacal silver nitrate solution. Wash the precipitate and determine the nitrogen in it by the Kjeldahl method. The uric acid nitrogen is separately determined and deducted.

Salkowski, Autenrieth, and Barth's m., (for oxalic acid), precipitate the oxalic acid by means of calcium chloride. Dissolve the precipitate in hydrochloric acid, extract the oxalic acid with ether, and reprecipitate it as calcium oxalate.

Satterthwaite's m., artificial respiration produced by alternating pressure and relaxation upon the abdomen.

Scherer's m., (for proteins), precipitate the protein by boiling with dilute acetic acid, wash, dry, and weigh.

Schlossmann's m., to prevent polymerization, 10 percent of glycerin is added to formaldehyde before it is volatilized by heat.

Schuller's m., a method of performing artificial respiration by rhythmic raisings of the thorax by means of the fingers hooked under the ribs.

Schweninger's m., reduction of obesity by the restriction of fluids in the diet.

Scott and Wilson's m., (for acetone and acetoacetic acid), distil the acetone into an alkaline solution of basic mercuric cyanide, filter, and titrate the precipitate with potassium thiocyanate.

Sectional m., segmentation m., a method of filling a root canal in which 2 to 3 mm. cut sections of gutta-percha cones are packed in the canal individually until it is filled.

Shaffer's m., (for creatinine), Folin's method (9), adapted to very dilute solutions.

Shaffer-Hartmann m., a chemical method for determining glucose levels in the blood, utilizing a cupric reagent incorporating potassium iodate and iodide and based on the amount of iodate reduced by the cuprous oxide to iodide, and thus on the amount of reducing sugars present.

Shaffer and Marriott's m., (for acetone bodies), precipitate the urine with basic lead acetate and ammonia. Distil off the acetone (acetone and diacetic acid). Oxidize the residue with potassium bichromate and distil again (beta-hydroxybutyric acid). Titrate the distillates with standard iodine and thiosulfate solutions.

Shohl and Pedley's m., (for calcium in urine), oxidize the urine with ammonium persulfate, precipitate the calcium as oxalate, add H_2SO_4 to the precipitate, and titrate with potassium permanganate.

Siffert m., a method for computing the volume of the gallbladder by tracing the gallbladder shadow on transparent paper and comparing it with a standard.

Silver point (cone) m., a method of filling a root canal in which a prefitted silver point is sealed into the apex of the root canal;

irregularities in the canal not sealed with the point are obliterated with gutta-percha by lateral condensation or segmentation, or by a root canal paste or sealer.

Single cone m., a method of filling the root canal of a tooth with a single, well-fitting gutta-percha cone or silver point in conjunction with a sealer cement or paste.

Sippy m., a regimen of treatment of peptic ulcer based on neutralization of hydrochloric acid by frequent feedings and the use of alkalies in carefully regulated but adequate quantities.

Sjoqvist's m., quantitative estimation of the urea in the urine by means of a baryta mixture.

Sluder m., removal of the tonsils by means of a tonsil guillotine.

Smellie's m., delivery of the aftercoming head with the body of the child resting on the forearm of the obstetrician.

Sodium, m. for, see Kramer and Gittleman s m.

Somogyi m., 1. (for blood glucose), a modification of the Shaffer-Hartmann method in which the cuprous oxide reduces an arsenomolybdate reagent, yielding a more stable end product. 2. (for amylase activity), a method based on the disappearance of the blue color given by iodine and amylose (linear fraction of starch) after amylase in serum, urine, etc., is allowed to act on starch.

Sorensen's m. (for amino acids by solution of formaldehyde titration), titrate the urine for total acidity using phenolphthalein as indicator, add fresh solution of formaldehyde (15 ml. of formalin, 30 ml. of water, and sufficient sodium to make it faintly alkaline to phenolphthalein), and titrate again.

Specific gravity, m. for, see Hammerschlag's m. and Fishberg's m. and see under tests.

Split cast m., 1. A procedure for placing indexed caste on a dental articulator to facilitate their removal and replacement on the instrument. 2. The procedure of checking the ability of a dental articulator to receive or be adjusted to a maxillomandibular relation record. Called also split cast mounting.

Stammer's m., (for glucose in blood), precipitate blood proteins by boiling with acid sodium sulfate and treatment with dialyzed iron. In a test tube place 20 ml of blood filtrate, 2 drops of a 20 percent solution of sodium hydroxide and 1ml of a 0.0075 percent solution of methylene blue. Boil until the blue color is discharged. The length of time required indicates the amount of sugar present. Time is counted from the beginning of vigorous boiling: thirty-seven seconds indicates 0.3 percent sugar; sixty seconds, 0.225 percent; one minute twenty-five seconds. 0.175 percent; one minute fifty-five seconds, 0.125 percent; and two minutes forty-five seconds, 0.075 percent.

Stas-Otto m., a method of separating alkaloids and similar amino compounds.

Stehle's m., (for urea), decompose the urea in a van Slyke pipet by sodium hypobromite and measure the nitrogen; called also gasometric m.

Stockholm and Koch's m., (for total sulfur in biological material), the material is disintegrated by heating in strong sodium hydroxide, then oxidized with 30 percent H_2O_2 and then with nitric acid, and bromine. Precipitate the sulfuric acid with barium, wash, dry, ignite, and weigh.

Sugar, m' for, see glucose (dextrose), m's for.

Sulfates, ethereal, m's for, see Folin's m. (10), Raiziss and Dubin's m. and Rosenheim and Drummond's m.

Sulfates, inorganic, m's for, see Folin's m. (11), Raiziss and Dubin's m. and Rosenheim and Drummond's m.

Sulfur, total, m's for, see Denis and Leche's m., Folin's m. (14), Osborne and Folin's m. and Stockholm and Koch's m.

Sumner's m., (for sugar in urine), heat 1 ml of urine and 3 ml of Sumner's dinitrosalicylic acid reagent, dilute to 25 ml and compare the color with that of a standard sugar solution similarly treated.

Suspension m., a method of intracavitary irradiation of the bladder wall by instilling a radioactive solution or suspension directly into the bladder by means of a catheter.

Taylor and Hulton's m., (for total nitrogen), similar to Folin and Farmer's method except that small amounts of sulfuric acid are used and the ammonia is nesslerized in the original tube without being aerated over into acid.

Thane's m., a method of locating the fissure of Rolando. Its upper end is about one-half inch behind the middle of a line uniting the inion and the glabella, and its lower end about one-quarter inch above and one and one-quarter inches behind the external angular process of the frontal bone.

Thezac-Porsmeur m., heliotherapy of suppurating wounds by concentrating the sun's rays on the part by means of a large double convex lens mounted on a cylinder of canvas three feet long.

Thyroid activity, m. for, see thyroid function tests, under tests.

Tisdall's m., (for phenols in urine), extract the phenolic substances from the urine with ether and then shake them from the ether with 10 percent NaOH. Neutralize and proceed as in the Folin and Denis method (5).

Total acidity, m. for, see Folin's m. (13).

Total fixed base, m. for, see Fiske's m.

Total nitrogen, m. for, see nitrogen, total, m.'s for.

Total sulfur, m. for, see sulfur, total, m.'s for.

Tracy and Welker's m., (for deproteinizing urine), a method depending on the use of aluminum hydroxide cream.

Trillat's m., volatilization of formaldehyde in an autoclave under pressure to prevent polymerization.

Trueta m., see closed plaster m.

Tryptic activity, m. for, see Gross's m.

Tswett's m., any of a diverse group of techniques used to seperate mixtures of substances based on differences in the relative affinities of the substances for two different media, one (the mobile phase) a moving fluid and the other (stationary phase or sorbent) a porous solid or gel or a liquid coated on a solid support; the speed at which each substance is carried along by the mobile phase depends on its solubility (in a liquid mobile phase) for vapour pressure (in a gas mobile phase) and on its affinity for the sorbent.

Tuffier's m., anesthesia produced by injection of a local anesthetic into the subarachnoid space around the spinal cord.

Uranium acetate m., (for phosphorus), add sodium acetate and acetic acid to the urine, heat to boiling, and titrate with a special uranium acetate solution.

Urea, m's for, see Benedict's m. (3), Clark and Collip's m. (2), Folin's m. (15), Folin and Wu's m. (6), Karr's m., Krogh's m., Marshall's m., Myers' m., Sjoqvist's m., Stehle's m., and van Slyke and Cullen's m. (2). See also urea test, under tests.

Urease m's, see Marshall's m. and van Slyke and Cullen's m. (2), and see under tests.

Uric acid, m's for, see Folin and Wu's m. (7), Heintz's m., Hunter and Given's m. Krueger and Schmidt's m., Ruhemann's m., and Salkowski's m. See also uric acid test under tests.

Urobilinogen, m. for, see Wallace and Diamond's m. and see urobilin test, under tests.

Van Gehuchten's m., fixing of a histologic tissue in a mixture of glacial acetic acid 10 parts, chloroform 30 parts, and alcohol 60 parts.

van Slyke's m., (for amino-nitrogen), the unknown is treated with nitrous acid in a special apparatus and the nitrogen liberated is measured.

van Slyke and Cullen's m., 1. (for the carbon dioxide in blood, or for the alkali reserve of blood), freshly prepared oxalated plasma is brought into equilibrium with the carbon dioxide of expired air, add is then added to a measured amount of the blood, and the carbon dioxide is pumped out and measured. 2. (for urea), the urea is changed into ammonium carbonate by means of the enzyme urease. The ammonia is aerated over into standard acid, and the excess titrated.

van Slyke and Fitz's m., (for alkali reserve), collect the urine for a two-hour period between meals; note amount and determine the ammonia and the titratable acid by Folin's methods. The plasma carbon dioxide capacity (C) may be calculated from the formula C = 80-5, $\sqrt{D \div W}$ where D = rate of excretion per twenty-four hours, and W = body weight in kilograms.

van Slyke and Meyer's m., (for amino acid nitrogen), precipitate the proteins of the blood by means of alcohol and then proceed by van Slyke's nitrous acid method.

van Slyke and Palmer's m., (for organic acids in urine), remove carbonates and phosphates and titrate with acid from the turning point for phenolphthalein to the turning point for tropeolin 00.

Vertical condensation m., a method of filling a root canal by alternately heating and vertically condensing gutta-percha until the apical third of the canal is filled; the coronal portion of the canal is then filled with warmed 2 to 4 mm sections of gutta-percha cones.

Volhard and Arnold's m., (for chlorides), acidify the urine with nitric acid and add a known amount of silver nitrate. Titrate excess of silver nitrate with ammonium sulfocyanate, using ferric thiocyanate as indicator.

Volhard and Harvey's m., (for chlorides); similar to the method of Volhard and Arnold except that the silver chloride is not filtered out, the excess of silver nitrate being titrated in the original mixture.

von Furth and Charnass'm., (for lactic acid in blood), remove the glucose and convert the lactic acid into acetaldehyde by permanganate. Combine the aldehyde with sodium bisultite and determine the bound sulfite iodometrically.

Walker's m., (for iron in foods), ignite sample, cool, and dissolve in dilute HNO_3. Filter, oxidize, filtrate with H_2O_2, add potassium thiocyanate, and compare color with standard iron solution, similarly treated.

Wallace and Diamond's m., (for urobilinogen), add Ehrlich's aldehyde reagent to a series of dilutions of the urine, note the highest dilution which shows a faint pink coloration, and express the result in terms of this dilution.

Wallhauser and Whitehead's m., the use of autogenous gland filtrate in the treatment of Hodgkin's disease.

Waring's m., a method of sewage disposal by subsurface irrigation; called also Waring's system.

Weber's m., (for guanidine), a colorimetric method based on the reaction of guanidine with an alkaline nitroprusside-ferricyanide reagent.

Welcker's m., determination of the total blood volume by bleeding and then washing out the blood vessels.

Welker's m. (for purine bodies): remove the phosphates with magnesia mixture, then precipitate the purine bodies with silver nitrate and ammonium hydroxide. Determine nitrogen in the precipitate by Kjeldahl's method.

Welker and Marsh's m., (for clarifying milk), a method using aluminum hydroxide.

Westergren m., (for erythrocyte sedimentation rate [ESR]), the standard method for ESR, used since 1924; four volumes of whole blood are mixed with one volume of sodium citrate anticoagulant-diluent solution and placed in a Westergren tube, a straight pipette 2.5 mm in internal diameter and graduated in millimeters from 0 to 200, filling to the 0 mark; the tube is left standing undisturbed in a vertical position, and the fall of the level of red cells in exactly one hour is recorded (in mm/hr).

Whipple's m., the use of liver in pernicious anemia.

White-horn's m., (for chlorides in blood), to the protein-free blood filtrate, add nitric acid, then heat, and add an excess of silver nitrate. Titrate excess silver with thiocyanate, using ferric ammonium sulfate as indicator.

Wiechowski and Handorsky's m., (for allantoin), precipitate the urine writs phosphotungstic acid, with lead acetate, and with silver acetate to remove chlorides, ammonia, and basic substance. Then add sodium acetate and 0.5 percent mercuric acetate to precipitate the allantoin, which may be weighed submitted to a Kjeldahl, or titrated with ammonium thiocyanate.

Wintrobe m., (for erythrocyte sedimentation rate [ESRI EDTA]) anticoagulated whole blood is placed in a Wintrobe hematocrit tube, the tube is left standing undisturbed in a vertical position, and the fall of the level of red cells in exactly one hour is recorded (in mm/hr). The volume of packed red cells can then be determined using the same tube.

Wintrobe and Landsberg's m., (for the sedimentation rate of red blood cells), determine the amount of sedimentation after one hour, then centrifuge and measure the volume of the packed red cells. Correct the first reading by the second by means of a table.

Wolter's m., (for iron), add nitric acid to urine, evaporate to dryness, ignite, oxidize the iron wits hydrogen peroxide, add potassium iodide and starch, and titrate excess of iodine with one-hundredth normal thiosulfate.

Wynn m., a procedure for repair of bilateral cleft lips by means of a long, narrow triangular flap.

Ziefal-Neelsen m., a stain for acid-fast organisms. A heat fixed smears is flooded with carbolfuschin, heated for 5 minutes, cooled, and washed. The slide is decolorized with acid alcohol, washed, and counterstained with methylene blue. Acid-fast organisms appear red against a blue background.

Zsigmondy'e gold number m., see colloidal gold test.

8
Pressures

Pressure: Stress or strain, whether by com-pression, pull, thrust, or shear.

After p., a sense of pressure which lasts for a short period after removal of the actual pressure.

Arterial p., the pressure of the blood within the arteries.

Atmosphere p., the pressure exerted by the atmosphere; it is about 15 pounds to the square inch at the level of the sea.

Back p., the pressure caused by the damming back of the blood in a heart chamber and its tributaries, due to an obstructive heart valve or failing myocardium.

Biting p., occlusal p.

Blood p., the pressure of the blood on the walls of the arteries, dependent on the energy of the heart action, the elasticity of the walls of the arteries, and the volume and viscosity of the blood. The maximum pressure occurs near the end of the stroke output of the left ventricle of the heart and is termed maximum or systolic pressure. The minimum pressure occurs late in ventricular diastole and is termed minimum or diastolic pressure. Mean blood pressure is the average of the blood pressure levels. Basic blood pressure is the pressure during quiet rest of basal conditions. See also hypertension and hypotension.

Brain p., the capillary venous pressure in the brain.

Capillary p., the blood pressure in the capillaries.

Central venous p. (CVP), the venous pressure as measured at the right atrium, done by means of a catheter introduced through the median cubital vein to the superior vena cava, the distal end of the catheter being attached to a manometer.

Cerebrospinal p., the pressure or tension of the cerebrospinal fluid., normally 100 to 150 mm. As measured by the manometer.

Diastolic p., see blood p.

Donders' p., increase of manometric pressure with the instrument placed on the trachea on opening the chest of a dead body; due to collapse of the lung.

Endocardial p., pressure of blood within the heart.

Hydrostatic p., the pressure at any level on water at rest due to the weight of the water above it.

Intra-abdominal p., the pressure between the viscera within the abdominal cavity.

Intracranial p., the pressure in the space between the skull and the brain., i.e., the pressure of the subarachnoidal fluid.

Intraocular p., the pressure of the fluids of the eye against the tunics. It is produced by continual renewal of the fluids within the interior of the eye, and is altered in certain pathological conditions (e.g., glaucoma). It may be roughly estimated by palpation of the eye or measured, directly or indirectly, with specially devised instruments, the tonometers.

Intrathecal p., pressure within in a sheath, particularly the pressure of the cerebrospinal fluid within the one ventricle of the heart.

Mean circulatory filling p., a measure of the average (arterial and venous) pressure necessary to cause filling of the circulation with blood; it varies with blood volume and is directly proportional to the rage of venous return and thus to cardiac output.

Negative p., a pressure less than that, of the atmosphere.

Occlusal p., pressure exerted on the occlusal surface of the teeth when the jaws are brought into opposition. Called also Biting p.

Oncotic p., the osmotic pressure due to the presence of colloids in a solution; in the case of plasma-interstitial fluid interaction. It is the force that tends to counterbalance the capillary blood pressure.

Osmotic p., effective, that part of the total osmotic pressure of a solution which governs the tendency of its solvent to pass through a semipermeable bounding membrane or across another boundary.

Partial p., the pressure exerted by each of the components of a gas.

Perfusion p., the difference between the arterial and venous pressures at the brain level.

Positive p., pressure greater than that of the atmosphere.

Positive end-expiratory p. (PEEP), a method of mechanical ventilation in which pressure is maintained to increase the volume of gas remaining in the lungs at the end of expiration thus reducing the shunting of blood through the lungs and improving gas exchange; done in acute respiratory failure to allow reduction of inspired O_2 concentrations.

Pulmonary capillary wedge p., intravascular pressure as measured by a introduced into the pulmonary artery; it permits indirect measurement of the mean pressure.

Pulse p., the difference between the systolic and diastolic pressures.

Selection p., an effect produced by a given gene that determines the frequency of a given allele; it may be advantageous for survival (positive selection pressure) or disadvantageous (negative selection pressure).

Solution p., the force which tends to bring into solution the molecules of a solid contained in the solvent.

Systolic p., see blood p.

Venous p., the blood pressure in a vein, usually utilized to reflect filing pressure to the ventricle.

9
Procedures

Procedure: A series of steps by which a desired result is accompanied.

Anderson p., reconstruction of the hypopharynx and cervical esophagus by the use of bilateral rectangular flaps.

Glenn p., see under operation.

Gomori-Takamatsu p., a method for localizing the alkaline phosphate enzyme; a tissue secretion is incubated in a buffered solution containing the substance releases phosphoric acid, and it combines with calcium and precipitated as calcium phosphate. This colorless precipitate is converted to brown cobalt sulfide, which is readily visualized with the microscope.

Hartmann's p., resection of a diseased portion of the colon, with the proximal end of the colon brought out as a colostomy and the distal stump or rectum being closed by suture. Bowel continuity can later be restored called also Hartmann's colostomy or operation.

Janetta p., a microsurgical procedure for relief of trigeminal nerve and blood vessel compressing the nerve.

Push-back p., see under technique*.

V-Y p., a method of repairing a skin defect in which a V-shaped flap is made proximal to the defect; the flap is transferred to the defect, and the secondary defect thus created is closed to produced a Y-shaped scar.

*See Appendix

10

Phenomena

Phenomenon: Any sign or objective symptom; any observable occurrence or fact.

Anderson's p., clumps of red blood cells in the stools of amebic dysentery; seen on microscopic examination.

Aqueous-influx p., entrance into conjunctival or subconjunctival vessels of clear fluid (aqueous humor), deriving from an aqueous vein during compression of its recipient vessel by a glass rod. Called also Ascher's positive glass-rod phenomenon. Cf: blood-influx p.

Arm p., see Pool's p., def. 2.

P. of Arthus., the development of an inflammatory lesion, characterized by induration, erythema, edema, hemorrhage, and necrosis, a few hours after intradermal injection of antigen into a previously sensitized animal producing precipitating antibody. The lesion results from the precipitation of antigen-antibody complexes which cause complement activation and the release of complement fragments that are chemotactic for neutrophils; large number of neutrophils infiltrate the site and cause tissue destruction by release of lysosomal enzymes.

Ascher's positive glass-rod p., see Aqueous-influx p.

Ascher's negative glass-rod p., see Blood-influx p.

Aschner's p., slowing of the pulse following pressure on the eyeball; it is indicative of cardiac vagus irritability, a slowing of from 5 to 13 beats is normal; one of from 13 to 50 or more is exaggerated; one of from 1 to 5 is diminished. If ocular compression produces acceleration of the heart the reflex is called inverted.

Ashman's p., aberrant ventricular activation resulting in a short cardiac cycle following a normal or long cycle; it is associated with supraventricular premature beats and with atrial fibrillation.

Aubert's p., an optical illusion in which a bright vertical line in a dark room tilts to one side when an observer tilts his head to the opposite side.

Austin Flint p., Austin Flint murmur; a presystolic murmur at the apex in aortic regurgitation.

Autokinetic visible light p., the apparent spontaneous movement of a pin-point source of light as seen by certain susceptible persons when they gaze steadily at it in a completely blacked-out room.

Babinski's p., dorsiflexion of the large toe and spreading of the other toes instead of plantar flexion of all the toes when the sole is stimulated; it is a sign of damage to the corticospinal tract.

Becker's p., increased pulsation of the retinal arteries in Graves' disease.

Bell s. p., an outward and upward rolling of the eyeball on the attempt to close the eye; it occurs on the affected side in peripheral facial paralysis (Bell's palsy).

Berry-Dedrick p., the transformation of fibroma viruses into myxoma viruses.

Blood-influx p., filling of conjunctival or subconjunctival vessels with blood during compression by a glass rod of the recipient vessel of an aqueous vein. This and the aqueous-influx phenomenon, depending on minute pressure differences between blood and aqueous humor, differ in glaucomatous eyes and those with normal intraocular pressure. Called also Aschner's negative glass-rod p.

Bordet-Gengou p., complement fixation—the consumption of complement upon reaction with immune complexes containing complement fixing antibodies.

Brake p., the tendency of a muscle to maintain itself in its normal resting position; called also Rieger's p.

Break-off p., a state of disconnectedness or unreality experienced by high-altitude pilots. Its symptomatic sensations are apparently indescribable in understandable physical terms, but the condition could be the result of a loss of all the physical sense perceptions.

Chase-Sulzberger p., see Sulzberger-Chase p.

Cheek p., in meningitis if pressure is exerted on both cheeks just under the zygomas there is reflex upward jerking of both arms with simultaneous bending of both elbows.

Cogwheel p., when a hypertonic muscle is passively stretched it resists, and this resistance sometimes takes the form of an irregular jerkiness; called also Negro's p.

Collie p., when pure neon is enclosed in a glass tube with a globule of mercury and shaken it glows with a bright, orange-red color, and when the globule rolls it appears to be followed by a flame.

Cushing's p., a rise in systemic blood pressure as a result of an increase in intracranial pressure.

Danysz's p., decrease of the neutralizing influence of an antitoxin when a toxin is added to it in divided portions instead of all at once.

Dawn p., the early-morning increase in plasma glucose concentration and thus insulin requirement in a patient with insulin-dependent diabetes mellitus.

Debre's p., absence of measles rash at the site of injection of convalescent measles serum which has not prevented the appearance of the eruption.

Dejerine-Lichtheim p., see Lichtheim sign.

Dental p., thermal and tactile sensations in the gums with toothache, produced by repeated faradic stimulation of hyperesthetic lines on the body (Calligaris).

Denys-Le-clef p., phagocytosis taking place in a test tube on mixing therein leukocytes, bacteria, and immune serum specific for the bacteria.

d'Herelle's p., see Twort-d'Herelle p.

Diaphragm p., Diaphragmatic p., the movement of the diaphragm as seen through the walls of the body, called also phrenic phenomenon and phrenic wave.

Doll s head p., an abnormal extraocular muscle manifestation of many ophthalmologic syndromes and conditions: the eyes depress as the head is bent backward.

Doppler p., the relationship of the apparent frequency of the waves, as of sound, light, and radiowaves, to the relative motion of the source of the waves and the observer, the frequency increasing as the two approach each other and decreasing as they move apart.

Duckworth's p., arrest of breathing before stoppage of the heart's action in certain fatal brain conditions.

Erb's p., see Erb's sign, def. 1.

Erben's p., slowing down of the pulse upon bending the head and trunk strongly forward, said to indicate vagal excitability.

Face p., Facia'lis p., see Chvostek's sign.

Fall-and-rise p., the drop in the number of bacteria that occurs at the beginning of drug treatment and the gradual rise that follows, even while treatment continues.

Felton's p., immunologic unresponsiveness or tolerance to pneumococcal polysaccharide induced in mice by administration of large doses of the antigen.

Fern p., the appearance of a fernlike pattern in the dried specimen of cervical mucus, an indication of the presence of estrogens.

Fick's p., a fogging of vision, with the appearance of halos around light, occurring in individuals wearing contact lenses.

Finger p. (in hemiplegia), 1. extension of all the fingers or of the thumb and index finger, on pressure against the pisiform bone; called also Gordon's sign. 2. see Souques' p.

First set p., the immunological reaction of the body against a tissue or organ in a host not previously sensitized against the graft antigens.

Friedreich's p., the tympanic note of skodaic resonance in pleuritis with effusion varies in pitch during inspiration and expiration, being raised on inspiration.

Galassi's pupillary p., see Orbicularis papillary p.

Gartner's p., the degree of fulness of the veins of the arm as it is raised to varying heights indicates the degree of pressure in the right atrium.

Gengou p., complement fixation, see Bordet p.

Gerhardt's p., see under signs.

Glass-rod p., positive, see Aqueous-influx p.

Glass-rod p., negative, see Blood-influx p.

Goldblatt p., ischemic tubular atrophy, a characteristic of renovascular hypertension.

Gowers' p., see under sign (def. 2).

Grasset's p., Grasset-Gaussel p., inability of a patient to raise both legs at the same time, though he can raise either alone; seen in incomplete organic hemiplegia.

Gunn's p., see under syndrome.

Gunn's pupillary p., see Swinging flashlight sign.

Halisteresis p., selective withdrawal of bone salt from already calcified tissue.

Hamburger p., chloride shift—the exchange of chloride (Cl^-) and bicarbonate (HCO_3^-) between the plasma and red blood cells which takes place whenever bicarbonate is generated or decomposed within the red blood cells.

Hammerschlag's p., abnormal fatigability toward continuous sounds of gradually decreasing intensity.

Hata p., increase in severity of an infectious disease when a small dose of a chemotherapeutical remedy is given.

Hecht p., see Rumpel-Leede p.

Hektoen p., when antigens are introduced into the animal body in allergic states, there may exist an increased range of new antibody production which may include production of antibodies concerned in previous infections and immunizations.

Hering's p., a faint murmur heard with the stethoscope over the lower end of the sternum for a short time after death.

Hertwig-Magendie p., skew deviation—downward eye fixates.

Hip-flexion p., in paraplegia, when the patient attempts to rise from a lying position, he flexes the hip of the paralyzed side.

Hochsinger's p., pressure on the inner side of the biceps muscle produces closure of the fist in tetany.

Hoffmann's p., increased excitability to electrical stimulation in the sensory nerves; the ulnar nerve is usually tested.

Holmes' p., Holmes-Stewart p., see Rebound p.

Houssay p., hypoglycemia and marked increase in sensitiveness to insulin produced by hypophysectomy in depancreatized experimental animals.

Hunt's paradoxical p., in dystonia musculorum deformans, if the examiner attempts forcible plantar flexion of the foot that is in dorsal spasm there is produced increase of the dorsal spasm, but if the patient is ordered to extend the foot he will perform plantar flexion.

Jaw-winking p., see Gunn's syndrome.

Kienbock's p., paradoxical diaphragm contraction—the hemidiaphragm on one side rises on inspiration and falls on expiration.

Koch's p., if a guinea pig which has been previously infected with tuberculosis organisms is reinjected intracutaneously, the skin over the injected area undergoes necrosis and a superficial ulcer develops. The ulcer heals quickly and infection of regional lymph nodes is retarded. The phenomenon demonstrates development of ability to localize tubercle bacilli.

Koebner's p., a cutaneous response seen in certain dermatoses, e.g.. psoriasis, lichen plannus. and infectious eczematoid dermatitis, manifested by the appearance on uninvolved skin of lesions typical of the skin disease at the site of trauma, on scars, or at points where articles of clothing (e.g., a belt) produce pressure. Called also isomorphic effect.

Kohnstamm's p., after movement—spontaneous elevation of the arm by the idiomuscular contraction after benumbing it by powerful pressure against a rigid object.

Kuhne's muscular p., see Porret's p.

LE p., the process by which the LE cell is formed.

Leede-Rumpel p., see Rumpel-Leede p.

LeGrand-Geblewics p., a nickering colored light (40 to 50 per second) observed indirectly is perceived as a constant white light.

Leichtenstern's p., see under sign.

Lewis' p., hydrophagocytosis—the absorption by macrophages of plasma surrounding them.

Liacopoulos p., nonspecific immunosuppression to an antigen induced by administration of large doses of an unrelated antigen.

Liesegang's p., the peculiar periodic formation of a precipitate in concentric banded rings, waves, or spirals, when two electrolytes diffuse into and meet in a colloid gel.

Litten's diaphragm p., a movable horizontal depression of the lower part of the sides of the thorax, seen in respiration.

Lucio's p., a local exacerbation reaction occurring in diffuse lepromatous leprosy, characterized histologically by ischemic necrosis of the epidermis as a result of necrotizing vasculitis of small blood vessels of the subpapillary plexus, and clinically by the eruption of crops of small erythematous lesions with central necrosis; the eschar may be shed, revealing ulceration, with eventual scar formation of erythema nodosum leprosun*.

Lust's p., abduction with dorsal flexion of the foot on tapping the external popliteal nerve just below the head of the fibula; indicative of spasmophilia.

*See Appendix

Marcus Gunn p., see Gunn'syndrome, under syndrome.

Marcus Gunn pupillary p., see Swinging flashlight sign.

Meirowsky p., darkening of existing melanin, perhaps by oxidation, beginning within seconds and complete within minutes to a few hours after exposure to long-wave ultraviolet radiation.

Mills-Reincke p., the mortality from all diseases decreases as a result of water purification.

Muscle p., the tendency of striated muscle to contract in hard lumps upon tapping.

Narsaroffs p., the difference in rectal temperature before and after a cold bath gradually decreases as cold baths are repeated.

Negro's p., see Cog-wheel p.

Neisser-Wechsberg p., complement deviation—inhibition of complement mediated immune hemolysis in the presence of excess antibody.

Orbeli p., when the response of a nerve-muscle preparation is diminishing because of fatigue, stimulation of the sympathetic nerve increases the height of the contractions.

Orbicularis p., unilateral contraction of the pupil followed by dilatation after closure or attempted closure of the eyelids that are forcibly held apart.

Paradoxical diaphragm p., one hemidiaphragm moves upward on inspiration and downward on expiration, opposite to the movements on the contralateral side: seen in phrenic nerve paralysis and eventration.

Paradoxical p., of dystonia, see Hunt's paradoxical p.

Paradoxical pupillary p., reversed pupillary reflex—any abnormal papillary reflex opposite of that which occurs normally, e.g., stimulation of the retina by light dilates the pupil.

Peroneal-nerve p., see Lust's p.

Pfeiffer's p., the lysis of vibrio cholerae when injected into the peritoneal cavity of an immunized guinea pig; the term is also used to describe the *in vitro* lysis of cholera vibrios or other bacteria when incubated with specific antibody and complement.

Phi p., the perception of the sequential flashing of a stationary row of lights as a moving light.

Phrenic p., see Diaphragm p.

Piltz-Westphal p., see Orbicularis papillary p.

Pool's p., 1. See Schlesinger's sign. 2. Contraction of the muscles of the arm following the raising of the arm above the head with the forearm extended, so as to cause stretching of the brachial plexus; seen in postoperative tetany.

Porret's p., the passage of a continuous current through a living muscle fiber causes an undulation proceeding from the positive toward the negative pole.

Psi p., psyche, an experience or effect that appears to be produced without physical agency or intermediation.

Purkinje'a p., as the intensity of illumination decreases and the eye becomes scotopic, the region of maximum visual acuity shifts from red-yellow to blue-green, the reds becoming less luminous, the blues more luminous. Called also Purkinje's effect and shift

Queckenstedt's p., see under signs.

Radial p., the involuntary dorsal flexion of the wrist which occurs on palmar flexion of the fingers.

Raynaud's p., intermittent bilateral attacks of ischemia of the fingers or toes and sometimes of the ears or nose, marked by severe pallor, and often accompanied by paresthesia and pain; it is brought on characteristically by cold or emotional stimuli and relieved by heat, and is due to an underlying disease or anatomical abnormality. When the condition is idiopathic or primary it is termed Raynaud's disease.

Rebound p., a manifestation of loss of coordination between groups of antagonistic muscles of the extremities in cerebellar dysfunction. It may be demonstrated by having the patient extend both arms horizontally, the examiner then tapping both outstretched arms sharply.

The normal arm returns to position promptly, whereas the affected arm overshoots the original position and may oscillate several times before achieving it or, the patient rests his elbow on a table and tries to flex his arm against the resistance of the examiner. When the resistance is suddenly withdrawn, the affected arm rebounds to the patient's chest, whereas the normal arm flexes only slightly, the flexion being arrested by contraction of antagonistic muscles (the triceps).

Reclotting p., thixotropy—the property exhibited by certain gels, of becoming fluid when shaken or stirred, and then becoming semisolid again.

Release p., the unhampered activity of a lower center when a higher inhibiting control is removed.

Rieger's p., see Brake p.

Ritter-Rollet p., flexion of the foot upon a gentle electric stimulation, and its extension upon energetic stimulation.

Rumpel-Leede p., the appearance of minute subcutaneous hemorrhages below the area at which a rubber bandage is applied not too tightly for ten minutes upon the upper arm; characteristic of scarlet fever and hemorrhagic diathesis.

Rust's p., in caries or cancer of the upper cervical vertebrae, the patient supports his head with his hands when rising from or assuming a lying position; see also under syndrome.

Satellite p., the more luxuriant development of a colony of microorganisms when in the neighborhood of a foreign colony, as shown by *Haemophilus influenzae* when contaminated by *Staphyloccus pyogenes var. aureus*.

Schellong-Strisower p., fall of systolic blood pressure on assuming an erect posture from the lying down position.

Schlesinger's p., see under signs.

Schramm's p., visibility with the cystoscope of a whole or part of the posterior urethra; seen in spinal cord disease.

Schuller' p., in hemiplegia due to organic lesion, the patient walks sideward more easily to the affected side than to the healthy side.

Schultz-Charlton p., when scarlet fever antitoxin or scarlet fever convalescent serum is injected into area of the skin showing a bright red rash, a blanching of the skin at the site of the injection occurs. Serum from scarlet fever patients does not produce this reaction.

Second-set p., the accelerated and intensified rejection by the recipient of a second graft of tissue from the same donor as a consequence of the primary immune response (i.e., antibody production and cell-mediated immunity) induced by the first graft, called also second-set rejection.

Sherrington p., the response of the hind limb musculature on stimulation of a motor nerve which has previously been degenerated.

Shot-silk p., an opalescent effect, as of changeable silk, sometimes seen in retinas of young persons.

Shwartzman p., it is generalized and localized; generalized—a generalized reaction following two intravenous injection of endotoxin separated by 24 hours; it is characterized by widespread hemorrhages, bilateral cortical necrosis of the kidneys, and a marked fall of leukocytes and platelet counts and usually results in the death of the animal localized—a localized vascular reaction consists of vascular necrosis, petechial hemorrhages, and leukocyte infiltration that occurs at the site of an orignal subcutaneous injection of endotoxin approximately 24 hr after an intravenous injection of the same or another endotoxin given at the site other than the original injection site.

Simonsen p., a graft-versus-host reaction produced by injection of lymphocytes from adult chickens into chick embryos; the principal features are splenomegaly and hemolytic anemia.

Sinkler's p., in an extremity with spastic paralysis, sharp flexion of the toe may be followed by flexion of the knee and hip.

Somogyi p., a rebound phenomenon occurring in diabetes: over treatment with insulin induces hypoglycemia, which initiates the release of epinephrine, ACTH, glucagon, and growth hormone, which stimulate lipolysis, gluconeogenesis, and glyconeogenesis, and glycogenolysis, which, in turn, result in a rebound hyperglycemia and ketosis. Called also Somogyi effect.

Soret p., when a solution is maintained for some time in a temperature gradient, a difference in concentration develops along the temperature gradient.

Souques' p., a phenomenon seen in incomplete hemiplegia, consisting of involuntary extension and separation of the fingers when the arm is raised; called also finger p.

Springlike p., see Andre-Thomas sign.

Staircase p., treppe—a phenomenon o gradual increase in the extent of muscular contraction following rapidly repeated stimulation.

Staub-Traugott p., after a glucose load is administered, subsequent loads, given after a short interval, are disposed of at an accelerated rate.

Straus' p., when material containing virulent glanders bacilli is inoculated into the peritoneal cavity of male guinea pigs, scrotal lesions develop.

Strumpell p., dorsiflexion and supination of the foot on flexing the extended leg against resistance offered by the examiner.

Sulzberger-Chase p., abolition of dermal contact hypersensitivity to sensitizing agents, e.g. picryl chloride, produced by prior oral feeding of the agent.

Theobald Smith's p., guinea pigs which have been used for standardizing diphtheria antitoxin and have thus been injected with a small dose of blood serum become highly susceptible to the serum and may die very promptly if given a rather large second dose of the same serum a few weeks later.

Toe p., see Babinski's p.

Tongue p., a slight blow upon the tongue produces a contraction with the appearance of deep depressions; seen in tetany. Called also Schultze's sign and tongue test.

Trousseau's p., spasmodic contractions of muscles provoked by pressure upon the nerves which go to them; seen in tetany.

Twort-d'Herelle p., the phenomenon of transmissible bacterial lysis; bacteriophagia. When to a broth culture of typhoid or dysentery bacilli there is added a drop of filtered broth emulsion of the stool from a convalescent typhoid or dysentery patient, complete lysis of the bacterial culture will occur in a few hours. If a drop of this lysed culture is added to another culture of the bacilli, lysis will take place exactly as in the first. A drop of this culture will then dissolve a third culture, and so on through hundreds of transfers d'Herelle attributed this phenomenon to the action of an ultramicroscopic parasite of bacteria, which he named the bacteriophage.

Tyndall p., the rendering visible of a transverse beam of light through its being broken up by solid particles suspended in a liquid or gas.

Wedensky's p., on applying a series of rapidly repeated stimuli to a nerve, the muscle contracts quickly in response to the first stimulus and then fails to respond further; but if the stimuli are applied to the nerve at a slower rate, the muscle responds to all of them.

Wenckebach p., the generation of impulses by the sinus node of the heart at a constant rate while the P-R interval grows progressively longer during several beats until an atrial complex is not followed by a ventricular complex.

Westphal's p., 1. (AKO Westphal) see Orbicularis papillary p 2. (CFO Westphal) see under signs.

Westphal-Piltz p., see Orbicularis pupillary p.

Wever-Bray p., cochlear microphonics—the electrical potential generated in the hair O cells of the organ of Gorti in response to acoustic stimulation.

Williams' p., the tympanic note of skodaic resonance in pleuritis with effusion varies in pitch with the opening and closing of the patient's mouth.

11
Paralyses

Paralysis: Loss or impairment of motor function in a part due to lesion of the neural or muscular mechanism; also, by analogy, impairment of sensory function (sensory paralysis). In addition to the types named below, paralysis is further distinguished as traumatic, syphilitic, toxic, etc., according to its cause; or as obturator, ulnar. etc., according to the nerve, part, or muscle specially affected. Other varieties, also hemiplegia, palsy, paraplegia, and paresis.

Abducens p., paralysis of the external rectus muscle of the eye due to lesion of the abducens nerve, with internal strabismus and diplopia.

Abducens-facial p., congenital, see Moebius' syndrome.

P. of accommodation, paralysis of the ciliary muscles so as to prevent accommodation of the eye.

Acoustic p., nerve deafness.

Acute ascending spinal p., acute febrile polyneuritis, see Guillain-Barre syndrome.

Acute atrophic p., an acute viral disease, occurring sporadically and in epidemics, and characterized clinically by fever, sore throat headache, and vomiting, often with stiffness of the neck and back. In the minor illness there may be the only symptom. The major illness, which may or may not be preceded by involvement of the central nervous system, stiff neck, pleocytosis in the spinal fluid, and perhaps paralysis. There may be subsequent atrophy of groups of muscles, ending in the contraction and permanent deformity.

Acute bulbar p., bulbar paralysis usually caused by acute vascular lesions of the brain, most commonly hemorrhage or thrombosis; called also acute bulbar polioencephalitis.

Acute infectious p., epidemic poliomyelitis—poliomyelitis occurring in epidemic form.

Acute wasting p., see Acute atrophic p.

P. Agitans, a form of parkinsonism of unknown etiology usually occurring in late life, although a juvenile form has been described. It is a slowly progressive disease characterized by mask-like facies, a characteristic tremor of resting muscles, a slowing of voluntary movements, a festinating gait, peculiar posture, and weakness of the muscles. There may be excessive sweating and feelings of heat. Pathologically, there is degeneration within the nuclear masses of the extrapyramidal system and a characteristic loss of melanin-containing cells from the substantia nigra and a corresponding reduction in dopamine levels in the corpus striatum. Called also Parkinson's disease and shaking palsy.

p. Agitans, juvenile (of Hunt), a condition developing in early life, usually familial but occasionally occurring sporadically, marked by increased muscle tonus with the characteristic attitude and facies of paralysis agitans, due to progressive degeneration of the globus pallidus; involvement of the substantia nigra and pyramidal tracts may occur. Called also paleostriatal syndrome, pallidal atrophy, pallidal syndrome, and Ramsay Hunt syndrome.

Alcoholic p., paralysis caused by habitual drunkenness.

Alternate p., alternating p., alternate hemiplegia that which affects a part on one side of the body and another part on the opposite side.

Ambiguo-accessorius p., see Schmidt's syndrome.

Ambiguo-accessorius-hypoglossal p., see Jackson's syndrome.

Ambiguo-hypoglossal p., see Tapia's syndrome.

Ambiguospinothalamic p., see Avellis' syndrome

Anesthesia p., paralysis following anesthesia.

Anterior spinal p., anterior poliomyelitis—inflammation of the anterior horns of the gray substance of the spinal cord.

Arsenical p., paralysis due to arsenical poisoning.

Ascending p., spinal paralysis that progresses cephalad.

Association p., see Bulbar p.

Asthenic bulbar p., myasthenia gravis pseudoparalytica—a disorder of neuromuscular function due to presence of antibodies to acetylcholine receptors at the neuromuscular junction; clinically there is fatigue and exhaustion of the muscular system with a tendency to fluctuate in severity and without sensory disturbance or atrophy. The disorder may be restricted to muscle group or become generalized with severe weakness, and in some cases, ventilatory insufficiency. It may affect any musle of the body, but especially those of the eyes, face, lips, tongue, throat, and neck.

Asthenobulbospinal p., myasthenia gravis, see Asthenic bulbar p.

Atrophic spinal p., anterior poliomyelitis, see anterior spinal p.

Avellis's p., see under syndromes.

Bell's p., unilateral facial paralysis of sudden onset, due to lesion of the facial nerve and resulting in characteristic distortion of the face.

Bilateral p., diplegia; paralysis on both sides.

Birth p., paralysis due to injury received at birth.

Brachial p., paralysis of an arm from lesion of the brachial plexus; see Erb-Duchenne p. and Klumpke-Dejerine p.

Brachiofacial p., paralysis affecting the face and an arm.

Brown-Sequard's p., 1. See Brown-Sequard's syndrome. 2. A flaccid paralysis seen in disorders of the urinary tract.

Bulbar p., paralysis due to changes in the motor centers of the medulla oblongata: a chronic, usually fatal disease, moot commonly affecting persons over 50 years old but also occurring in the course of amyotrophic lateral sclerosis, syringobulbia, and multiple sclerosis. It is marked by progressive paralysis and atrophy of the muscles of the lips, tongue, mouth, pharynx, and larynx, and is due to degeneration of the nerve nuclei of the floor of the fourth ventricle. Called also labioglossopharyngeal p., labioglossolaryngeal p., and Duchenne's p.

Bulbospinal p., myasthenia gravis, see Asthenobulbospinal p.

Cage p., a complex nutritional deficiency sometimes seen in captive primates, which is said to resemble osteomalacia.

Central p., any paralysis due to a lesion of the brain or spinal cord.

Centrocapsular p., that which is due to lesions of the internal capsule.

Cerebral p., any paralysis due to an intracranial lesion; a persistent qualitative motor disorder appearing before the age of three years, due to nonprogressive damage to the brain.

Chastek p., progressive ataxia and paralysis in silver foxes due to thiamine deficiency following the substitution of raw fish for meat in the diet.

Circumflex p., paralysis of the circumflex nerve.

Complete p., entire loss of motion, sensation, and function.

Compression p., paralysis caused by pressure on a nerve, as by a crutch or during sleep.

Congenital abducens-facial p., see Moebius syndrome.

Congenital oculofacial p., see Moebius syndrome.

Conjugate p., loss of ability to perform some of the parallel ocular movements.

Cortical p., paralysis dependent upon a lesion of the brain cortex.

Crossed p., cruciate p., paralysis affecting one side of the face and the opposite side of the body.

Crural p., that which chiefly affects the thigh or thighs.

Crutch p., paralysis of one or both arms, due to pressure of the crutch in the axilla.

Cruveilhier's p., progressive muscular atrophy—see Aran-Duchenne disease.

Decubitus p., paralysis due to pressure on a nerve from lying for long time in one position.

Dejerine-Klumpke p., see Klumpke's p.

Diaphragmatic p., unilateral paralysis of the diaphragm.

Diphtheric p., Diphtheritic p., a partial paralysis which often follows diphtheria, chiefly affecting the soft palate and throat muscles.

Divers' p., paralysis occurring in deep-sea divers as a result of too rapid reduction of pressure.

Duchenne's p., 1. see Bulbar paralysis. 2. see Erb-Duchenne paralysis.

Duchenne-Erb p., Erb-Duchenne p.

Epidemic infantile p., see Acute infectious p.

Erb's p., 1. Erb-Duchenne paralysis. 2. Erb's spastic paraplegia. 3. pseudohypertrophic muscular dystrophy – see Duchenne muscular disease, Erb's disease.

Erb-Duchenne p., the upper-arm type of brachial paralysis; paralysis of the upper roots of brachial plexus due to destruction of the fifth and sixth cervical roots and characterized by absence of involvement of the small hand muscles.

Essential p., see Acute Atrophic p.

Facial p., weakening or paralysis of the facial nerve, as in Bell's palsy.

False p., pseudoparalysis—apparent loss of muscular power, without true paralysis marked by defective coordination of movements or by repression of movements on account of pain.

Familial periodic p., see Periodic p.

Felton's p., see under phenomenon.

Flaccid p., paralysis with loss of tone of the muscles of the paralyzed part and absence of tendon reflexes. Cf: spastic p.

Fowl p., see Marek's disease.

Functional p., a temporary paralysis which is apparently not caused by a nerve lesion.

P. of Gaze., paralysis due to pathological processes which implicate the supranuclear oculomotor centers or pathways and result in either lateral or vertical gaze paralysis.

General p., General p. of the insane, parenchymatous neurosyphilis in which chronic meningoencephalitis causes gradual loss of cortical function, resulting in progressive dementia and generalized paralysis, which generally occurs 10 to 20 years after the initial infection of syphilis.

Ginger p., see Jamaica ginger p.

Glossolabial p., glossopharyngolabial p., see Bulbar p.

Gubler's p., see Millard-Gubler syndrome.

Hereditary cerebrospinal p., (hemiplegia, diplegia, paraplegia, or tetraplegia), a hereditary condition which develops usually in early middle life, characterized by gradually developing paralyses which may be manifest in the upper or lower extremities, in the two extremities, or one side, or in all four extremities.

Histrionic p., paralysis of certain muscles of the face, producing a facial expression of some emotion.

Hyperkalemic periodic p., see Familial periodic p.

Hypoglossal p., paralysis due to a lesion of the hypoglossal nucleus or the hypoglossal nerve at any point.

Hypokalemic periodic p., see Familial periodic p.

Hysterical p., apparent loss of power of movement in a part, in the absence of an organic neurological cause.

Immune p., Immunologic p., immunologic unresponsiveness induced by administration of large doses of antigen; now called immunologic tolerance.

Incomplete p., partial paralysis or paresis.

Indian bow p., paralysis of the thyroarytenoid muscles.

Infantile p., see Acute atrophic p.

Infantile, cerebral, ataxic p., a condition which is dependent upon faulty development of the frontal regions of the brain, is present at birth, affects all extremities, and is not definitely progressive; called also diataxia infantilis cerebralis and cerebral diataxia.

Infantile cerebrocerebellar diplegic p., a condition developing in infants affecting all extremities, and due to combined failure of development or destruction of the reciprocating portions of the cerebrum and the cerebellum.

Infantile spastic p., see Cerebral p.

Infantile spinal p., the classic form of acute anterior poliomyelitis, in which the appearance of flaccid paralysis, usually of one or more limbs, makes the diagnosis quiet definite.

Infectious bulbar p., a highly contagious disease affecting the central nervous system of swine, catties, dogs, cats, rats, and other animals; in swine the infection usually runs the milder course than in other species. Caused by a herpes virus, it is characterized by sudden onset, severe pruritus, late paralysis, and death within three to four days after onset.

Ischemic p., local paralysis due to an impairment of the circulation, as in certain cases of embolism or thrombosis; called also Volkmann's ischemic paralysis.

Jake p., see Jamaica ginger p.

Jamaica ginger p., paralysis of the extremities, especially of the legs, following the use of Jamaica ginger as a beverage; called also Jake paralysis, jake neuritis, ginger paralysis, Jamaica ginger polyneuritis.

Juvenile p., general paralysis in young persons.

Klumpke's p., Klumpke-Dejerine p., the lower-arm type of brachial paralysis; atrophic paralysis of the muscles of the arm and hand, from lesion of the eighth cervical and first dorsal nerves. It often occurs in infants delivered by breech extraction.

Kussmaul's p., Kussmaul-Landry p., acute febrile polyneuritis, see Barre-Guillain syndrome.

Labial p., Labioglossolaryngeal p., Labioglossopharyngeal p., see Bulbar p.

Lambing p., pregnancy toxemia in ewes, see Pregnancy disease.

Landry's p., acute febrile polyneuritis, see Barre-Guillain syndrome.

Laryngeal p., paralysis of one of the laryngeal muscles.

Lead p., paralysis caused by lead poisoning, due to a peripheral neuritis, and marked by wrist-drop.

Lingual p., paralysis of the tongue.

Lissauer's p., an apoplectiform type of dementia paralytica, see General p.

Local p., paralysis of one muscle or of a group of muscles.

Masticatory p., paralysis of the muscles of mastication.

Medullary tegmental p's., paralyses due to lesions of the medullary tegmentum: they include alternate hemiplegia, Tapia's syndrome, syndrome of Babinski-Nageotte, and Cestan's syndrome.

Millard-Gubler p., see under syndrome.

Mimetic p., paralysis of the facial muscles.

Mixed p., combined motor and sensory paralysis.

Motor p., paralysis of voluntary muscles.

Musculospiral p., paralysis of the extensor muscles of the wrist and fingers, most often due to compression of the musculospiral (radial) nerve, and, depending upon the site of the nerve injury, sometimes accompanied by weakness of extension of the elbow; called also radial p. and Saturday night palsy.

Myopathic p., paralysis due to disease of the muscle itself.

Narcosis p., paralysis during anesthesia, caused by pressure, cold, curare, etc.

Normokalemic periodic p., see Familial periodic p.

P. notario'rum., writers' cramp—muscle cramp in hand caused by excessive use in writing.

Nuclear p., any paralysis due to a lesion in a nucleus of origin.

Obstetric p., see Birth p.

Ocular p., it is combination of amourosis, cycloplegia, and ophthalmoplegia, Amaurosis—blindness, especially blindness occurring without apparent lesion of the eye, as from disease of the optic nerve, spine or brain, Cycloplegia—paralysis of the cilliary muscle; paralysis of accommodation, ophthalmoplegia—paralysis of the eye muscles.

Oculofacial p., congenital p., see Moebius' syndrome.

Oculomotor p., paralysis of the oculomotor nerve.

Organic p., paralysis due to lesion of nerve tissue.

Parotitic p., paralysis accompanying mumps.

Parturient p., a form of paralysis affecting cows near delivery; usually accompanied by hypocalcemia, it is due to metabolic disorder.

Periodic p., familial, an autosomal dominant trait marked by recurring attacks of rapidly progressive flaccid paralysis; there are three types; (i) associated with a fall in serum potassium levels (hypokalemic periodic p.) (ii) associated with a rise therein (hyperkalemic periodic p.; called also adynamia episodica hereditaria): and (iii) with normal levels (normokalemic periodic p.).

Peripheral p., loss of power due to some lesion of the nervous mechanism between the nucleus of origin and the muscle.

Peroneal p., crossed leg palsy—palsy of the peroneal nerve caused by sitting with one leg crossed over another.

Phonetic p., paralysis of the muscles of speech.

Post-diphtheric p., see Diphtheric paralysis.

Posthemiplegic p., residual weakness after a stroke.

Posticus p., paralysis of the posterior cricothyroid muscle.

Pott s p., which is due to vertebral caries or spinal tuberculosis.

Pressure p., paralysis, generally temporary, caused by pressure on a nerve trunk.

Progressive bulbar p., see Bulbar p.

Pseudobulbar p., spastic weakness of the muscles innervated by the cranial nerves, i.e. the muscles of the face, pharynx, and tongue, due to bilateral lesions of the corticospinal tract; it is often accompanied by uncontrolled weeping or laughing. Called also supranuclear p. and spastic bulbar palsy.

Pseudohypertrophic muscular p., see Duchenne disease, Erb's disease.

Radial **p.**, 1. See musculospiral p. 2. A condition usually affecting horses, but also other domestic animals, in which paralysis of certain muscles of the elbow and knee occurs as a result of injury to the radial nerve. Called also dropped elbow.

Ramsay Hunt p., see Juvenile paralysis agitans.

Range p., see Marek's disease.

Reflex p., one ascribable to peripheral irritation; in some cases secondary changes occur in the spinal cord, and the paralysis ceases to be truly reflex.

Remak's p., paralysis of the extensor muscles of the fingers and wrist; called also Remak's type.

Rucksack p., a disorder of motor and sensory function of the upper extremities as a result of damage to the brachial plexus caused by the wearing of a backpack.

Saturday night **p.**, see Musculospiral p.

Sensory p., loss of sensation resulting from a morbid process.

Serum p., peripheral nerve paralysis following administration of serum.

Sleep p., paralysis occurring at awakening or sleep onset; extension of sleep atonia into the waking state.

Spastic p., paralysis marked by spasticity of the muscles of the paralyzed part and increased tendon reflexes, due to upper motor neuron lesions. Cf: flaccid p.

Spastic spinal p., lateral sclerosis of the spinal cord.

Spinomuscular p., paralysis due to lesion of the gray matter of the spinal cord, or the nerves originating therefrom.

Supranuclear p., see Pseudobulbar p.

Tick p., a progressive ascending flaccid motor paralysis which follows the bite of certain ticks (Dermacentor andersoni.) in children and in domestic animals in Oregon, British Columbia, and other parts of the world. A similar paralysis sometimes follows the bites of species of *Ixodes, Haemaphysalis,* and *Rhipicephalus.*

Todd's p., postepileptic hemiplegia or monoplegia lasting for a few minutes or hours, or occasionally for several days, after the epileptic attack.

Trigeminal p., paralysis due to a lesion of the trigeminal (fifth) nerve, marked by sensory loss in the face and weakness of the muscles of mastication.

p. Vacil'lans, chorea—the ceaseless occurrence of a wide variety of rapid highly complex, jerky movements that appear to be well coordinated but are performed involuntarily.

Vasomotor p., cessation of vasomotor control.

Volkmann's ischemic p., see Ischemic p.

Waking p., a form of hypnogogic helplessness that follows waking, especially in some cases of narcolepsy.

Wasting p., spinal muscular atrophy, see Aran-Duchenne disease, Cruveilhier disease.

Weber's p., see under syndrome.

Writers' p., writers' cramp, see p. notario'rum.

12

Operations

Operation: Any act performed with instruments or by the hands of a surgeon; a surgical procedure.

Abbe o., attachment of a triangular, full-thickness flap from the median portion of the lower lip to fill a defect in the upper lip.

Abbe's o., 1. A lateral intestinal anastomosis made with rings of catgut. 2. Division of an esophageal stricture by string friction. 3. (obs.) Intracranial resection of the second and third divisions of the fifth nerve for trigeminal neuralgia.

Adams' o., 1. Subcutaneous intracapsular division of the neck of the femur for ankylosis of the hip. 2. Subcutaneous division of the palmar fascia at various points for Dupuytren's contracture. 3. Excision of a wedge-shaped piece from the eyelid for relief of ectropion.

Akin o., resection of the medial prominence of the first metatarsal head and cuneiform osteotomy of the proximal phalanx of the great toe, done for hallux valgus.

Albee's o., operation for ankylosis of the hip, consisting of cutting off the upper surface of the head of the femur and freshening a corresponding point on the acetabulum, and permitting the two freshened surfaces to rest in contact.

Albee-Delbet o., an operation for fracture of the neck of the femur, done by drilling a hole through the trochanter and the neck and head of the femur and inserting a bone peg in this hole.

Albert's o., excision of the knee to secure ankylosis for the cure of flail joint.

Alexander's o., Alexander-Adams o., shortening of the round ligaments to repair displacement of the uterus.

Alouette's o., amputation at the hip with a semicircular outer flap to the great trochanter and a large internal flap from within outward.

Ammon's o., 1. Blepharoplasty (plastic surgery of the eyelid) by a flap from the cheek. 2. Dacryocystotomy—surgical creation of new opening in the lacrimal sac. 3. For epicanthus—resection of a spindle-shaped piece of skin over the bridge of the nose, undermining the flaps of the epicanthal fold and closing with sutures.

Amussat's o., a long transverse incision for exposure of the colon.

Anagnostakis' o., an operation for entropion; also an operation for trichiasis.

Aries-Pitanguy o., an operation to reduce mild to moderate macromastia.

Asch's o., an operation for deflection of the nasal septum by reinserting resected pieces of cartilage and holding them in place with a splint; of historical interest.

Babcock's o., extirpation of the saphenous vein by inserting a long probe with an acorn tip and drawing out the vein by invagination; done for eradication of varicose veins.

Baldy's o., Baldy-Webster o., see Webster's o.

Barkan's o., goniotomy—an operation for glaucoma characterized by an open angled and normal depth of anterior chamber; it consists of opening of Schlemm's canal under direct vision secured by a contact glass.

Barker's o., 1. An excision of the hip joint by an anterior cut. 2. A special method of excising the astragalus by an incision extending from just above the external malleolus forward and inward to the dorsum of the foot.

Barraquer's o., phacoerysis—removal of lens in cataract by means of suction with an instrument known as erysiphake.

Barsky's o., an operation for repair of a cleft hand with a missing central ray and a deep central V-shaped cleft, consisting in closing the cleft, bringing the ring and index fingers closer together, and correcting the associated syndactyly, if present.

Barton's o., an operation for ankylosis consisting of sawing through the bone and removing a V-shaped piece.

Basset's o., a method of dissecting the inguinal glands in operation for cancer of the vulva.

Bassini's o., repair of inguinal hernia, with high ligation of the sac, reinforcement of the floor of the canal, and placement of the spermatic cord under the external oblique anastomosis.

Battle's o., an operation for appendicitis in which the rectus muscle is temporarily retracted.

Beer's o., a flap method for cataract.

Belsey Mark IV o., an operation for gastroesophageal reflux performed through a thoracic incision; the fundus is wrapped 270 degrees around the circumference of the esophagus, leaving its posterior wall free.

Berger's o., interscapulothoracic amputation—amputation of the upper extremity, including the scapula and clavicle.

Berke's o., an operation for ptosis of the upper eyelid, consisting of (i) a modification of the Blaskovics operation, with resection of the levator muscle through a skin incision and excision of excess muscle, (ii) a modification of the Motais' operation, with suspension of the ptotic lid from the superior rectus muscle.

Bevan's o., an operation for an undescended testicle, by which the testicle is brought down permanently into the scrotum.

Bier's o., osteoplastic amputation of the leg with a bone flap cut out of the tibia and fibula above the stump.

Biesenberger's o., a reduction mammoplasty using transposition of the nipple consisting in excision of the lateral portion of the mammary gland, with the rotation of the remainder glandular pedicle attached to the nipple and formation of the skin brassierie.

Bigelow's o., litholapaxy—the crushing of a calculus in the bladder, followed at once by the washing out of the fragments.

Billroth's o., 1. Partial resection of the stomach with anastomosis of the severed end of the duodenum to the end of the resected stomach (Billroth I), or with anastomosis of the resected stomach to the jejunum (Billroth II). 2. Excision of the tongue by making a transverse incision below the symphysis of the jaw and joining it by two incisions, one on each side, parallel to the body of the mandible, with preliminary ligation of the lingual arteries.

Blair-Brown o., repair of a cleft lip by the use of a lateral flap one-half the length of the lip.

Blalock-Hanlon o., a palliative operation for transposition of the great vessels consisting in the creation of an interatrial septal defect.

Blalock-Taussig o., the anastomosis of the subclavian artery to the pulmonary artery in order to shunt some of the systemic circulation into the pulmonary circulation; performed as palliative treatment of congenital cardiac anomalies (tetralogy of Fallot).

Blaskovic's o., an operation for ptosis of the upper eyelid, consisting of excision of the levator muscle and the tarsus through a conjunctival approach.

Bozeman's o., hysterocystocleisis—an operation of turning the cervix uteri into the bladder and suturing it; done for the relief of vesicouterovaginal fistula or for ureterouterine fistula.

Bricker's o., the surgical creation of an ileal conduit with a flat stoma for the collection of urine; the flat contour is achieved by suturing the ileal mucosa to the skin.

Brock's o., transventricular closed valvotomy—correction of pulmonary valvular stenosis by passage of a valvulotome through the wall of the right ventricle into the pulmonary artery to open the valve.

Brophy's o., one for cleft palate (with or without cleft lip), consisting of the forcible approximation of the freshened palate margins, which are held in position by special sutures supported by lead plates.

Browne's o., a urethroplasty for hypospadias repair, in which an intact strip of epithelium is left on the ventral surface of the penis to form the roof of the urethra, and the floor of the urethra is formed by epithelialization from the lateral wound margins.

Brunschwig's o., a technique of pancreatoduodenectomy.

Buck's o., cuneiform excision of the patella and the ends of the tibia and fibula.

(Von) Burow's o., a method of excising triangles of skin at the base of the pedicle of a skin flap to facilitate advancement.

Caldwell-Luc o., 1. The operation of opening into the maxillary sinus by way of an incision into the supradental fossa opposite the premolar teeth. Usually done to remove tooth roots or abnormal tissue from the sinus. 2. In compound zygomaticomaxillar fractures, the packing of the maxillary sinus by approaching the antrum through the canine fossa of the maxilla above the tooth apices, thus allowing reduction of displaced fragments of the zygoma by upward and outward pressure. Also called Luc's o.

Carpue's o., the Indian method of rhinoplasty, see Indian o.

Cecil's o., 1. A two-stage urethroplasty for hypospadias repair, with construction of a new urethral segment buried in the scrotum, followed by separation of the new urethra from the scrotum. 2. A three-stage urethroplasty for repair of urethral stricture, with excision of the strictured area through an incision on the ventral surface of the penis, followed by the steps of the operation used for hypospadias repair.

Chopart's o., amputation of the foot with the calcaneus, talus, and other parts of the tarsus being retained.

Colonna's o., 1. A reconstruction operation for intracapsular fracture of the femoral neck. 2. Capsular arthroplasty of the hip.

Commando's o., an operation for management of oral cancer, consisting in resection of the primary lesion and the regional lymphatic nodes.

Conway's o., a method of correcting severe macromastia, consisting in partial breast amputation and free transplantation of the nipple and areolae.

Cosmetic o., one intended to remove or correct a deformity in an esthetically acceptable manner.

Cotte's o., removal of the presacral nerve.

Cotting's o., an operation for ingrowing toenail, consisting in cutting off the side of the toe down to and including the ingrowing edge of the nail.

Daviel's o., extraction of cataract through a corneal incision without cutting the iris.

Denis Browne o., see Browne's o.

Denonvilliers' o., plastic correction of a defective ata nasi by transferring a triangular flap from the adjacent side of the nose.

Dieffenbach's o., plastic closure of triangular defects by displacing a quadrangular flap toward one side of the triangle.

Dittel's o., enucleation of an enlarged prostate through an external incision; of historical interest.

Doleris'o., an operation for retrodeviation of the uterus by shortening the round ligaments and fixing them on either side by an opening in the rectus muscle just above the spine of the ilium.

Duhamel's o., the treatment of congenital megacolon (Hirschsprung's disease) by a modification of the pull-through procedure and establishment of a longitudinal anastomosis between the proximal ganglionated segment of the colon and the rectum leaving the latter *in situ*.

Dührssen's o., vaginofixation of the uterus.

Duplay's o., a method of urethroplasty for repair of hypospadias, employing a buried skin strip.

Dupuy-Dutemps o., blepharoplasty of the lower lid with tissue from the opposing lid.

Dupuytren's o., amputation of the arm at the shoulder joint.

Elliot's o., a method of trephining the sclerocornea for the relief of increased tension in glaucoma.

Emmet's o., 1. A method of repairing a lacerated perineum. 2 Trachelorrhaphy, or suture of the edges of a lacerated cervix uteri. 3. Surgical creation of a vesicovaginal fistula to secure drainage of the bladder in cystitis.

Equilibrating o., tenotomy (cutting of an extraocular tendon for strabismus) of the direct antagonist of a paralyzed eye muscle.

Esser's o., epithelial inlay—a method of securing epithelialization of an unhealed deep wound. A mold of the wound cavity is taken and covered with a Thiersch's graft of epidermis, the whole being inserted in the wound cavity, and the edges then approximated with sutures. The mold is removed after 10 days, leaving the cavity completely epithelialized.

Estes' o., implantation of an ovary into a uterine cornu; performed for sterility when the tubes are absent.

Estlander's o., 1. Resection of one or more ribs in empyema so as to allow the chest wall to collapse and close the abnormal cavity; of historical interest. 2. Rotation of a triangular flap from the side of the lower lip to fill a defect in the lateral upper lip.

Eversbusch's o., an operation for ptosis of the upper eyelid, consisting of resection of the levator muscle through a skin incision.

Exploratory o., surgical incision into an area of the body followed by inspection and palpation of organs and tissues to determine the cause of unexplained symptoms.

Fergusson's o., an incision for excision of upper jaw; it runs along the junction of the nose with the cheek, around the ala of the nose to the median line, and descends to bisect the upper lip.

Finney's o., reconstruction of pyloric channel by means of a longitudinal incision through the pylorus and adjacent walls of the stomach and duodenum and the establishment of inverted U-shaped anastomosis between the stomach and duodenum.

Flap o., any operation involving the raising of a flap of tissue. In periodontics, an operation to secure greater access to granulation tissue and osseous defects, consisting of detachment of the gingivae, the alveolar mucosa, and/or a portion of the palatal mucosa.

Fothergill's o., see Manchester's o.

Franco's o., suprapubic cystotomy—the operation of cutting the bladder by an incision just above the symphisis pubis.

Frank's o., see Ssabanejew-Frank o.

Frazier-Spiller o., division of the sensory root of the gasserian ganglion for relief of trigeminal neuralgia.

Fredet-Ramstedt o., pyloromyotomy—the operation for congenital stenosis of the pylorus, performed by longitudinally incising the thickened serosa and muscularis down to the mucosa.

Freund's o., resection of cartilages of the chest wall to restore elasticity and improve respiratory mechanics; of historical interest.

Freyer's o., a method of performing suprapubic enucleation of the hypertrophied prostate; of historical interest.

Frost-Lang o., insertion of a gold ball to take the place of an enucleated eyeball.

Fukala's o., removal of the lens of the eye for the treatment of marked myopia.

Fuller's o., perineal incision and drainage of the seminal vesicles; of historical interest

Gifford's o., delimiting keratotomy—incision of the cornea in the ulcus serpens by a cut tangential to the advancing border of the ulcer and made to emerge at a corresponding point in the other side.

Gigli's o., lateral section of the os pubis by means of Gigli's wire saw; done in difficult labor.

Gilliam's o., an operation for retroversion of the uterus by drawing a loop of each round ligament through the abdominal wall and fixing the loops to the abdominal fascia.

Gillies' o., 1. An operation for correction of ectropion utilizing a split-thickness skin graft and a mold. 2. A technique for reducing fractures of the zygoma and zygomatic arch through an incision in the temporal region above the hairline.

Glenn's o., an operation for congenital cyanotic heart disease, consisting of anastomosis of the superior vena cava to the right pulmonary artery.

Gonin's o., treatment of retinal detachment by thermocautery of the fissure in the retina performed through an opening in the sclera.

Grade's o., removal of the cataractous lens by a scleral cut, with laceration of the capsule and iridectomy.

Gritti's o., amputation of the leg through the knee, using the patella as an osteoplastic flap over the end of the femur.

Grondahl-Finney o., esophagogastroplasty in which the orifice between the esophagus and stomach is enlarged.

Guyon's o., amputation above the malleoli.

Halsted's o., 1. An operation for inguinal hernia with transposition of the spermatic cord above the external oblique aponeurosis. 2. Radical mastectomy—removal of the breast, pectoral muscles, axillary lymph nodes, and associated skin and subcutaneous tissue in treatment of breast cancer.

Hancock's o., a modification of Pirogoff's amputation (amputation of the foot at the ankle, part of the calcaneus being left in the lower end of the stump) a part of the astragalus being retained in the flap, the lower surface being sawed off, and the cut surface of the calcaneus being brought into contact with it.

Hartley-Krause o., excision of the gasserian ganglion and its roots to relieve trigeminal neuralgia; of historical interest.

Hartmann's o., resection of a diseased portion of the colon, with the proximal end of the colon brought out as colostomy and the distal stump or rectum being closed by suture. Bowel continuity can later be restored.

Haultaim's o., a modification of the Huntington's operation (qv) for replacement of a chronically inverted uterus, involving a posterior incision in the uterus through the cervical ring.

Heath's o., division of the ascending rami of the lower jaw with a saw for ankylosis, performed within the oral cavity; rarely done.

Heine's o., cyclodialysis in glaucoma.

Heineke-Mikulicz o., reconstruction of the pyloric channel by incising the pylorus longitudinally and suturing the incision transversely.

Heller's o., cardiomyotomy for relief of obstruction of the esophagogastric junction.

Herbert's o., displacement of a wedge-shaped flap of sclera in order to form a filtering cicatrix in glaucoma.

Hey's o., disarticulation of the metatarsus from the tarsus, with removal of a part of the medial cuneiform bone.

Hibbs'o., a spinal fusion operation done by fracturing the spinous processes of the vertebrae and pressing the tip of each downward to rest in the denuded area caused by the fracture of its elbow below.

Hochenegg's o., total excision of the rectum with preservation of the anal sphincter; of historical interest.

Hoffa's o., Hoffa-Lorenz o., see Lorenz's o.

Holth's o., excision of the sclera by punch operation.

Horsley's o., excision of an area of motor cortex for relief of athetoid and convulsive movements of an upper extremity; of historical interest.

Huggins' o., orchiectomy performed for cancer of the prostate.

Hunter's o., litigation of an artery in the proximal side of an aneurysm, above the first collateral; of historical interest.

Huntington's o., transabdominal repair of a chronically inverted uterus. It is done by grasping the invaginated portion of the uterus with forceps; as the uterus is pulled up, additional forceps are placed sequentially lower down, and upward traction is applied. After the uterus is in place, the position is maintained by packing through the vagina.

Indian o., the reconstruction of a nose by a flap of skin taken from the forehead, with its pedicle at the root of the nose.

Interposition o., see Watkins' o.

Interval o., an operation performed during the interval between two acute attacks of a disease, as in appendicitis.

Irving's sterilization o., a method of tubal ligation in which the uterine tubes are ligated and severed.

Italian o., taglia cotian rhinoplasty—the reconstruction of a nose by a flap of skin taken from the arm, the flap remaining attached to the arm until union has taken place.

Jaboulay's o., interpelviabdominal amputation—amputation of the thigh with excision of the lateral half of the pelvis.

Kader's o., gastrostomy by which the feeding tube is introduced through a valve-like flap which closes on withdrawal of the tube.

Kasai's o., portoenterostomy—surgical anastomosis of the jejunum to an intrahepatic biliary radicle; done to establish a conduit from the intrahepatic bile ducts to the intestine in biliary atresia or stenosis or common duct tumor.

Kazanjian's o., 1. A technique of surgical extension of the buccal vestibular sulcus of edentulous ridges to increase their height and to improve denture retention. 2. The use of extraskeletal fixation for support in compound zygomaticomaxillary fractures—a small hole is drilled through the infraorbital rim, and a stainless steel wire is inserted with both ends brought out through the wound, where they are twisted together into a loop or hook. Rubber band traction between the suspension wire and an outrigger on a head cap provides support for the zygomatic fragments.

Keller's o., sagittal resection of the medial prominence of the first metatarsal head and excision of the base of the proximal phalanx of the great toe; done for halius valgus.

Kelly's o., 1. (Howard A Kelly) an operation for correction of urinary incontinence (usually due to stress) in women, in which the site of the internal urethral sphincter is identified by means of a balloon catheter, and the connective tissue between the vagina and the urethra and the floor of the bladder are sutured to form a wide shelf of firm tissue to support the urethra and bladder. 2. (J D Kelly) arytenoidopexy—surgical fixation of the arytenoids cartilage or muscle.

Killian's o., excision of the anterior wall of the frontal sinus, with removal of the diseased tissue, and formation of a permanent communication with the nose.

Killian-Freer o., submucous resection of the nasal septum, including the septal cartilage, vomer, and perpendicular plate of the ethmoid.

King's o., arytenoidopexy—surgical fixation of the arytenoid cartilage or muscle.

Knapp's o., (for cataract), the formation of a peripheral opening in the capsule behind the iris, without iridectomy.

Kocher's o., 1. A method of excising the ankle joint by a cut below the outer malleolus, division of the peroneal tendons, removal of the diseased tissues, and suture of the divided tendons. 2. A method of reducing a subcoracoid dislocation of the humerus. 3. Excision of the tongue through an incision extending from the symphysis of the jaw to the hyoid bone and thence to the mastoid process. 4. See under maneuver. 5. A method of pylorectomy.

Körte-Ballance o., anastomosis of the facial and hypoglossal nerves.

Kraske's o., removal of the coccyx and part of the sacrum for access to a carcinoma of the rectum.

Krause's o., extradural excision of the gasserian ganglion for trigeminal neuralgia; of historical interest.

Krimer's o., uranoplasty in which mucoperiosteal flaps from each side of the palatal cleft are sutured together at the median line.

Krönlein's o., resection of the outer wall of the orbit for the removal of an orbital tumor without excising the eye.

Küstner's o., replacement of an inverted uterus through an incision made in the cervix and uterus along the posterior surface.

Lagrange's o., sclerectoiridectomy—an operation or excision of a portion of the sclera and of the iris for glaucoma.

Landolt's o., the formation of a lower eyelid with a double pedicle or bridge flap of eyelid skin taken from the upper lid.

Lane's o., the operation of dividing the ileum near the cecum, closing the distal portion and anastomosing the proximal end with the upper part of the rectum or lower part of the sigmoid, thus eliminating the colon from the fecal current.

Lapidus' o., Silver's o., with wedge resection and fusion of the innermost cuneometatarsal joint and establishment of a bridge between the bases of the first and second metatarsals; done for hallux valgus.

Larrey's o., a method of disarticulation of the humerus at the shoulder joint by an incision extending from the acromion about three inches down the arm, splitting the deltoid muscle, and from this point going round the arm to the center of axilla.

Latzko's o., 1. Incision through the abdominal and uterine walls for delivery of fetus. 2. A method of repairing a vesicovaginal fistula by using mucosa denuded from the posterior wall of the vagina as a flap to cover the fistula.

Le Fort's o., Le Fort-Neugebauer o., the operation of uniting the anterior and posterior vaginal walls along the middle line for the repair of prolapse of the uterus.

Lempert's fenestration o., an operation for otosclerosis, consisting of drilling a small window into the lateral semicircular canal and then placing a flap of skin over the fistula.

Lisfranc's o., a division of the foot between tarsus and metatarsus.

Liston's o., an operation for excision of the upper jaw.

Lizars' o., excision of the upper jaw by a curved incision extending from the angle of the mouth to the malar bone.

Lorenz's o., an operation for congenital dislocation of the hip, consisting in reduction of the dislocation, and keeping the head of the femur fixed against the rudimentary acetabulum until a socket is formed.

Lowsley's o., an operation for repair of simple epispadias, consisting in closing the glandular cleft urethra, splitting the glans, and burying the repaired urethra deep in the soft tissue so that the orifice will be positioned at the normal site.

Luc's o., see Caldwell-Luc o.

Macewen's o., an operation for the radical cure of hernia by closing the internal ring with a pad made of the hernial sac.

Madlener's o., a method of sterilization in the female, in which the middle portion of the fallopian tube is crushed with a clamp, which is then replaced with a ligature of nonabsorbable material.

Magnet o., removal of a fragment of steel or iron from the eyeball by means of a powerful magnet.

Major o., a surgical procedure of major magnitude and risk.

Manchester's o., an operation for uterine prolapse comprising dilation and curettage, anterior repair, amputation of the vaginal portion of the cervix, shortening of the cardinal ligaments and posterior colpoperineorrhaphy.

Marshall-Marchetti-Krantz o., an operation for the correction of stress incontinence, the anterior portion of the urethra, vesical neck, and bladder being sutured to the posterior surface of the pubic bone.

Mastoid o., mastoidectomy—excision of the mastoid cells or the mastoid process of the temporal bone.

Matas' o., endoaneurysmorrhaphy—operation for aneurysm by opening the aneurysmal sac and narrowing the internal lumen by suture; of historical importance.

Maydl's o., 1. Colostomy in which the colon is drawn out through the wound and maintained in position by placing a glass rod beneath it until adhesions have formed; of historical interest. 2. Insertion of the ureters into the rectum for exstrophy of the bladder; of historical interest.

Mayo's o., 1. Excision of the pyloric end of the stomach, followed by closure of both duodenum and stomach and the construction of an independent posterior gastrojejunostomy. 2. For umbilical hernia; the hernial mass is excised and the abdominal aponeuroses are overlapped transversely; of historical interest. 3. Subcutaneous removal of varicose veins with a long-handled stripper terminating in a small ring angled with the shaft of the instrument.

McBride's o., resection of the medial prominence of the first metatarsal head, medial capsulorrhaphy, resection of the fibular sesamoid, and transfer of the adductor tendon to the neck of the first metatarsal; done for hallus valgus.

McBurney's o., an operation for inguinal hernia: the sac is exposed, ligated, and cut off at the internal ring; the skin is turned in and stitched to the underlying tendinous and ligamentous structures.

McGill's o., suprapubic transvesical prostatectomy—removal of the prostate through an incision above the pubis and through the urinary bladder; of historical interest.

Meller's o., an operation for excision of the tear sac.

Mikulicz's o., 1. Removal of the sternocleidomastoid muscle for torticollis. 2. See Heineke-Mikulicz pyloroplasty. 3. Tarsectomy in which the heel, os calcis, and astragalus are removed, the articular surfaces of the tibia, fibula, cuboid, and scaphoid are excised, and the foot brought into line with the leg; also called Vladimiroff's o. 4. Enter-ectomy in stages, including exteriorization of the section of intestine to be resected, usually the colon; resection of the exteriorized loop; elimination of the fecal fistula by crushing the spur between the two barrels of the anastomosis; and closure of the fecal fistula.

Miles'o., abdominoperineal resection for cancer of the lower sigmoid and rectum, which includes permanent colostomy, removal of the pelvic colon, mesocolon, and adjacent lymph nodes, and wide perineal excision of the rectum and anus.

Millin-Read o., an operation for the correction of stress incontinence employing the suprapubic approach.

Minor o., a surgical operation which is not serious in its magnitude or risk.

Mitchell's o., Silver's o., with distal osteotomy of the first metatarsal; done for hallux valgus.

Moschcowitz's o., an operation for the repair of a femoral hernia by the inguinal approach.

Motais'o., an operation for ptosis, consisting of transplanting the middle portion of the tendon of the superior rectus muscle of the eye lid into the upper lid.

Mules'o., evisceration of the eyeball, with insertion of an artificial vitreous.

Mustard's o., creation of an intra-atrial baffle using pericardial tissue to correct the anatomic defect in transposition of the great vessels.

Naffziger's o., excision of the superior and lateral walls of the orbit for exophthalmos.

Nissen's o., fundoplication—mobilization of the lower end of the esophagus and plication of the stomach around it (fundus wrapping), in the treatment of reflux esophagitis that may be associated with various disorders, such as hiatal hernia.

Ober's o., medial subtalar syndesmotomy for club foot.

Olshausen's o., the operation of fixing or suturing the uterus to the abdominal wall for the cure of retroversion.

Ombrédanne's o., trans-scrotal orchiopexy.

Open o., an operation in which the tissues and organs are exposed to view through a surgical incision.

Partsch's o., a technique for marsupialization of a dental cyst.

Patey's o., modified radical mastectomy—total mastectomy with axillary node dissection, but with preservation of pectoral muscles.

Péan's o., 1. (obs) vaginal hysterectomy bit by bit. 2. Hip joint amputation in which the vessels are ligated as the operation goes on.

Phelps' o., an open and direct incision through the sole and inner side of the foot, done for talipes.

Phemister o., use of an onlay graft of cancellous bone without internal fixation, for treatment of a stable but ununited fracture.

Plastic o., one in which the shape of a part or the character of its covering is altered by transplantation of tissue, etc.

Polya's o., anastomosis of the transected end of the stomach to the side of the jejunum following subtotal gastrectomy.

Pomeroy's o., a method of sterilization in the female, in which the fallopian tube is picked up about two inches from the uterine cornua, a chromic catgut ligature tied around the loop without crushing it, and the tied loop is then resected.

Potts' o., anastomosis between the aorta and the pulmonary artery as palliative treatment of congenital pulmonary stenosis.

Radical o., one involving extensive resection of tissue for the complete extirpation of disease.

Ramstedt's o., see Fredet-Ramstedt o.

Rastelli's o., an operation to correct such cardiac anomalies as transposition of the great vessels (with pulmonary stenosis), truncus arteriosus, and pulmonary arterial atresia, in which a graft is used to carry blood from the right ventricle to the pulmonary artery.

Regnoli's o., excision of the tongue through a median opening below the lower jaw; reaching from the chin to the hyoid bone.

Ridell's o., obliteration of the frontal sinus by removal of the anterior wall and floor and sometimes posterior walls of the sinus: for treatment of malignant tumors.

Roux-en-Y o., any Y-shaped anastomosis in which the small intestine is included; after division of the small intestine segment, the distal end is implanted in other organ, such as the stomach or esophagus, and the proximal end into the small intestine below the anastomosis to provide drainage without reflux.

Saemisch's o., transfixion of the cornea and of the base of the ulcer for the cure of hypopyon.

Scanzoni's o., see under maneuver.

Schauta's o., radical hysterectomy by the vaginal route.

Schede's o.,1. Resection of the thorax for chronic empyema. 2. An operation for varicose veins of the leg, done by a circular incision, rolling one cuff up and another down, so as to reach and remove the varices. 3. Excision of the necrosed part of a bone, all dead bone and diseased tissue being scraped away, and the cavity permitted to fill with blood clot, the latter being kept moist and aseptic with a cover of gauze and rubber tissue and eventually becoming organized.

Scheie's o.,1. Scleral cauterization with peripheral iridectomy for treatment of glaucoma. 2. A technique for needling and aspiration of cataract.

Schönbein's o., staphyloplasty in which a flap of mucous membrane from the posterior wall of the pharynx is stitched to the velum palati, shutting off the nose from the mouth.

Sédillot's o., 1. A method of staphylorrhaphy—surgical correction of a midline cleft in the uvula and soft palate. 2. A flap operation for restoring the upper lip.

Senning's o., surgical creation of two interatrial channels for crossing the systemic and pulmonary venous circulations in transposition of the great vessels.

Serre's o., an operation for correction of skin contractures that distort the angle of the mouth, involving switching of a skin and subcutaneous tissue flap from one lip to another.

Silver's o., resection of the medial prominence of the first metatarsal head, medial capsulorrhaphy of the first metatarsophalangeal joint, and sectioning of the adductor tendon; done for hallux valgus.

Sistrunk's o., a surgical procedure for removal of thyroglossal cysts and sinuses.

Smith's o., extraction of an immature cataract with an intact capsule.

Soave's o., the treatment of congenital megacolon (Hirschsprung's disease) by endorectal pull-through, with normal colon connected to the anus through a rectum denuded of mucosa.

Spinelli's o., the operation of splitting the anterior wall of the prolapsed inverted uterus, reversing the organ, and restoring it to the correct position.

Ssabane jew-Frank o., a method of performing gastrostomy by pulling a cone of the stomach through an incision in the left rectus muscle and suturing it to the skin.

Stacke's o., the removal of the mastoid and the contents of the tympanum, so that the antrum, attic, tympanum, and meatus form a single cavity.

State's o., the treatment of congenital megacolon (Hirschsprung's disease) by end-to-end anastomosis of the colon from above the aganglionic segment to the upper part of the rectum.

Stein's o., an operation for reconstruction of the lower lip with flaps taken from the upper lip.

Stokes's o., Gritti-Stokes amputation—a modification of Gritti's amputation (amputation of the leg through the knee, using patella as an osteoplastic flap over the end of the femur) using an oval anterior flap.

Strombeck's o., a one-stage breast reduction operation that includes transposition of the nipple in a medial or lateral pedicle.

Sturmdorf's o., conical excision of the diseased endocervix.

Swenson's o., an operation for congenital megacolon (Hirschsprung's disease), consisting in removal of the rectum and the aganglionic segment of the bowel, with preservation of the anal sphincters, by the pull-through surgical technique.

Syme's o., amputation of the foot at the ankle joint, with removal of both malleoli.

Tagliacotian o., see Italian o.

Talma's o., omentopexy in treatment of ascites; of historical interest.

Tanner's o., an operation for bleeding esophageal varices in which the terminal end of the esophagus, the cardia, and the proximal portion of the stomach are freed of all external vascular and ligamentous connections, and the stomach is transected below the cardia.

Teale's o., amputation with preservation of a long rectangular flap of muscle and integument on one side of the limb and a short rectangular flap on the other.

Thiersch's o., removal of thin split-thickness skin grafts by means of a razor, skin-graft cutting knife, or a dennatome.

Torek's o., 1. An operation for an undescended testicle. 2. An operation for the excision of the thoracic part of the esophagus; of historical interest.

Torkildsen's o., ventriculocisternostomy—surgical establishment of communication between the third ventricle and cisterna magna for drainage of cerebrospinal fluid in hydrocephalus.

Toti's o., dacryocystorhinostomy—surgical creation of a communication between the lacrimal sac and the nasal cavity.

Trendelenburg's o., 1. Excision of varicose veins. 2. Ligation of the great saphenous vein for varicose veins. 3. Synchondroseotomy—an operation for exstrophy of the bladder done by cutting through the sacroiliac ligaments and forcibly drawing together the iliac bones. 4. Transthoracic pulmonary embolectomy.

Van Hook's o., ureteroureterostomy—end-to-end anastomosis of the two portion of transected ureter.

Vineberg's o., implantation of the internal mammary artery into the myocardium to enhance the growth of collateral circulation.

Vladimiroff o., see Mikulicz's o., def. 3.

Voronoff's o., transplantation into a man of the testes of an anthropoid ape, in the hope of rejuvenating the recipient.

Water's o., a form of extraperitoneal cesarean section.

Waterston's o., anastomosis between the ascending aorta and right pulmonary artery as palliative treatment of congenital pulmonary stenosis.

Watkins' o., an operation for prolapse and procidentia uteri in which the bladder is separated from the anterior wall of the uterus so that the uterus is left in a position to support the entire bladder. Also called interposition o.

Webster's o., for retrodisplacement of the uterus; the round ligaments are passed through the perforated broad ligaments and fixed to the back of the uterus.

Wertheim's o., radical hysterectomy; removal of the uterus, tubes, parametrium, tissues surrounding the upper vagina, and pelvic lymphatics.

Whipple's o., radical pancreatoduodenectomy with removal of the distal third of the stomach, the entire duodenum, and the head of the pancreas, with gastrojejunostomy, chledochojejunostomy, and pancreatic jejunostomy.

White's o., castration for hypertrophy of the prostate.

Whitehead's o., treatment of hemorrhoids by excision.

Whitman's o., 1. An operation for arthroplasty of the hip joint. 2. A method of astragalectomy.

Witzel's o., insertion of a tube in the gastric lumen, the tube being implanted so as to create a serosal tunnel of stomach as it enters the gastric lumen.

Wölfler' o., anterior gastrojejunostomy for pyloric obstruction; of historical interest.

Young's o., 1. An operation for penile epispadias, with formation of a new urethral tube. 2. Perineal prostatectomy—removal of the prostate through an incision in the perenium.

Ziegler's o., V-shaped iridectomy for forming an artificial pupil.

13
Triads

Triad (group of three): 1. Any trivalent element, 2. A group of three entities or objects, as an association of three symptoms.

Acute compression t., see Beck's t.

Adrenomedullary t., the symptoms produced by activation of the adrenal medulla: tachycardia, vasoconstriction and sweating.

Andersen's t., see under syndrome.

Beck's t., three symptoms characteristics of cardiac compression: (i) a high venous pressure, (ii) a low arterial pressure, and (iii) a small quiet heart.

Bezold's t., prolonged bone conduction and lessened perception of low tones, indicating otosclerosis.

Charcot's t., 1. Nystagmus, intention tremor, and staccato speech, often seen in multiple sclerosis. 2. The symptoms of billiary colic, jaundice, and fever and chills characteristic of intermittent cholangitis.

Dieulafoy's t., hypersensitiveness of the skin, reflect muscular contraction, and tenderness at McBurney's point in appendicitis.

Grancher's t., lessened vesicular quality of breathing, skodaic resonance, and increased vocal fremitus; seen in early pulmonary tuberculosis.

Hepatic t's., the grouping of the tributaries of the hepatic artery, vein, and bile duct at the angles of the lobules of the liver.

Hutchinson's t., diffuse interstitial keratitis, labyrinthine disease, and Hutchinson teeth, seen in inherited syphilis.

Kartagener's t., see under syndrome.

T. of Luciani., asthenia, atonia, and astasia, the three major symptoms of cerebellar disease.

Oscler's t., telangiectasis, capillary fragility, and hereditary hemorrhagic diathesis.

Portal t's., see Hepatic t's.

T. of Retinal Cone., the tip of two horizontal cell dendrites and one midget cell dendrite. Enclosed a synaptic invagination of a retinal cone pedicle.

Saint's t., hiatus hernia, colonic diverticula. And cholelithiasis, occurring concomitantly.

T. of Schultz, jaundice, gangrenous stomatitis, and leukopenia,

T. of skeletal muscle, a pair of terminal cisterns in close apposition to the T tubule, running transversely across a myofibril of skeletal muscle; in mammalian muscle there are two triad to each sarcomere, situated at the A band-1 band junction.

Whipple's t., the essential clinical features of insulin- producing tumors (i) spontaneous hypoglycemia (blood sugar levels below 50 mg per 100 ml.), (ii) accompanied by central nervous or vasomotor system symptoms, and (iii) relief of symptoms by the oral or intravenous administration of glucose.

14

Factors

Factor: 1. Any of several substances or activities that are necessary to produce a result, e.g., a coagulation factor. Often, use of the term "factor" indicates that the chemical nature of the substance or its mechanism of action is unknown, as in endocrinology, where "factors" are renamed as "hormones" when their chemical nature is determined. 2. Any of the numbers of algebraic symbols multiplied together to form a product 3. A coefficient or conversion factor, a number by which a quantity is multiplied to produce a change of units of measurement. 4. A gene (hereditary factor).

F. A., C3 (in the alternative complement pathway): it is of following subtypes and having functions as follows; C3a: an anaphylatoxins generated by C3 convertases, C3b: a constituent of the classic pathway C5 convertase and of the alternative pathway of C3 and C5 convertases generated by C3 convertases in both pathways and also continuously generated in the circulation in the small amounts required to initiate the alternative pathway: it is initiated by the action of factor H, factor I, and a proteolytic enzyme, possibly plasmin, producing C3c and C3d. C3b is also an opsonin having receptors on erythrocytes, B-lymphocytes, granulocytes and macrophages. C3b, Bb: an alternative pathway C3 convertase generated by the interaction of factor B and factor D with C3b deposited on activators of alternate pathway and thus protected from inactivation by factor I and factor H C3b, P, Bb: a more stable alternative pathway C3 convertase generated by addition of factor P to C3B, b C3b$_n$, Bb: an alternative pathway C5 convertase generated by addition of one or more C3b fragments to CSb Bb C3b$_n$, P, Bb: a more stable alternative pathway C5 convertase containing factor P.

Accelerator f., see Factor V, under coagulation fs.

Activation f., see Factor XII, under coagulation fs.

Adrenocorticotropic releasing f. (ACTH-RF)., see corticotropin releasing f.

Angiogenesis f., a substance that causes the growth of new blood vessels, found in tissues with high metabolic requirements such as cancers and the retina. It is also released by hypoxic macrophages at the edges or outer surface of a wound and initiates revascularization in wound healing.

Animal protein f., an element in animal proteins found to be essential to maximal growth of animals: vitamin B_{12}. Abbreviated as APF.

Antiachromotrichia f., pantothenic acid.

Antiacrodynia f., pyridoxine.

Antialopecia f., inositol.

Antianemia f., cyanocobalamin.

Antianemia f. for chicks, a vitamin, folic acid, in spinach and other green leaves, which prevents anemia in chicks.

Antiblack tongue f., niacin.

Anticanities f., Antidermatitis f. of chicks, pantothenic acid. **Antidermatitis f.** of rats, pyridoxine.

Anti-egg white f., biotin

Antigen-specific T-cell helper f., a soluble factor produced by helper T cells that activates other lymphocytes that are specific for the stimulating antigen; it may itself bind antigen.

Antigen-specific T-cell suppressor f., a soluble factor produced by suppressor T cells following immunization; it produces antigen-specific suppression of the immune response and may itself bind antigen.

Antigray hair f., pantothenic acid.

Antihemophilic f., 1. see Factor VIII, under coagulation fs. Abbreviated AHF. 2. (USP) a sterile freeze-dried powder containing the Factor VIII fraction obtained from suitable whole-blood donors.

Antihemophilic f., cryoprecipitate (USP), a sterile, frozen concentrate of human antihemophilic factor prepared from the Factor VIII—rich cryoprotein fraction of human venous plasma obtained from suitable whole-blood donors from a single unit of plasma derived from whole blood or by plasmapheresis, collected and processed in a closed system. Called also human antihemophilic f.

Antihemophilic f., see human, antihemophilic f., def. 2.

Antihemophilic f. A., see Factor VIM, under coagulation fs.

Antihemophilic f. B., see Factor IX, under coagulation fs.

Antihemophilic f. C., see Factor XI, under coagulation fs.

Antihemorrhagic f., vitamin K.

Antineuritic f., thiamine.

Antinuclear f. (ANF), antibodies directed against nuclear antigens (ANA); ANA against a variety of different antigens are almost invariably found in systemic lupus erythematosus, and are frequently found in rheumatoid arthritis, scleroderma, and Sjögren's syndrome, and mixed connective tissue disease. ANA can be detected by immunofluorescent staining. Serologic tests are also used to determine antibody titers against specific antigens.

Antipellagra f., niacin.

Anti-pernicious anemia f., cyanocobalamin.

Antirachitic f., vitamin D.

Antiscorbutic f., ascorbic acid.

Antisterility f., vitamin E.

Antixerophthalmia f., Antixerotic f., vitamin A.

Atrial natriuretic f. (ANF), a peptide secreted by specific endocrine cells in the right atrium of the mammalian heart that, in response to atrial dilatation or increased intravascular fluid volume, exerts a natriuretic effect on the kidney.

f. B, a complement component C3 proactivator which participates in the alternative pathway of complement activation. The factor

B-C3b complex is split by factor D, which leads to formation of C3 convertase, which in turn acts in the alternative pathway.

Basophil chemotactic f. (BCF), a lymphokine produced by activated lymphocytes that is chemotactic for basophils, possibly responsible for the influx of basophils into sites of inflammation (Jones-Mote reaction).

B cell differentiation fs. (BCDF), factors derived from T cells that stimulate B cells to differentiate into antibody-secreting cells. Cf: B lymphocyte stimulatory fs.

B cell growth fs. (BCGF), factors derived from T cells that stimulate B cells to proliferate *in vitro* but (unlike B cell differentiation factors) do not stimulate antibody secretion. Cf: B lymphocyte stimulatory fs.

B-lymphocyte stimulatory fs. (BSF), a system of nomenclature for factors that stimulate B cells, replacing individual factor names (e.g., B cell differentiation factor). Each factor is designated by BSF and a number, BSF1, BSF2, etc., with the letter p prefixed to the number for factors that have not been purified or whose structure has not been identified, e.g., BSP-p1.

Bittner milk f., mouse mammary tumor virus—a virus causing mammary adenocarcinoma in mouse of certain genotype and influenced by estrogenic stimulation; it is usually transmitted from the mother to the offspring through milk.

Blastogenic f. (BF), see lymphocyte mitogenic f.

Bone f., in periodontal disease, the systemic influence on alveolar bone loss in response to local inflammatory processes.

Bx f., aminobenzoic acid.

C f., a factor found in the soluble part of cytoplasm which promotes the contraction of mitochondria.

C3 nephritic f. (C3 NeF), an autoantibody specific for the alternative complement pathway C3 convertase C3b, Bb found in the serum of many patients with type II membrano proliferative glomerulonephritis. It stabilizes the C3b, Bb complex and prevents its inactivation by factor H, resulting in chronic fluid phase alternative pathway activation.

CAMP f., see under tests.

Castle's f., see Intrinsic factor.

Chemotactic f., a substance that induces chemotaxis. Called also chemoattractant and chemotactin.

Chick antidermatitis f., pantothenic acid.

Chick antipellagra f., pantothenic acid.

Chick growth f s., strepogenin—a factor present in casein and certain other protein which is essential to optimal growth of animals.

Christmas f., see Factor IX, under coagulation fs.

Chromotrichial f., aminobenzoic acid.

Citrovonun f., folinic acid.

Clonal inhibitory f., Cloning inhibitory f. (CIF), see growth inhibitory fs.

Coagulation fs., substances in the blood that are essential to the clotting process and hence, to the maintenance of normal hemostasis. They are designated by Roman numerals, to which the notation "a" is added to indicate the activated state. Platelet factors, designated by Arabic numerals, also play a role in coagulation.
Factor I, fibrinogen: a high molecular weight plasma protein which is converted to fibrin through the action of thrombin. Deficiency of this factor results in afibrinogenemia or hypofibrinogenemia. Several molecular forms of this factor have been recognized.
Factor II, prothrombin: a protein present in the plasma that, in theoretical hematology, is converted to thrombin by extrinsic prothrombin converting principle. More than one molecular form has been detected. Deficiency of this factor leads to hypoprothrombinemia.
Factor III, tissue thromboplastin: a material derived from several sources in the body (brain, lung, etc.) and importan in the formation of extrinsic prothrombin converting principle in the extrinsic pathway of blood coagulation. Called also tissue factor.
Factor IV, calcium: a factor required in many phases of blood coagulation.
Factor V, proaccelerin: a heat- and storage-labile material, present in plasma but not in serum, functioning in both the intrinsic and extrinsic

pathways of blood coagulation. Deficiency of this factor, an autosomal recessive trait, leads to a rare hemorrhagic tendency, known as Owren's disease or parahemophilia, which varies greatly in severity. Called also accelerator globulin (AcG) and labile factor.

Factor VI, a factor (accelerin) previously thought to be an activated form of Factor V. It no longer is considered in the scheme of hemostasis, and hence, it is assigned neither a name nor a function at this time.

Factor VII, proconvertin: a heat-and storage-stable factor participating only in the extrinsic pathway of blood coagulation. Deficiency of this factor, which deficiency may be hereditary (autosomal recessive) or acquired (associated with vitamin K deficiency), results in a hemorrhagic tendency. Called also, autoprothrombin I, serum prothrombin corversion accelerator (SPCA), and stable factor.

Factor VIII, antihemophilic factor (AHF): a relatively storage-labile factor participating only in the intrinsic pathway of blood coagulation. Deficiency of this factor, when transmitted as a sex-linked recessive trait, causes classical hemophilia (hemophilia A). More than one molecular form of this factor has been discovered. Called also antihemophilic globulin (AHG) and antihemophilic factor A.

Factor IX plasma thromboplastin component (PTC) a relatively storage-stable substance involved only in the intrinsic pathway of blood coagulation. Deficiency of this factor results in a hemorrhagic syndrome called hemophilia B or Christmas disease, which is similar to classical hemophilia (hemophilia A). More than one molecular form has been discovered. A transient form, known as hemophilia B Leyden, is clinically indistinguishable from ordinary hemophilia, but the bleeding tendency abates after puberty. Called also autoprothrombin II, Christmas factor and antihemophilic factor B.

Factor X, Stuart factor: a storage-stable factor that participates in both the intrinsic and extrinsic pathways ot blood coagulation. Deficiency of this factor may cause a systemic coagulation disorder (Factor X deficiency). Also called autoprothrombin C, Prower factor, Stuart-Prower factor, and thrombokinase.

Factor XI, plasma thromboplastin antecedent (PTA): a stable factor involved in the intrinsic pathway of blood coagulation. Deficiency of this factor results in a systemic blood-clotting defect called hemophilia C or Rosenthal's syndrome, that may resemble classical hemophilia. Called also antihemophilic factor C.

Factor XII, Hageman factor: a stable factor activated by contact with glass or other foreign surfaces, which initiates the intrinsic process of blood coagulation *in vitro*. Deficiency of this factor results in prolonged *in vitro* blood clotting but overt clinical bleeding is rare. Also called glass, contact, or activation factor.

Factor XIII, fibrin stabilizing factor (FSF): a factor that polymerizes fibrin monomers so that they become stable and insoluble in urea, thus enabling fibrin to form a firm blood clot. Deficiency of this factor produces a clinical hemorrhagic diathesis. Called also fibrinase and Laki-Lorand factor (LLF). The inactive form is also known as protransglutaminase, and the active form as transglutaminase. Platelet factor 1, adsorbed Factor V from the plasma, Platelet factor 2, an accelerator of the thrombin fibrinogen reaction, attached to platelets, Platelet factor 3, a substance, probably a lipoprotein, extracted from platelets, which contributes to the interaction of plasma coagulation proteins in the generation of intrinsic prothrombin converting principle, Platelet factor 4, an intracellular protein component of blood platelets capable of neutralizing the antithrombic activity of heparin in the fibrinogen-fibrin reaction and the inhibitory effect of heparin in the thromboplastin generation test.

Colony-stimulating f. (CSF), a glycoprotein lymphokine produced by blood monocytes, tissue macrophages, and stimulated lymphocytes required for differentiation of stem cells into granulocyte and monocyte cell colonies, and which may be required in granulopoiesis. It has been used as an experimental cancer agent.

Conglutinogen activating f. (KAF), factor I. contact f., see Factor XII, under coagulation fs.

Cord f., a mycoside produced by those strains of *Mycobacterium tuberculosis* that characteristically grow in long serpentine cords.

Corticotropin releasing t. (CRF), a factor or hormone (43 amino acids) elaborated by the hypothalamus at the median eminence, which stimulates the release of corticotropin by the anterior pituitary gland. Called also corticotropin releasing hormone.

Crystal-induced chemotactic f. (CCF), a glycoprotein, mol. wt. 8400, produced by neutrophils upon ingestion of monosodium urate or calcium pyrophosphate crystals that is directly chemotactic for neutrophils and is thought to be involved in the inflammatory process in gouty arthritis.

Curling f., griseofulvin.

f. D, a protein of the alternate complement pathway;

Day's f., folic acid.

Decay-activating f. (DAF), an intrinsic red blood cell protein that prevents the assembly of convertase on the cell surface, thus protecting it from injury by autologous complement.

Diabetogenic f., a substance of unknown constitution associated with extracts of growth hormone from the anterior pituitary which, when injected into normal dogs, causes them to become diabetic.

Diffusion f., hyaluronidase—1. Any of three enzymes (hyaluronate lyase, hyaluronoglucosaminidase, and hyaluronidase) that catalyze the breakdown of hyaluronic acid. These enzymes are found in mammalian testicular and spleen tissue, in bee and snake venom, and in certain species of *Clostridium*, *Staphylococcus*, and *Streptococcus*. Called also Durans-Reynals factor, invasion, and diffusion or spreading factor. 2. A pharmaceutical preparation suitable for injection (NF), which is a sterile, dry, soluble, enzyme product prepared from mammalian testes and capable of hydrolyzing mucopolysaccharides of the type of hyaluronic acid, used to aid absorption and dispersion of other injected drugs and fluids, for hypodermoclysis, and for improving resorption of radiopaque media.

Duran-Reynals f., hyaluronidase, see Diffusion factor.

Elongation f., one of two soluble proteins (EF-1 and EF-2) involved in the addition of each amino acid to the growing polypeptide chain in protein synthesis.

Eluate f., pyridoxine.

Eosinophil chemotactic f. (ECF), 1. Eosinophil chemotactic f. of anaphylaxis. 2. A lymphokine produced by activated lymphocytes that is chemotactic for eosinophils.

Eosinophil chemotactic f. of anaphylaxis (ECF-A)., eosinophil chemoattractants released by basophils and mast cells in immediate hypersensitivity reactions. ECF-A activity is associated with two acidic tetrapeptides (Ala-Gly-Ser-Glu and Val-Gly-Ser-Glu) and with less well characterized larger peptides, which are chemotactic for eosinophils and, to a lesser degree, for neutrophils. Some ECF-A activity is due to arachidonic acid metabolites (leukotriene B, 12-HETE and 12-HHT). Called also eosinophil chemotactic f (ECF).

Epidermal growth f., a protein extractable from the submaxillary glands of male mice that stimulates proliferation of cells of ectodermal and mesodermal origin and inhibits gastric secretion; it is very similar or identical to urogastrone.

Erythrocyte maturation f. (EMF), a former name for vitamin B_{12} (cyanocobalamin).

Erythropoietic stimulating f. (ESF), a name given to a factor in the body which stimulates the production of erythrocytes; probably identical with erythropoietin.

Extrinsic f., vitamin B_{12} (cyanocobalamin).

F (fertility) f., F plasmid—a conjugative plasmid found in F^+ (male) bacterial cells that lead with high frequency to its transfer and much less often to transfer of the bacterial chromosome. A cell possessing the F plasmid (F^+, male) can form a conjugation bridge (F pilus) to a cell lacking the F plasmid (F^- female), through which genetic material may pass from one cell to another.

Fermentation Lactobacillus casei f., pteropterin—pteroyltriglutamic acid, or folic acid, conjugated to two glutamic residues.

Fibrin stabilizing f., see Factor XIII, under coagulation fs.

Filtrate f., filtrate f. II, pantothenic acid.

Follicle-stimulating hormone releasing f. (FRF, FSH-RF), gonadotropin releasing hormone,

Galactopoietic f., prolactin.

Gastric anti-pernicious anemia f., gastric intrinsic f., intrinsic f.

Glass f., see Factor XII, under coagulation fs.

Glucose tolerance f., a biologically active complex of chromium and nicotinic acid that facilitates the reaction of insulin with receptor sites on tissues.

Gonadotropin releasing f. (GnRF), a decapeptide hormone elaborated by the median eminence of the hypothalamus that stimulates the release of follicle stimulating hormone and luteinizing hormone from the anterior pituitary gland. A preparation of the acetate and hydrochloride salts of the same principles obtained from pig, sheeps or other species is used in differential diagnosis of hypothalamic, pituitary, and gonadal dysfunction, and in the treatment of certain forms of female and male infertility and hypogonadism.

Growth hormone releasing f. (GRF, GH-RF), a peptide hormone elaborated by the median eminence of the hypothalamus, which stimulates the release of growth hormone from the anterior pituitary gland. Called also growth hormone releasing hormone (GH-RH) and somatotropin releasing-hormone (SRF).

Growth inhibitory fs., lymphokines, clonal inhibitory factor (CIF) and proliferation inhibitory factor (PIF) that inhibit the growth of certain target cells, permanently at higher concentrations and temporarily at lower concentrations. Both inhibitory factors and lymphotoxin may be activities of the same substance.

f. H, a glycoprotein that binds to C3b (see complement) and acts as an alternative pathway complement inhibitor by interfering with the binding of factor B to C3b; it also acts as a cofactor in the conversion of C36 to C3bi by factor I.

Hageman f. (HF), see Factor XII. under coagulation fs.

High-molecular-weight neutrophil chemotactic f. (HMW-NCF), see neutrophil chemotactic f.

Histamine releasing f., a lymphokine that produces basophil degranulation.

Hydrazine-sensitive f. (HSF), C3 (in the alternative complement pathway); see factor A.

Hyperglycemic-glycogenolytic f., see glucagons—a polypeptide secreted by the α cells of the islet of Langerhans in response to hypoglycemia or to stimulation by growth hormone of the anterior pituitary. It induces glycogenolysis in the liver by inducing activation of liver phosphorylase.

f.I, a plasma enzyme that inactivates C3b (see complement) by cleaving it to form C3bi; factor H is required as a cofactor (or its activity).

f. II, 1 see under coagulation fs. **2.** pantothenic acid.

f. III, see under coagulation fs.

Immunoglobulin-binding f. (IBF), a lymphokine having the ability to bind IgG complexed with antigen and prevent complement activation, possibly Fc receptors shed from T cells.

Inhibiting fs, factors elaborated by one structure (as by the hypothalamus) that inhibit the release of hormones by another structure (as by the anterior pituitary gland), including melanocyte-stimulating hormone inhibiting factor and prolactin inhibiting factor (presumably peptides). The term is applied to substances of unknown chemical structure, while substances of established chemical identity are called inhibiting hormones.

Initiation f., one of three soluble proteins (IF-1, IF-2, and IF-3) involved in the binding of mRNA and the first aminoacyl-tRNA to the small ribosomal subunit and the attachment of the small subunit to the large subunit at the beginning of protein synthesis.

Insulin-like growth fs (IGF)., insulin-like substances in serum that do not react with insulin antibodies; they are growth hormone dependent and possess all the growth-promoting properties of the somatomedins. Called also nonsuppressible insulin-like activity.

Intermediate lobe inhibiting f., see melanocyte stimulating hormone inhibiting f.

Intrinsic f., a glycoprotein secreted by the parietal cells of the gastric glands, necessary for the absorption of vitamin B_{12} (cyanocobalamin, extrinsic factor). Lack of intrinsic factor, with consequent deficiency of vitamin B_{12}, results in pernicious anemia.

f. IV, see under coagulation fs.

f. IX, see under coagulation fs.

Labile f., see Factor V, under coagulation fs.

Lactobacillus casei f., folic acid.

Lactobacillus lactis Dorner f., cyanocobalamin.

Lactogenic f., prolactin.

Laki-Lorand f., see Factor XIII, under coagulation fs.

LE f., an antibody having a sedimentation rate of 7S that reacts with leukocyte nuclei in the LE cell test, now referred to as antinuclear antibody (q v).

Leukocyte inhibitory f. (LIF), a lymphokine that inhibits the migration of polymorphonuclear leukocytes but not macrophages.

Liver filtrate f., pantothenic acid.

Liver Lactobacillus casei f., folic acid.

LLD f., cyanocobalamin.

Luteinizing hormone releasing f. (LRF, LH-RF), a factor elaborated by the hypothalamus at the median eminence, which stimulates the release of luteinizing hormone by the anterior pituitary gland.

Lymph node permeability t. (LNPF), a vasoactive factor, distinct from histamine, serotonin, bradykinin, and kallikrein, that is released without immunologic stimulus from many tissues, including lymph nodes, spleen, kidney, liver, and muscle.

Lymphocyte activating f., interleukin—1. a macrophage-produced interleukin that induces the production of interleukin-2 by T-cells that have been stimulated by antigen or mitogen. 2 Types exist designated as α and β. IL-1 or a similar protein is also produced by epithelial cells and stimulates fibroblast proliferation and release of proteolytic enzymes and prostaglandin in inflammatory processes. IL-1 also appears to be identical to endogenous pyrogen.

Lymphocyte blastogenic f. (BF), see lymphocyte mitogenic f.

Lymphocyte mitogemc fs (LMF), a nondialyzable heat-stable macromolecule, mol. wt. approximately 20,000 to 30,000, released by lymphocytes stimulated by specific antigen, that causes nonstimulated lymphocytes to undergo blast transformation and cell division. Called also lymphocyte blastogenic f. (BF) and lymphocyte transforming f. (LTF).

Lymphocyte transforming f. (LTF), see lymphocyte mitogenic f.

Lysogenic f., bacteriophage—a virus that lyses bacteria.

Macrophage-activating f. (MAF), a lymphokine that, after a 72-hour incubation period, induces or increases macrophage adherence, phagocytosis, oxygen consumption, and bactericidal and tumoricidal activity. MAF and MIF (macrophage inhibitory factor) appear to be activities of the same macromolecule.

Macrophage chemotactic t. (MCF), a lymphokine produced by activated lymphocytes that is chemotactic for macrophages.

Macrophage-derived growth f., a substance released by macrophages below the surface of a wound that induces the proliferation of fibroblasts with consequent deposition of collagen, fibronectin, and glycosaminoglycan.

Macrophage growth f. (MGF), glycoproteins that permit macrophages harvested from peritoneal exudates to proliferate in liquid-suspension cultures and form colonies consisting solely of mononuclear phagocytes.

Macrophage inhibitory f., migration inhibiting t. (MIF), a lymphokine that causes temporary inhibition of macrophage migration, lasting about 24 hours.

Melanocyte stimulating hormone inhibiting f. (MIF), a tripeptide, Pro-Leu-Gly-NH$_2$, formed in the hypothalamus by enzymatic cleavage of oxytocin that inhibits the release of MSH by the intermediate lobe of the pituitary gland in fish and amphibians.

Melanocyte stimulating hormone releasing f. (MRF, MSH-RF), a hypothalamic factor or factors of undetermined chemical nature reported to cause release of MSH from the pituitary gland in lower animals.

Milk f., mouse mammary tumor virus, see Bittner milk f.

Mitogenic f., see lymphocyte mitogenic f.

Mouse antialopecia f., inositol.

Mouse mammary tumor f., see Bittner milk f.

MSH inhibiting f., see melanocyte-stimulating hormone inhibiting f.

Mullerian regression f., Mullerian duct inhibitory f., a factor postulated to be present in the male embryo which inhibits development of the wolffian ducts.

Multiple f's, in heredity, two or more genes or environmental variants that act in combination to produce a certain trait.

Myocardial depressant f. (MDF), a peptide formed in response to a fall in systemic blood pressure that has a negatively inotropic effect on myocardial muscle fibers.

N f., a factor occurring in yeast, meat, liver, and wheat germ, the absence of which from an otherwise complete diet causes rats to voluntarily consume more alcohol than they do when factor N is present in the diet.

Necrotizing f., necrotoxin—a toxin that kills tissue cells, e.g., the exotoxins secreted by the species of *Clostridium* and *Staphylococcus aureus*.

Nerve growth f., a protein consisting of two identical polypeptide chains associated with two gamma subunits (enzymes) and two alpha subunits; first isolated from mouse sarcoma and later from snake venom and mouse salivary glands, it stimulates the growth of sensory and sympathetic nerve cells and of the adrenal medulla and has been found to be secreted by a variety of normal and neoplastic cells, including those of man. Abbreviated as NGF.

Neutrophil chemotactic f. (NCF), 1. A poorly characterized chemotactic factor, mol. wt. approximately 750,000. that attracts neutrophils but not eosinophils or monocytes and is released by basophils or mast cells in immediate hypersensitivity reactions. Called also high-molecular-weight neutrophil chemotactic f. (HMW-NCF). 2. A lymphokine produced by activated lymphocytes that is chemotactic for neutrophils.

Osteoclast activating f. (OAF), a lymphokine that stimulates bone resorption: it is a small protein unrelated to parathyroid hormone and may be involved in the born-resorption associated with multiple myeloma and other hematologic neoplasms or inflammatory disorders such as rheumatoid arthritis and periodontal disease.

f. P, properdin—a nonimmunoglobulin gammaglobulin component of the alternative pathway; it complexes with C3b and stabilizes alternative pathway C3 convertase.

Pellagra-preventive f., niacin.

Platelet fs, factors important in hemostasis which are contained in or attached to the platelets. See platelet factors 1, 2, 3, and 4, under coagulation fs.

Platelet activating f. (PAF), a substance released by basophils and mast cells in immediate hypersensitivity reactions and macrophages and neutrophils in other inflammatory reactions that is an extremely potent mediator of bronchoconstriction and of the platelet aggregation and release reactions. It differs from other known biochemical mediators in being a phospholipid. Called also PAF-ac ether or AGEPC (acetyl glyceryl ether phosphoryl choline).

Platelet-derived growth f., a substance contained in the alpha granules of platelets and capable of inducing proliferation of vascular endothelial cells, vascular smooth muscle cells, fibroblasts, and glia cells; its action contributes to the repair of damaged vascular walls.

PP f., niacin.

Prolactin inhibiting t. (PIF), a factor elaborated by the hypothalamus at the median eminence, which inhibits the secretion of prolactin by the anterior pituitary gland.

Prolactin releasing f. (PRF), a factors elaborated by the hypothalamus at the median eminence, which stimulates the release of prolactin by the anterior pituitary gland. In human subjects, thyrotropin releasing hormone can also act as prolactin releasing factors.

Proliferation inhibitory f. (PIF), see growth inhibitory fs.

Prower f., see Factor X, under coagulation fs.

R f., R plasmid—a conjugative factor in bacterial cells that promotes resistance to agents such as antibiotics, metal ions, ultraviolet radiation, and bacteriophage. R plasmids are large with two functionally distinct parts; a resistance transfer factor (RTF), consisting of genes for autonomous replication and conjugation; and a resistance determinant (R determinant) containing genes for resistance (R genes).

Rat acrodynia f., pyridoxine.

Recruitment f., see lymphocyte mitogenic t.

Releasing f., one of two soluble proteins (RF-1 and RF-2) involved in the release of the completed polypeptide chain from the ribosome when a termination codon is encountered during protein synthesis (see translation); RF-1 recognizes the termination codons UAA or UAG and RF-2 recognizes UAA or UGA.

Releasing f., factors elaborated in one structure (as in the hypothalamus) that affect the release of hormones from another structure (as from the anterior pituitary gland), including corticotropin releasing factor, melanocyte stimulating hormone releasing factor, and prolactin releasing factor. The term is applied to substances of unknown chemical structure, while substances of established chemical identity are called releasing hormones.

Resistance-inducing f., see Rubin's test (def. 2), under tests.

Resistance transfer f., the portion of an R plasmid in a bacterial cell that contains the genes for conjugation and replication.

Rh f., Rhesus f., antigens (agglutinogens) present on the membrane of red blood cells; the most complex of all human blood groups because the genes differ by determining a different number of 33 antigens thus far described and do so by remarkably different quality. Blacks show the greatest degree of diversity, Orientals the least. The major antigen, $Rh1(Rh_0D)$, is highly immunogenic and, before the development of passive immunization prophylaxis, was responsible for serious hemolytic diseases of the newborn. Two other pairs of alternative antigens are inherited without Rh1; these are $Rh21(rh°,C^G)$ and Rh4(hr', c) and Rh3 (rh", E) and Rh5 (hr", e).

Rheumatoid f., (RF), antibodies directed against antigenic determinants, i.e., Gin, in the Fc region of IgG, found in the serum of about 80 percent of patients with classical or definite rheumatoid arthritis; but in only about 20 percent of patients with juvenile rheumatoid arthritis; rheumatoid factors may be IgM, IgG, or IgA antibodies, although serologic tests measure only IgM. Rheumatoid factors also occur in other connective tissue diseases and infectious diseases (Sjögren's syndrome, systemic lupus erythematosus, sarcoidosis, subacute bacterial endocarditis, infectious hepatitis, leprosy).

Risk f., a clearly defined occurrence or characteristic that has been associated with the increased rate of a subsequently occurring disease.

f. S, biotin.

Separation f., the ratio of the relative concentration of two isotopes after processing, to their relative concentration before processing.

Sex f., see F plasmid.

Simon's septic f., decrease of eosinophils and increase of neutrophils in the blood in pyogenic infections.

Skin reactive f. (SRF), a lymphokine derived from antigen-stimulated lymphocytes that augments the delayed hypersensitivity skin reaction, increasing capillary permeability and infiltration of monocytes perhaps a mixture of other lymphokines.

Somatotropin releasing t. (SRF), see Growth hormone releasing f.

Specific macrophage arming f. (SMAF), a lymphokin reported to be a nonimmunoglobulin factor produced by activated T cells that is capable of activating macrophages so that they are capable of specifically recognizing and killing tumor cells.

Spreading f., hyaluronidase, see Diffusion f.

Stable f., see Factor VII, under coagulation fs.

Stuart f, Stuart-Prower f., see Factor X, under coagulation fs.

Sulfation f., a formerly used term for somatomedin.

T-cell growth f., interleukin 2—an interleukin produced by T-cells in response to antigenic or mitogenic stimulation and signal carried by interleukin 1. It stimulates the proliferation T cells bearing specific receptors for IL-2, which are only expressed by antigenetically stimulated T cells. IL-2 also seems to induce production of interferon-Y. It is used as a anticancer drug in wide variety of solid malignant tumors.

Thyrotropin-releasing f. (TRF), a tripeptide hormone elaborated by the median eminence of hypothalamus or obtained by synthesis which stimulates the release of thyrotropin from the anterior pituitary gland. In human subjects, it also acts as a prolactin releasing factor. A preparation is used in the diagnosis of mild hyperthyroidism, and Graves' disease, and differentiating among primary, secondary and tertiary hypothyroidism.

Transfer f. (TF), a dialyzable extract obtained from lysates of peripheral blood lymphocytes that is capable of transferring antigen-specific cell-mediated immunity (delayed type hypersensitivity) from donor to recipient and also has nonspecific immunostimulatory activity; it appears to contain both protein and RNA but not DNA and consist of small molecules (mol. wt. less than 10,000). TF is nonantigenic and does not transfer humoral immunity. Clinical trials have shown promising results in treatment of immunodeficiency diseases, including Wiskott-Aldrich syndrome, severe combined immunodeficiency disease, and ataxia-telangiectasia, and in fungal infections refractory to chemotherapy, including disseminated mucocutaneous candidiasis and disseminated coccidioidomycosis; the use of TF in viral infections, parasitic diseases, and cancer is also under investigation.

Trapp's f., the last two figures expressive of the specific gravity of urine; when multiplied by 2 they give the number of parts of solids per 1000.

Tumor-angiogenesis f., a factor produced by cancer cells of solid tumors that stimulates the growth of blood vessels into the tumor.

Tumor necrosis t. (TNF), a lymphokine produced by macrophages capable of causing *in vivo* hemorrhagic necrosis of certain tumor cells, but not affecting normal cells. It is the same substance as cachectin. It has been used as an experimental anticancer agent.

V f., an accessory substance required for the growth of certain species of *Haemophilus*, replaceable by nicotinamide-adenine dinucleotide (NAD) or nicotinamide-adenine dinucleotide phosphate (NADP) and present in red blood cells. Cf: Xf.

f. V, see under coagulation fs.

f. VI, see under coagulation fs.

f. VII, see under coagulation fs.

f. VIII, see under coagulation fs.

von Willebrand's f., the attribute of Factor VIII (see under coagulation fs) necessary for the adhesion of platelets to vascular elements. Deficiency of this factor results in the prolonged bleeding time seen in von Willebrand's disease. Called also factor VIII vwf.

f. W, biotin.

Wills f., folic acid.

f. X, see under coagulation fs.

X f., an accessory substance required for the aerobic growth of certain species of *Haemophilus* replaceable by hemin or other iron porphyrin compounds, and present in red blood cells. It is heat stable and not destroyed by autoclaving. Cf: V f.

f. XI, see under coagulation fs.

f. XII, see under cogulation fs.

f. XIII, see under coagulation fs.

Yeast eluate f., pyridoxine.

Yeast filtrate f., pantothenic acid.

Appendix

DSM-III R: Diagnostic and statistical manual of mental disorders of the American psychiatric Association 3rd edition revised (1987).

Parapertussis: An acute respiratory disease clinically in distinguishable from mild or moderate pertussis caused by Bordetelia parapertussis.

Theaaurismosis: Obsolete term for amyloidosis.

Paracoccidioidomycosis: An often fetal infection caused by *Para-coccidioides brasiliensis*. The primary infection begins in the lungs and mucosa and may extent to the adjacent skin tonsils, gastrointestinal lymphatics, liver and spleen.

Keratogis follicularis: Slowly progressive autosomal dominant disorder of keratinization characterized by pinkish or tan or skin colored papules on the seborrheic areas of the body that coalesce to form plaques which may become crusted and secondarily infected; over time the lesion may become darker and may fuse to form papullomatous and warty malodorous growth.

Larva migrans visceral: A condition caused by prolonged migration of larvae of nematodus in human tissues other than skin, characterized by persistent hypereosinophilia, hepatomegaly and frequently by pneumonitis caused by *Toxocara canis* which do not complete their lifecycle in man.

Amaurotic familial idiocy: A term for several lipidoses differing biochemically in clinical manifestation, the congenital form may be lethal within less than one month from birth; adisialoganglioside G (f_{23}) is present in tissue and there is a three-fold concentration of cholesterol in the brain the infantile type is Tay-Sach's disease.

The juvenile type is a neuronal ceroid lipofusunosis with on set between five and ten years. A prolonged course and death during late adolescence. It is relatively common among Scandinavians and shows a salt and pepper pigmentary degeneration (a typical retinitis pigmentosa) than cerebellar ataxia, polymyotonia and dementia called also Vogt-Spielmeyer disease.

Erythema nodosum leprosum: A recurrent Arthuslike lepra reaction occurring during the course of chemotherapy in lepromatous leprosy; sometimes in the borderline form and occasionally spontaneously usually characterized histologically by vasculitis and clinically by the appearance of crops of small erythematous tender cutaneous nodules or plaques which are distributed especially on extremities and face. It may be associated with severe systemic symptoms and visceral manifestation

Plam chin reflex: Twitching of chin produced by stimulation (Scrat-ching) the palm.

Push back technique: A surgical design procedure designed to reposition to the soft palate posteriorly and reestablish venopharyngeal competence.

q.v.   Which see (L. quod vide)
o.b.s. Obsolete
c.f.   Compare.

READER SUGGESTIONS SHEET

Please help us to improve the quality of our publications by completing and returning this sheet to us.

Author/Title: **Doshis' A to Z Series on Syndromes** *By Sachin M Doshi, Sanket M Doshi, Ankur M Doshi*

Your name and address:

Phone and Fax:

e-mail address:

How did you hear about this book? [please tick appropriate box (es)]

☐ Direct mail from publisher ☐ Conference ☐ Bookshop
☐ Book review ☐ Lecturer recommendation ☐ Friends
☐ Other (please specify) ☐ Website

Type of purchase: ☐ Direct purchase ☐ Bookshop ☐ Friends

Do you have any brief comments on the book?

Please return this sheet to the name and address given below.

JAYPEE BROTHERS
MEDICAL PUBLISHERS (P) LTD
EMCA House, 23/23B Ansari Road, Daryaganj
New Delhi 110 002, India